Glencoe

DOSAGE CALCULATIONS

for

MEDICAL CAREERS

With
Interactive
CD-ROM

Kathryn A. Haddix
James E. Whaley

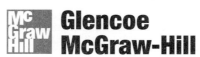

Glencoe
McGraw-Hill

New York, New York   Columbus, Ohio   Woodland Hills, California   Peoria, Illinois

Library of Congress Cataloging-in-Publication Data

Haddix, Kathryn A.
    Glencoe Dosage Calculations for Medical Careers / Kathryn A. Haddix, James E. Whaley.
        p. ; cm.
    Includes index.
    ISBN 0-02-802189-4 (pbk. : alk. paper)
    1. Pharmaceutical arithmetic—Problems, exercises, etc. I. Whaley, James E. (James
Earl) II. Title.
    [DNLM: 1. Pharmaceutical Preparations—administration & dosage—Problems and
Exercises. 2. Mathematics—Problems and Exercises. QV 18.2 H126g 2001]
    RS57 .H334 2001
    615'.1'0151—dc21

                                                            2001023222

Glencoe/McGraw-Hill

A Division of The **McGraw·Hill** Companies

Dosage Calculations for Medical Careers

Send all inquiries to:
Glencoe McGraw-Hill
8787 Orion Place
Columbus, OH 43240-4027

ISBN 0-02-802189-4

  2 3 4 5 6 7 8 9 079 06 05 04 03 02 01

Co-developed by
Glencoe/McGraw-Hill
and Visual Education Corporation
Princeton, NJ

WARNING NOTICE: The clinical procedures, medicines, dosages, and other matters described in this publication are based upon research of current literature and consultation with knowledgeable persons in the field. The procedures and matters described in this text reflect currently accepted clinical practice. However, this information cannot and should not be relied upon as necessarily applicable to a given individual's case. Accordingly, each person must be separately diagnosed to discern the patient's unique circumstances. Likewise, the manufacturer's package insert for current drug production information should be consulted before administering any drug. Publisher disclaims all liability for any inaccuracies, omissions, misuse, or misunderstanding of the information contained in this publication. Publisher cautions that this publication is not intended as a substitute for the professional judgment of trained medical personnel.

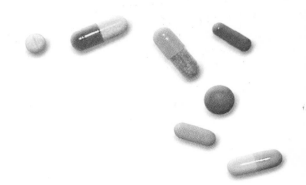

PREFACE

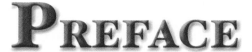

Dosage Calculations for Medical Careers teaches the skills and techniques students need to calculate the amount of medication they should administer to patients. It also teaches students to interpret both physician's orders and drug labels. The textbook is written especially for students preparing to be medical assistants, licensed practical nurses, pharmacy technicians, paramedics, and other health care workers.

Correct dosage calculations play a large role in ensuring that medications are administered accurately and safely. This book is published at a time when the medical community is under close scrutiny by the public to determine the level of medication errors and their effect on patient safety. *Dosage Calculations For Medical Careers* offers several responses to the public's concerns.

First, the text carefully guides students through all the steps that they need to find the correct amount of medication to administer to patients. The early chapters provide a detailed review of the basic arithmetic and algebra skills that are needed. In later chapters, students have the option of reviewing how important formulas were developed.

Students learning to calculate dosages come from a variety of mathematical backgrounds. Rather than requiring students to relearn skills they already have, the text recognizes that various approaches will work better for different students within a classroom. Therefore, students may pick among several options: ratio proportions, fraction proportions, the formula method, and dimensional analysis. Students are shown how these different approaches lead to the same results. They are then encouraged to select the method that they find most comfortable.

One of the major advances we introduce in this text is a fresh approach to the formula method. Traditionally, the formula

$$\frac{desired\ dose}{dosage\ unit} \times dose\ on\ hand = amount\ to\ administer$$

or

$$\frac{D}{Q} \times H = A$$

has been used to calculate the amount to administer. We have adjusted this formula slightly, instead using

$$D \times \frac{H}{Q} = A$$

for this calculation.

The adjusted formula has two key advantages. First, the formula is a building block for students who prefer to use dimensional analysis for their calculation. Second, the adjusted formula is easier for students to learn and less likely to introduce errors. The reason is that $\frac{H}{Q}$ is simply the reciprocal of the dosage strength listed on the drug label. Thus, students don't have to find D, H, and Q as separate values. Instead, they can determine the desired dose and then look directly to the drug label. This approach will dramatically reduce calculation errors, thereby improving patient safety.

Unlike many other texts, *Dosage Calculations for Medical Careers* pays attention to the fastest growing segment of our society, the geriatric population. We introduce students to concerns about patient education and polypharmacy. We also set the stage for further study of drug orders that involve creatinine clearance. We believe this topic will be of increasing importance in years to come, especially for those students who will work in nursing homes, other long-term health facilities, and hospices. In addition, *Dosage Calculations for Medical Careers* gives special attention to pediatric concerns. Students learn to calculate orders based on body weight as well as body surface area.

Text Organization

Dosage Calculations for Medical Careers is organized into thirteen chapters, along with a pretest and a comprehensive evaluation, or posttest.

The *Pretest* gives students an opportunity to review the basic math skills they will need for the book. The content of the Pretest parallels much of the content of Chapters 1 and 2.

Chapter 1 provides a comprehensive review of Roman numerals, fractions, and decimals. These skills are basic building blocks for all that follows. *Chapter 2* continues the math review by introducing percents, ratios, and proportions. The concept of solution strengths for both dry and liquid medications is also introduced. In both of these chapters, word problems draw on medical settings.

Chapter 3 reviews weights and measures. It introduces the metric system as well as apothecary and household systems. Time and temperature conversions are also included. Special attention is given to the conversion factors that will become so important in later chapters.

Chapter 4 covers the equipment used to measure and administer medications. It looks first at equipment used for oral administration, then hypodermic syringes, and finally other means of delivering medication, including transdermal patches. The chapter includes a discussion of needle gauge and length.

Chapter 5 focuses on drug orders. It begins with the Seven Rights of medication administration and then shows the various ways that drug orders may be written. The chapter includes a full list of abbreviations used for drug orders as well as a list of look-alike and sound-alike drug names. The chapter also includes examples of drug orders that could be easily misread.

In turn, *Chapter 6* focuses on drug labels and package inserts. Students are taught to find a wide range of information common to all drug labels, and then specifically to oral and parenteral medications. The discussion of dosage strength is written to provide a building block for later calculations. In the exercises, students evaluate drug labels independently and then compare them.

Chapter 7 teaches techniques for calculating dosages. It builds on the proportions introduced in Chapter 2 and the conversion factors introduced in Chapter 3. The chapter first looks at finding the desired dose, using the conversion factor method and the ratio-proportion method. Once students can find the desired dose, they learn to calculate the amount to administer, using either the proportion method or the formula method. It is in Chapter 7 that the variation of the formula method, $D \times \frac{H}{Q} = A$, is first used.

Chapter 8 then shows how to use dimensional analysis to combine the two main calculations—desired dose and amount to administer—into one calculation. Students are again reminded that the various approaches all lead to the same result. Students should select the method with which they are most comfortable. In both Chapters 7 and 8, background text that explains how methods are developed is provided in a second color. Students and instructors may use or ignore this additional text as they please.

Chapter 9 focuses on oral dosages. Tablets and capsules are discussed in depth, along with information about breaking or crushing them. Liquid oral medications are also discussed. The methods of calculation introduced in Chapters 7 and 8 are applied throughout the chapter to oral dosages.

Chapter 10 applies techniques learned in Chapters 7 and 8 to calculations of parenteral dosages. The chapter discusses reconstituting powders and provides information about expiration dates of reconstituted solutions. Insulin is covered next, including information about how to measure and combine different insulins. The chapter concludes with a look at other medication routes, including parenteral medications that are not delivered by injection (e.g., inhalants, rectal medications, and transdermal systems).

Chapter 11 continues the discussion of parenteral medications, presenting information and calculations unique to intravenous medications. After introducing IV solutions and equipment, we turn our attention to calculating flow rates for electronic and manual regulation. Students also learn calculations for adjusting the flow rate, infusion times, and infusion volumes. We then discuss heparin calculations, followed by critical care calculations, including per minute and body weight orders as well as titrated medications.

Drug orders based on body weight are revisited in *Chapter 12*, which focuses on pediatric concerns. The chapter also introduces body surface area (BSA) calculations. We discuss in even greater depth concerns regarding intramuscular and intravenous medications as well as daily maintenance fluid needs.

Chapter 13 presents information and calculations focusing on geriatric concerns. Relevant physiological changes that occur with aging are discussed. The clinical significance of creatinine clearance is discussed in greater detail, setting the stage for students to learn Cockcroft's Equation in further study. An overview is also provided about the relationship between ideal and actual body weight. The chapter describes the process of working with geriatric patients and concludes with an overview of polypharmacy, an area of increasing importance to the medical community.

Following Chapter 13, students may take a *Comprehensive Evaluation* that tests the skills they learned from the entire textbook.

Ancillaries

Dosage Calculations for Medical Careers is accompanied by an *Instructor's Manual*. This guide provides detailed solutions to the Pretest and Comprehensive Evaluation, all the Review and Practice exercises, and all Chapter Review questions, including the Critical Thinking exercises, Case Studies, and Internet Activities. The *Instructor's Manual* includes a set of additional exercises for each chapter as well as the solutions to these exercises. It contains a set of more than two dozen overhead transparency masters for classroom use. The *Instructor's Manual* also lists the Error Alert and Critical Thinking on the Job features from the student edition.

Also included with the *Instructor's Manual* is a CD-ROM containing the ExamView Pro® test generator and an Instructor's PowerPoint Presentation. The PowerPoint Presentation allows instructors to illustrate and review key points from each chapter. ExamView Pro® allows instructors to create their own tests from the database of test questions.

A comprehensive CD-ROM is available to help students learn, review, and test their skills with *Dosage Calculations for Medical Careers*. This highly interactive multimedia CD corresponds directly with the textbook's 13 chapters. Students can review the content of each chapter at their own pace and view animation for further explanation of each Rule. *Review and Practice* exercises, along with *Chapter Review* exercises, allow students to check answers by a simple click of a button.

These tutorial tests provide feedback, scoring, and study recommendations. Answers to the *Chapter Review* questions are entered into the computer; upon completion, they can be printed for documentation. Students can even bookmark their study location upon exiting. Furthermore, when they have their computer on with an active Internet connection, they can complete each Internet activity. The reference portion of the CD provides quick access to essential information regarding *Dosage Calculations for Medical Careers*. And just for fun, students can navigate to the games section of the CD to practice *Dosage Calculations for Medical Careers* in an interactive way.

Features To Help You Study and Learn

Error Alerts

The text includes numerous *Error Alerts* designed to bring your attention to common mistakes that are often made when calculating dosages. These Alerts will help you avoid repeating these mistakes.

Critical Thinking on the Job

More than two dozen *Critical Thinking on the Job* features set up common problems that you are likely to encounter. You are then encouraged to *think before you act.*

To administer 500 mg of drug, calculate the amount of solution to administer:

$$500 \text{ mg} \times \frac{1 \text{ mL}}{280 \text{ mg}} = A$$

$$25 \overset{25}{\cancel{500}} \text{ mg} \times \frac{1 \text{ mL}}{280 \text{ mg}}_{14} = 25 \times \frac{1}{14} \text{ mL} = \frac{25}{14} = 1.786 \text{ mL}$$

Round 1.786 mL to the nearest tenth. Administer 1.8 mL of solution, using a standard syringe.

ERROR ALERT!
Select the correct instructions for the strength and route ordered.

The package insert for the last example specifies that a 500-mg vial of Maxipime can be reconstituted for both IM and IV use. Suppose a nurse mistakenly reconstitutes Maxipime 500 mg IM for 500 mg IV instead. The IV instructions indicate that the nurse use 5 mL of diluent, producing a solution strength of 100 mg/mL. Calculating the *amount to administer,*

$$500 \text{ mg} \times \frac{1 \text{ mL}}{100 \text{ mg}} = A$$

$$5 \overset{5}{\cancel{500}} \text{ mg} \times \frac{1 \text{ mL}}{100 \text{ mg}}_{1} = 5 \times 1 \text{ mL} = 5 \text{ mL}$$

The nurse administers two injections of 2.5 mL each. The patient's discomfort increases, and the number of injection sites available for future injections are reduced. Costs increase because more diluent and syringes than necessary are used. The risk of injection complications is doubled. Correctly reconstituted for IM use, 1.3 mL of diluent will be used to produce a solution with a dosage strength of 280 mg/mL. As the previous example showed, the IM injection will require only 1.8 mL of solution, not 5 mL.

CRITICAL THINKING ON THE JOB
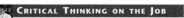

Recording Accurate Information

A medical assistant receives the following order: *Humatrope 2 mg IM TIW*

At 0800 on 10/15/01, the medical assistant prepares the medication to administer later that day. After reading the label, she draws up all of the diluent supplied with the medication and injects it into the vial. According to the drug label the remaining medication may be [used] for 14 days if protected from light. She [...] and signs it with her initials. The vial will not [...] to light in the refrigerator. Otherwise, the [...] assistant might wrap it in foil or place it inside [...]

Later that day, the medical assistant calculates the amount to administer, based on the label,

$$2 \text{ mg} \times \frac{1 \text{ mL}}{5 \text{ mg}} = A$$

$$2 \text{ mg} \times \frac{1 \text{ mL}}{5 \text{ mg}} = 2 \times \frac{1}{5} \text{ mL} = \frac{2}{5} \text{ mL} = 0.4 \text{ mL}$$

She uses a LoDose tuberculin syringe to administer the medication.

Think Before You Act

While the medical assistant has followed instructions carefully, she has mislabeled the vial. She used 5 mL of sterile diluent, not 1 mL. Her label should indicate 5 mg/5 mL so that her calculation is

$$2 \text{ mg} \times \frac{5 \text{ mL}}{5 \text{ mg}} = A$$

$$2 \text{ mg} \times \frac{\overset{1}{\cancel{5}} \text{ mL}}{5 \text{ mg}}_{1} = 2 \times 1 \text{ mL} = 2 \text{ mL}$$

She would administer this amount using a standard syringe. Because of her labeling error, the patient receives only $\frac{1}{5}$ the amount of medication ordered.

Parenteral Dosages **239**

PATIENT EDUCATION

Review with patients the following guidelines for taking tablets and capsules:

1. Perform all necessary calculations, so that you can tell patients how many pills to take.

2. Tell patients whether or not they need to take a medication with food. Encourage them to drink at least 8 ounces of water with any medication.

3. Tell patients who need to divide tablets that pharmacists can provide this service on request. If the patients will be dividing the tablets, demonstrate and advise them as follows:
   a. Wash hands before handling tablets.
   b. Grasp the tablet with the scored line between your fingers. Exert pressure in the same direction—downward or upward—with both hands, until the tablet breaks along the scored line.

c. You may use a knife or pill cutter to break the tablet. Place the tablet on a clean surface, place the blade in the scored line, and press directly downward until the tablet breaks.

4. For patients who have difficulty swallowing, offer the following suggestions:
   a. Drink water before taking pills, so your mouth is moist.
   b. Place whole tablets or capsules in a small amount of food, such as applesauce or pudding. The pill will go down when the food is swallowed. *Note: Also tell patients which foods should **not** be used.*
   c. Crush tablets by placing them on a spoon and pressing another spoon down on top of them. *Note: Warn patients not to crush any medication without first checking with the pharmacist or physician.*

REVIEW and PRACTICE

TABLETS AND CAPSULES

In Exercises 1–16, calculate the *amount to administer.* Unless otherwise noted, all scored tablets are scored in half.

1. Ordered: *Tegretol 400 mg po bid*
   On hand: Tegretol 200 mg unscored tablets   Administer:_____

2. Ordered: *Luvox 75 mg po qd*
   On hand: Luvox 50 mg scored tablets   Administer:_____

3. Ordered: *Seroquel 75 mg po tid*
   On hand: Seroquel 25 mg unscored tablets   Administer:_____

4. Ordered: *Tolectin 300 mg tid*
   On hand: Tolectin 200 mg scored tablets   Administer:_____

5. Ordered: *Isordil Titradose 15 mg*
   On hand: Isordil Titradose 10 mg deep-scored tablets   Administer:_____

6. Ordered: *Felbatol 600 mg po qd*
   On hand: Felbatol 400 mg scored tablets   Administer:_____

7. Ordered: *Decadron 1.5 mg po qd*
   On hand: Decadron 0.75 mg unscored tablets   Administer:_____

8. Ordered: *Coumadin 5 mg po qd*
   On hand: Coumadin 2 mg scored tablets   Administer:_____

212   *Chapter Nine*

Patient Education

We also have included several *Patient Education* boxes. These features encourage you to understand what information to communicate to patients and how to communicate it in a clear and professional manner.

Review and Practice

Most sections are followed by a *Review and Practice* set. In many cases, exercises are paired. Instructors may choose to assign either the even- or odd-numbered exercises. If you need additional practice, you can solve the corresponding exercises. Answers to all exercises appear at the back of the book. Worked-out solutions are in the *Instructor's Manual.*

Storage Information

Some drugs must be stored under specific conditions to maintain their potency and effectiveness. Storage information will appear on the drug's label. The label may have information about storage temperature, exposure to light, or the length of time the drug will remain potent after the container has been opened. Storage at the wrong temperature or exposure to light can trigger a chemical reaction that makes the drug unusable. (See Figures 6-13 and 6-14, letter I, for storage information.)

Manufacturing Information

Pharmaceutical manufacturers are strictly regulated by the U.S. Food and Drug Administration (FDA). FDA regulations state that every drug label must include the name of the manufacturer (Figure 6-15, letter J); an expiration date, abbreviated EXP, after which the drug may no longer be used (letter K); and the lot number (letter L).

Medications are produced in batches, known as lots. The lot number is a code that indicates when and where a drug was produced. It allows the manufacturer to trace problems linked to a particular batch. If a manufacturer has to remove an entire lot from the market because of contamination, suspected tampering, or unexpected side effects, the lot number helps identify which batch to recall.

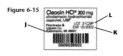

Figure 6-15

Rule 6-3

Never use a drug after the expiration date has passed.

Older drugs may become chemically unstable or altered. As a result, they may not provide the correct dosage strength. Worse, they could have an effect different from the intended one. Advise patients to check the expiration dates on all drug labels. If they have not used a product by the date listed, they should discard it. At an inpatient setting, the medication may need to be returned to the pharmacy, depending on the facility's policy.

Information About Reconstituting Drugs

Some drugs, such as antibiotics for pediatric use, are packaged in powder form. You reconstitute the drug (add liquid to the powder) shortly before administering it. Reconstituted medications remain potent for only a short amount of time. The label indicates the time period within which they can be safely administered (see Figures 6-16 and 6-17, letter M).

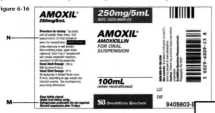

Figure 6-16

Drug Labels and Pac...

Labels

More than 250 full-color labels are integrated throughout the text, giving you practice finding the information you need from the drug label. We also have included excerpts from several package inserts as well as numerous sample Medication Administration Records, Physician's Orders, and Medication Cards.

Tables

More than thirty reference tables are in *Dosage Calculations for Medical Careers*. These tables concisely summarize key information. The listing of abbreviations that are commonly used in physician's orders is the most comprehensive one we have seen.

Equivalent Weight Measurements

Earlier you learned that 1 grain is equivalent to either 60 or 65 milligrams:

gr i = 60 mg *or* gr i = 65 mg

The relationship between grains and milligrams or grams is actually more complex. The conversion varies from 60 mg to 66.7 mg per gr. You will need to use information from the drug label or a drug reference to help you determine which equivalent measure to use for a given drug.

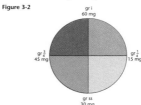

Figure 3-2

In cases where you use 60 mg as the equivalent measure, one way to remember the relationship between grains and milligrams is to think of a clock (see Figure 3-2). If each "minute" is one milligram, then an entire hour is one grain. This image of the clock may help you when you need to find the equivalent of $\frac{1}{2}$ grain (gr ss) or $\frac{1}{4}$ grain (gr $\frac{1}{4}$). Each half of an "hour" or grain is 30 "minutes" or milligrams. Similarly, each quarter of an "hour" or grain is 15 "minutes" or milligrams.

Table 3-8 summarizes important weight equivalent measures, including the relationship between kilograms and pounds (lb).

Table 3-8 Approximate Equivalent Measures for Weight

Metric	Apothecary
60 mg	gr i (1 grain)
30 mg	gr ss ($\frac{1}{2}$ grain)
15 mg	gr $\frac{1}{4}$
1 mg	gr $\frac{1}{60}$
1 g (1000 mg)	gr xv (15 grains)
0.5 g	gr viiss ($7\frac{1}{2}$ grains)
1 kg	2.2 lb

Converting Using Conversion Factors

A conversion factor expresses an equivalent measure. It helps you switch from one unit of measure to an equivalent one. Its numerator and denominator are equivalent. Both the factor and its reciprocal equal 1. For example, $\frac{1 \text{ mg}}{1000 \text{ mcg}}$ and $\frac{1000 \text{ mcg}}{1 \text{ mg}}$ are conversion factors that relate mg and mcg. Both factors equal 1. Similarly, $\frac{\text{gr i}}{60 \text{ mg}}$ and $\frac{60 \text{ mg}}{\text{gr i}}$ relate gr and mg.

You can use fraction proportions with conversion factors to convert a quantity from one unit of measure to another. (Recall from Chapter 2 that you cross-multiply to find a missing value in a fraction proportion.)

Systems of Weights and Measures **83**

Photographs and Art

The book includes numerous photographs and pieces of art to enhance the text. In most cases, images of syringes show uncapped syringes, ready for use. You should be aware, however, that for safety reasons syringes should remain capped when not in use.

Volume-control sets such as Buretrol, Soluset, and Volutrol are used with manual IV setups and electronic rate controllers to improve accuracy, especially for small volumes of medication or fluid (see Figure 11-11). They are calibrated in 1-mL increments, with a total volume capacity ranging from 100–150 mL. Medication is injected through an injection port into a burette—a chamber that holds a smaller controlled amount of fluid. An exact amount of IV fluid is added as a diluent to the burette chamber, where it is mixed. The fluid is delivered to the patient in microdrips. Burettes are often used in critical care or pediatric IVs because of their accuracy.

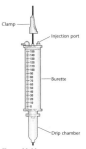

Figure 11-11
Volume control set.

Secondary Lines ("Piggybacks")

A secondary line, also known as a piggyback or IVPB, is an IV setup that attaches to a primary line (see Figure 11-12). It can be used to infuse medications or other compatible fluids on an intermittent basis, such as q6h. Although shorter than primary tubing, secondary tubing has the same basic components. IVPB bags are smaller, often holding 50, 100, or 150 cc of fluid. The ADD-Vantage® system from Abbott Laboratories is a secondary system. It uses a specially designed IV bag into which you add medication directly from the vial, often in powdered form. Any mixing takes place in the bag. The solution is then infused, with the medication vial remaining in place.

Peripheral and Central IV Therapy

Peripheral IV therapy accesses the circulatory system through a peripheral vein. Sites are usually located in the hand, forearm, foot, and leg. Because peripheral veins can be difficult to locate in small or premature infants, a peripheral IV line may be set up using a vein in the scalp.

Central IV therapy provides direct access to major veins. A central line is used when the patient needs large amounts of fluids, a rapid infusion of medication, infusion of highly concentrated solutions, or long-term IV therapy. Central lines can be inserted using a catheter through the chest wall or by threading a catheter through a peripheral vein. In newborn infants, a central line can be inserted into the umbilical vein or artery. These procedures are usually performed by a physician. Peripherally inserted central catheters (PICC) are inserted in arm veins and threaded into a central vein, often by specially trained nurses.

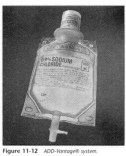

Figure 11-12 *ADD-Vantage® system.*

If you flush (or irrigate) an IV needle or catheter that is clogged, you may push a clot into the circulatory system, causing an embolism—an obstruction of a blood vessel that can be fatal. You also increase the risk of infection.

Calculating Flow Rates

An order for IV fluids indicates the flow rate—the amount of fluid that is to be infused over a certain time period. The amount of time listed in the physician's order may be expressed in hours or minutes. By controlling the flow rate, you control the speed with which medication is administered.

Rule 11-5

The flow rate can be expressed as $F = \frac{V}{T}$, where

F = flow rate
V = volume of fluid to infuse
T = time period of the infusion

EXAMPLE 1 Find the flow rate in mL/h.

Ordered: *1000 mL D5W to infuse over 8 h*

The volume to infuse (V) is 1000 mL. The time period of the infusion (T) is 8 hours.

$$F = \frac{V}{T} = \frac{1000 \text{ mL}}{8 \text{ h}} = \frac{\overset{125}{\cancel{1000}} \text{ mL}}{\underset{1}{\cancel{8}} \text{ h}} = \frac{125 \text{ mL}}{1 \text{ h}}$$

The flow rate is 125 mL/h.

Flow Rates for Electronic Regulation

Most electronic devices that regulate the flow of IV infusions measure the flow in milliliters per hour, or mL/h. Sometimes an order will call for an infusion to last less than an hour. However, you still calculate an hourly flow rate.

Rule 11-6

To find the flow rate F for electronic devices that measure an infusion in milliliters per hour, find $\frac{V}{T}$

$$\frac{\text{volume to infuse}}{\text{time period of infusion}} = \frac{V}{T}$$

where T = 1 hour and V is rounded to the nearest mL.

EXAMPLE 1 Find the flow rate.

Ordered: *500 mL 5%D 0.45%S over 3 hours by infusion pump*

The volume to infuse is 500 mL and the time period of infusion is 3 h.

$$\frac{\text{volume to infuse}}{\text{time period of infusion}} = \frac{500 \text{ mL}}{3 \text{ h}} = \frac{166.7 \text{ mL}}{1 \text{ h}}$$

Rounding to the nearest mL, the flow rate is 167 mL/h. You could also solve this problem using a fraction proportion.

$$\frac{500 \text{ mL}}{3 \text{ h}} = \frac{V}{1 \text{ h}}$$

$$500 \text{ mL} \times 1 \text{ h} = 3 \text{ h} \times V$$

$$\frac{500 \text{ mL}}{3} = V$$

$$166.67 \text{ mL} = V$$

Rules and Examples

The text makes extensive use of a *Rule* and *Example* format. Rules state important formulas and facts. The examples that follow illustrate the rules.

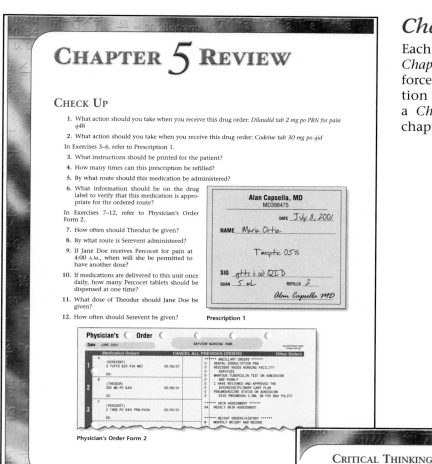

CHAPTER 5 REVIEW

CHECK UP

1. What action should you take when you receive this drug order: *Dilaudid tab 2 mg po PRN for pain q4h*

2. What action should you take when you receive this drug order: *Codeine tab 30 mg po qid*

In Exercises 3–6, refer to Prescription 1.

3. What instructions should be printed for the patient?

4. How many times can this prescription be refilled?

5. By what route should this medication be administered?

6. What information should be on the drug label to verify that this medication is appropriate for the ordered route?

In Exercises 7–12, refer to Physician's Order Form 2.

7. How often should Theodur be given?

8. By what route is Serevent administered?

9. If Jane Doe receives Percocet for pain at 4:00 A.M., when will she be permitted to have another dose?

10. If medications are delivered to this unit once daily, how many Percocet tablets should be dispensed at one time?

11. What dose of Theodur should Jane Doe be given?

12. How often should Serevent be given?

Alan Capsella, MD
MD398475

DATE July 8, 2001

NAME Maria Ortiz

Timoptic 0.5%

SIG gtts ii od QID

QUAN 5 mL   REFILLS 2

Alan Capsella MD

Prescription 1

Physician's Order
Date JUNE 2001   BAYVIEW NURSING HOME

Physician's Order Form 2

Chapter Review

Each chapter concludes with an extensive *Chapter Review* to help you apply and reinforce what you have learned. The first portion of each *Chapter Review* provides a *Check Up* of the basic skills from that chapter.

Each *Chapter Review* also contains a *Critical Thinking* exercise, a *Case Study,* and an *Internet Activity.* The *Critical Thinking* exercises require you to go beyond simple calculations. Each *Case Study* provides a real-world situation. Each *Internet Activity* helps you learn to use the Internet for research and training. Answers to all *Chapter Review* exercises are in the back of the book. Worked-out solutions are in the *Instructor's Manual.*

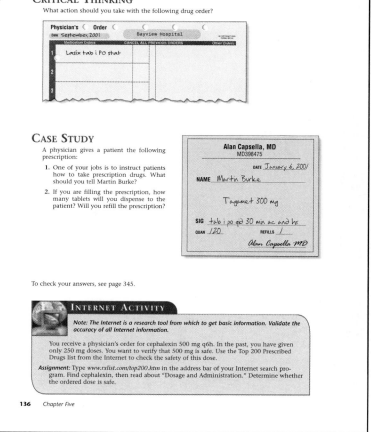

CRITICAL THINKING

What action should you take with the following drug order?

Physician's Order
Date September, 2001   Bayview Hospital
CANCEL ALL PREVIOUS ORDERS

1 Lasix tab i PO stat

CASE STUDY

A physician gives a patient the following prescription:

1. One of your jobs is to instruct patients how to take prescription drugs. What should you tell Martin Burke?

2. If you are filling the prescription, how many tablets will you dispense to the patient? Will you refill the prescription?

Alan Capsella, MD
MD398475

DATE January 6, 2001

NAME Martin Burke

Tagamet 300 mg

SIG tab i po qid 30 min ac and hs

QUAN 120   REFILLS 1

Alan Capsella MD

To check your answers, see page 345.

INTERNET ACTIVITY

Note: The Internet is a research tool from which to get basic information. Validate the accuracy of all Internet information.

You receive a physician's order for cephalexin 500 mg q6h. In the past, you have given only 250 mg doses. You want to verify that 500 mg is safe. Use the Top 200 Prescribed Drugs list from the Internet to check the safety of this dose.

Assignment: Type *www.rxlist.com/top200.htm* in the address bar of your Internet search program. Find cephalexin, then read about "Dosage and Administration." Determine whether the ordered dose is safe.

136 *Chapter Five*

Pretest

You may review your understanding of basic math skills by taking the pretest before you begin your study of dosage calculation.

PRETEST

The following test covers basic mathematical concepts you will need to understand and calculate dosages. This test will help you determine which concepts you need to review before continuing. You should already be able to perform basic operations—addition, subtraction, multiplication, and division—with whole numbers. The test covers Roman numerals, fractions, decimals, percent, ratios, and proportions.

Take 90 minutes to answer the following 50 questions. Then check your answers on page 329. Review the questions you answered incorrectly to learn more about any basic math weaknesses. Then, as needed, review that content in Chapters 1 and 2.

1. Write the answer to XVIII + IX in Arabic numbers. (Arabic numbers are those commonly used, such as 23 or 7056.)

2. Write the answer to 212 − 198 in Roman numerals.

3. Convert $\frac{14}{3}$ to a mixed number.

4. Convert $3\frac{7}{8}$ to an improper fraction.

Find the missing numerator in the following equations:

5. $\frac{2}{7} = \frac{?}{21}$

6. $1\frac{1}{8} = \frac{?}{16}$

7. Reduce $\frac{40}{100}$ to its lowest terms.

8. Which fraction has the greater value: $\frac{3}{8}$ or $\frac{2}{6}$?

Calculate the following. Reduce fractions to lowest terms and rewrite any improper fractions as mixed numbers.

9. $\frac{4}{5} + \frac{3}{8}$

10. $1\frac{1}{3} + \frac{5}{7}$

11. $\frac{7}{10} - \frac{1}{4}$

12. $8\frac{1}{4} - 2\frac{1}{3}$

$\frac{1}{9}$

1

COMPREHENSIVE EVALUATION

The following test will help you check your dosage calculation skills. Throughout the book you have learned a variety of methods for calculating dosages. In these questions, you should use the methods with which you are most comfortable and competent.

In Exercises 1–8, refer to MAR 1.

1. What dose of Neurontin should be administered?

2. By what route should Desyrel be administered?

3. When should Reglan be administered?

4. Why are no times listed for Ativan?

5. Are any of the orders incomplete? If so, what information is missing?

6. What is the likely reason that Reglan is administered half an hour before Neurontin?

7. If the order for Neurontin read q8h instead of TID, when would the second and third doses be administered?

8. If Ativan is administered at 1330, when can the patient receive another dose?

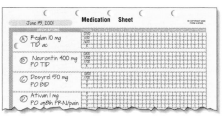

In Exercises 9–12, refer to Label A.

9. What is the generic name of the drug?

10. At what temperature should the drug be stored?

11. What is the dosage strength?

12. If an adult took twice the usual adult dose, how long would the container last?

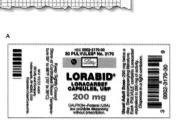

323

Comprehensive Evaluation

You may take the *Comprehensive Evaluation* following Chapter 13. You will find the answers to Review and Practice Sets and Chapter Reviews in the back of the book.

Reviewers

The following reviewers provided invaluable advice along the way. Their contribution helped shape all aspects of the text.

Linda S. Albrecht
Richland College
Dallas, Texas

Sylvia Banzone
Elk Grove, California

Ellon Barlow
Fayetteville Technical Community College
Fayetteville, North Carolina

Gail A. Chester, CMA
Community College of Southern Nevada
Las Vegas, Nevada

Barbara M. Dahl, CMA
Whatcom Community College
Bellingham, Washington

Deb Getting, BSN
Northwest Iowa Community College
Sheldon, Iowa

Margaret M. Gingrich, BSN, MSN
Harrisburg Area Community College
Harrisburg, Pennsylvania

Kris A. Hardy, CMA
Brevard Community College
Cocoa, Florida

Elizabeth Keene, CMA, BSN
Lansdale School of Business
North Wales, Pennsylvania

Rita Michelson, LPN
Middlesex Community College
Middletown, Connecticut

Lori Moseley, RN
Hill College
Cleburne, Texas

Bonnie Normile
Carnegie Technical Institute
Troy, Michigan

Warren Ruud
Santa Rosa Junior College
Santa Rosa, California

Mary E. Stassi, RN
St. Charles County Community College
St. Peters, Missouri

Wanda M. Webb, MSN
Hickory House Nursing Home
Honey Brook, Pennsylvania

Holly Ann Williamson, BSN
Lorenzo Walker Institute of Technology
Naples, Florida

Acknowledgments

Many pharmaceutical companies and drug equipment manufacturers provided us with drug labels, package inserts, and photographs of equipment for use throughout this text and the *Instructor's Manual*. We graciously acknowledge the assistance of the following companies:

Labels for Biaxin®, Biaxin® Filmtab®, Cartrol®, Cylert®, Depakene®, E.E.S.®, Eryped® Drops, Erythromycin, Iberet®-Liquid, Norvir®, Tranxene®, and Tricor® as well as 5% Dextrose and Lactated Ringer's Injection, and 0.9% Sodium Chloride Injection Courtesy: Abbott Laboratories, Abbott Park, IL

Alaris Medical Systems, San Diego, CA

Labels and excerpts from package labels for Epogen® and Neupogen® reprinted with permission of Amgen Inc.

Labels for Kantrex®, Nydrazid® Courtesy: Apothecon, A Bristol-Myers Squibb Co., Princeton, NJ 08540 USA

Labels for Prilosec® and Tonocard® Courtesy: AstraZeneca, L.P.

Label for 5% Dextrose Injection Courtesy: Baxter Healthcare Corporation

Label for Cipro® reprinted by permission of Bayer Corporation

Becton Dickinson and Company, Franklin Lakes, NJ 07417

Labels for CeeNu®, Cytoxan®, Maxipime®, and Megace® and excerpts from Package Inserts for Maxipime® Courtesy: Bristol-Myers Squibb Company

Label for Aricept® Copyright 1997, Eisai Inc. All rights reserved. Use with permission.

Labels for Aerobid®, Antilirium®, Celexa®, Sus-phrine®, and Tiazac® Courtesy: Forest Laboratories, Inc.

Labels and excerpts from Prescribing Information for Ceftin®, Ceptaz®, Fortaz®, Flonase®, Imitrex®, Lamictal®, Lanoxin®, Ventolin®, Wellbutrin®, Zantac®, Zinacef®, Zofran®, and Zovirax® reproduced with permission of Glaxo Wellcome Inc.

Label for Lasix® Courtesy: Hoechst Marion Roussel, Inc.

Hoffman-LaRoche, Inc., Nutley, NJ

Labels for Amicar® and Leucovorin® Calcium and excerpt of package insert for Leucovorin® Calcium Courtesy: Immunex Corporation

Actimmune® is a registered trademark licensed by InterMune Pharmaceuticals, Inc.

Label for Tigan® Courtesy: King Pharmaceuticals, Inc.

Labels for Dilaudid®, Dilaudid-HP®, Isoptin®, Synthroid®, and Vicodin Tuss® Copyright© Knoll Pharmaceutical. All Rights Reserved. Used by permission. Dilaudid®, Dilaudid-HP®, Isoptin®, Synthroid®, and Vicodin Tuss® are trademarks or registered trademarks of Knoll Pharmaceutical.

Labels for Atropine Sulfate, Ceclor®, Glucagon®, Humalog®, Humatrope®, Humulin®, Lente® Iletin®, Keflex®, Lorabid®, Mandol®, Oncovin®, Phenobarbital, Prozac®, and Seconal® copyright Eli Lilly and Company. Used with permission.

Label for Motrin® IB Gelcap, Courtesy: McNeil Consumer Healthcare, Fort Washington, PA

Medex, Dublin, OH

The labels for the products MEFOXIN® (cefoxitan for injection), PRIMAXIN® (imipenem and cilastatin for injection), and VASOTEC® I.V. (enalaprilat) are reproduced with permission of Merck & Co., Inc., copyright owner.

Labels for Brethine®, Clozaril®, Ritalin®, and Sandostatin® are used with the permission of Novartis Pharmaceuticals Corporation.

Labels for Novolin®, Prandin®, and Velosulin® Courtesy: Novo Nordisk Pharmaceuticals, Inc.

Labels and excerpt of package insert for Follistim® and Humegon® are reproduced with permission of Organon Inc.

Labels for Haldol® and Regranex® Gel 0.01%, Courtesy: Ortho-McNeil Pharmaceutical, Inc.

Labels for Pfizerpen®, Procardia®, Vistaril®, and Zithromax® Courtesy: Pfizer Inc.

Labels for Azulfidine®, Camposar®, Cleocin HCl®, Cleocin Pediatric®, Cleocin Phosphate®, Deltasone®, Depo-Provera®, Fragmin®, Halcion®, Heparin Sodium Injection®, Provera®, Vantin®, Xanax®, and Zinecard® Courtesy: Pharmacia Corp.

MS Contin® 30 mg tablets label reproduced with permission of The Purdue Frederick Company.

OxyContin® 20 mg tablets label reproduced with permission of Purdue Pharma L.P.

Retractable Technologies, Inc., Lewisville, TX

Labels for DDAVP® and Lovenox® Courtesy: Rhône-Poulenc Rorer

Labels for Rocephin® and Valium® Courtesy: Roche Products, Inc.

Label and package insert for Pediazole® used with permission of Ross Products Division, Abbott Laboratories Inc., Columbus, OH 43215. Copyright 1998 Ross Products Division, Abbott Laboratories Inc.

Labels for Codeine and Morphine Sulfate Courtesy: Roxane Laboratories, Inc.

Labels for Cedax®, Claritin®, Diprolene®, Intron® A, Proventil®, Vancenase®, and Vanceril® Inhaler reproduced with permission of the copyright owners Schering Corporation. All rights reserved.

Labels for Calciferol™, Clozaril®, Deponit®, Levsin®, Monoket®, and Univasc® Courtesy: Schwarz Pharma, Inc.

Labels for Amoxil®, Augmentin®, Compazine®, Engerix-B®, Famvir®, Kefzol®, Paxil®, Requip™, Stelazine®, and Thorazine® Courtesy: SmithKline Beecham Pharmaceuticals.

Label for Duphalac® reproduced with permission of Solvay Pharmaceuticals, Inc.

Labels for Lortab® and Theo-24® Courtesy: UCB Pharma, Inc.

Labels for Felbatol™ and Rynatan® reprinted with permission of Wallace Laboratories, Division of Carter-Wallace, Inc., Cranbury, New Jersey 08512

Label for Nitrostat® Courtesy: Warner-Lambert Company

CONTENTS

Chapter 1   Roman Numerals, Fractions, and Decimals

Chapter 2   Percents, Ratios, and Proportions

Chapter 3   Systems of Weights and Measures 71

Chapter 4   Equipment for Dosage Measurement 93

Chapter 5

Drug Orders 115

Chapter 6

Drug Labels and Package Inserts 137

Chapter 7   Methods of Dosage Calculations 161

Chapter 8   Dimensional Analysis 185

Chapter 9   Oral Dosages 205

Chapter 10   Parenteral Dosages 228

List of Tables

PRETEST

The following test covers basic mathematical concepts you will need to understand and calculate dosages. This test will help you determine which concepts you need to review before continuing. You should already be able to perform basic operations—addition, subtraction, multiplication, and division—with whole numbers. The test covers Roman numerals, fractions, decimals, percent, ratios, and proportions.

Take 90 minutes to answer the following 50 questions. Then check your answers on page 329. Review the questions you answered incorrectly to learn more about any basic math weaknesses. Then, as needed, review that content in Chapters 1 and 2.

1. Write the answer to XVIII + IX in Arabic numbers. (Arabic numbers are those commonly used, such as 23 or 7056.)

2. Write the answer to $212 - 198$ in Roman numerals.

3. Convert $\dfrac{14}{3}$ to a mixed number.

4. Convert $3\dfrac{7}{8}$ to an improper fraction.

Find the missing numerator in the following equations:

5. $\dfrac{2}{7} = \dfrac{?}{21}$

6. $1\dfrac{1}{8} = \dfrac{?}{16}$

7. Reduce $\dfrac{40}{100}$ to its lowest terms.

8. Which fraction has the greater value: $\dfrac{3}{8}$ or $\dfrac{2}{6}$?

Calculate the following. Reduce fractions to lowest terms and rewrite any improper fractions as mixed numbers.

9. $\dfrac{4}{5} + \dfrac{3}{8}$

10. $1\dfrac{1}{3} + \dfrac{5}{7}$

11. $\dfrac{7}{10} - \dfrac{1}{4}$

12. $8\dfrac{1}{4} - 2\dfrac{1}{3}$

1

13. $\frac{3}{5} \times \frac{1}{9}$

14. $3\frac{1}{5} \times 4\frac{3}{8}$

15. $\frac{2}{3} \div \frac{4}{5}$

16. $5\frac{1}{4} \div 2\frac{5}{8}$

17. Which number has the lesser value: 1.01 or 1.009?

18. Round 14.42 to the nearest whole number.

19. Round 6.05 to the nearest tenth.

20. Round 19.197 to the nearest hundredth.

21. Convert $3\frac{4}{5}$ to a decimal number. If necessary, round to the nearest hundredth.

22. Convert 0.045 to a fraction or a mixed number. Reduce to lowest terms.

Calculate the following.

23. 7.289 + 8.011

24. 0.012 + 0.9 + 4.2

25. 19.1 − 4.4

26. 100.03 − 0.6

27. 0.07 × 3.2

28. 0.4 ÷ 0.02

29. Convert 0.8% to a decimal number.

30. Convert 0.99 to a percent.

31. Convert 260% to a proper fraction or mixed number.

32. Convert $1\frac{1}{8}$ to a percent.

33. Convert 7:12 to a fraction.

34. Convert $\frac{10}{50}$ to a ratio. Reduce to lowest terms.

35. Convert 1:12 to a decimal. Round to the nearest hundredth, if necessary.

36. Convert 0.4 to a ratio. Reduce to lowest terms.

37. Convert 3:8 to a percent. Round to the nearest percent, if necessary.

38. Convert 0.5% to a ratio. Reduce to lowest terms.

Determine whether the following proportions are true.

39. 8:16::4:8

40. 5:9::8:12

Find the missing value in the following proportions.

41. 8:12::?:9

42. $\dfrac{2}{7} = \dfrac{?}{28}$

43. A nurse is instructed to give a patient $1\frac{1}{2}$ teaspoons of cough syrup four times a day. How many teaspoons of cough syrup will the nurse give each day?

44. A pharmacy technician tries to keep the equivalent of 12 bottles of a medication on hand. The hospital's first floor has $1\frac{1}{2}$ bottles, the second floor has $1\frac{3}{4}$ bottles, the third floor has $3\frac{1}{4}$ bottles, and the supply closet has 3 bottles. Is there enough medication on hand? If not, how much should the technician order?

45. A bottle contains 75 milliliters of a liquid medication. Since the bottle was opened, one patient has received 3 doses of 2.5 milliliters. A second patient has received 4 doses of 2.2 milliliters. How much medication remains in the bottle?

46. A tablet contains 0.125 milligram of medication. A patient receives 3 tablets a day for five days. How many milligrams of medication does the patient receive over the five days?

47. An IV bag contained 1000 mL of a liquid that was 10% drug. The liquid was administered to a patient and now there are 400 mL left in the bag. How many grams of drug remain in the bag?

48. 3% of the volume of a 200 mL solution contains active drug. How many mL of the solution contain active drug?

49. Write a ratio that represents that 500 mL of solution contains 5 mg of drug.

50. Write a ratio that represents that every tablet in a bottle contains 25 mg of drug.

ROMAN NUMERALS, FRACTIONS, and DECIMALS

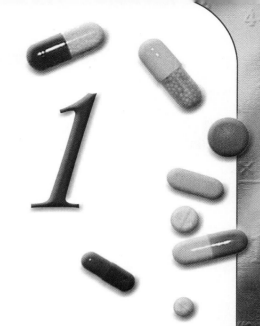

1

Objectives

When you have completed Chapter 1, you will be able to:

- **Recognize and work with Roman numerals as they relate to physicians' orders, prescriptions, and dosage calculations.**
- **Distinguish between the various formats of fractions and measure their relative values.**
- **Accurately add, subtract, multiply, and divide fractions.**
- **Convert fractions to mixed numbers and decimals.**
- **Recognize the format of decimals and measure their relative values.**
- **Accurately add, subtract, multiply, and divide decimals.**
- **Round decimals to the nearest tenth, hundredth, or thousandth.**
- **Identify common errors in working with Roman numerals, fractions, and decimals.**

Roman Numerals

In the Roman numeral system, letters are used to represent number values. Unlike the Arabic system that we use in everyday counting, the Roman system has no symbol for zero. Roman numerals are used less frequently in dosage calculations. Still, some practitioners use them in prescriptions and physicians' orders. You will need to understand Roman numerals to interpret physicians' orders, prescriptions, and drug dosages correctly. In medical settings, you will generally see and use only the Roman numerals that represent the values 1 through 30.

You can write Roman numerals as either uppercase or lowercase letters. In medical usage, iv, which represents the number 4, is generally written in lowercase to distinguish it from IV, the abbreviation for intravenous. Sometimes a line is written above lowercase letters. When the letter *i* is written with this line, the dot of the i appears above the line. Thus, the number four can be written IV, iv, or i͞v.

The building blocks of the Roman system are the letters I, V, X, L, C, D, and M. Only I, V, and X are needed to represent the values 1 through 30.

$$I = i = 1 \qquad C = c = 100$$
$$V = v = 5 \qquad D = d = 500$$
$$X = x = 10 \qquad M = m = 1000$$
$$L = = 50$$

Rule 1-1

When working with Roman numerals,

1. If a numeral appears twice in a row, count its value twice. If it appears three times in a row, count its value three times.

2. Do not use a numeral more than three times in a row. Use the largest numeral possible to represent a value.

EXAMPLE 1
a. ii = 1 + 1 = 2
b. XXX = 10 + 10 + 10 = 30

EXAMPLE 2
a. Write 5 as v, not iiiii.
b. Write 10 as X, not VV.

Rule 1-2

To combine Roman numerals,

1. If a numeral with a smaller value comes immediately after (to the right of) a numeral with a larger value, add their values.

2. If a numeral with a smaller value comes immediately before (to the left of) a numeral with a larger value, subtract the smaller value from the larger one.

3. Unless you are subtracting, write numerals with larger values before those with smaller ones.

EXAMPLE 1
a. vii = v + i + i = 5 + 1 + 1 = 7
b. XXVIII = X + X + V + I + I + I = 10 + 10 + 5 + 1 + 1 + 1 = 28

EXAMPLE 2
a. iv = v - i = 5 - 1 = 4   Do not write iiii.
b. IX = X - I = 10 - 1 = 9   Do not write VIIII.
c. XL = L - X = 50 - 10 = 40   Do not write XXXX.

EXAMPLE 3
a. Write 8 as viii. Do not write iiiv or iix.
b. Write 18 as XVIII. Do not write IIIVX or VXIII.

CRITICAL THINKING ON THE JOB

Understand the Order of Roman Numerals

A medication card lists a drug order of gr ix. (The abbreviation gr stands for grains. See Chapters 3 and 5.) A medical assistant reading the card thinks, "The Roman numeral i equals 1 and x equals 10, so I should give 11 grains of the drug."

Think Before You Act

The numeral with the smaller value comes immediately before the one with the larger value. Instead of adding i and x, the medical assistant should subtract i from x to calculate the correct dose of 9 gr.

In numbers that have a numeral placed between two others with larger values, you need to know when to add and when to subtract.

Rule 1-3

When a Roman numeral comes between two numerals with larger values, subtract the smaller numeral from the one to its right. Then add the remaining values.

EXAMPLE 1 Calculate the Arabic number for xiv.

In xiv, the numeral i is placed between two numerals with larger values. Subtract i from v first, then add.

$$xiv = x + iv = x + (v - i) = 10 + (4) = 14$$

EXAMPLE 2 Calculate the Arabic number for XXIX.

Do not look at this numeral as X + XI + X. Instead, subtract I from the X that follows it, so that

$$XXIX = X + X + IX = X + X + (X - I) = 10 + 10 + 9 = 29$$

Rule 1-4

To add or subtract Roman numerals, first change the numerals into Arabic numbers. Then perform the calculations.

EXAMPLE 1 **a.** vii + xiii = 7 + 13 = 20
b. XII + III = 12 + 3 = 15
c. XXIV − IX = 24 − 9 = 15
d. $\overline{vi}$ − $\overline{iv}$ = 6 − 4 = 2

The Roman numerals from 1 to 30 are the ones you are most likely to see in physicians' orders. Table 1-1, which summarizes these numerals, will help you practice converting them.

Table 1-1 Converting Roman Numerals

Roman Numeral	Arabic Number	Roman Numeral	Arabic Number	Roman Numeral	Arabic Number
I, i	1	XI, xi	11	XXI, xxi	21
II, ii	2	XII, xii	12	XXII, xxii	22
III, iii	3	XIII, xiii	13	XXIII, xxiii	23
IV, iv	4	XIV, xiv	14	XXIV, xxiv	24
V, v	5	XV, xv	15	XXV, xxv	25
VI, vi	6	XVI, xvi	16	XXVI, xxvi	26
VII, vii	7	XVII, xvii	17	XXVII, xxvii	27
VIII, viii	8	XVIII, xviii	18	XXVIII, xxviii	28
IX, ix	9	XIX, xix	19	XXIX, xxix	29
X, x	10	XX, xx	20	XXX, xxx	30

ROMAN NUMERALS

Convert the following Roman numerals to Arabic numbers:

1. VI   **2.** XII   **3.** IX

4. XIV   **5.** xxiv   **6.** xviii

Convert the following Arabic numbers to Roman numerals:

7. 13   **8.** 8   **9.** 23

10. 17   **11.** 29   **12.** 24

Write the answers to the following problems as Arabic numbers:

13. IV + XVII   **14.** xii + xiv

15. VIII + III   **16.** V + V

17. XXIII − VII   **18.** xvi − ix

19. XXI − III   **20.** XXX − V

To check your answers, see page 329.

Fractions

Fractions measure a portion or part of a whole amount. They are written in two ways: as common fractions or as decimals. In medical settings, you must often convert from one type of fraction to another.

Working With Common Fractions

A common fraction represents equal parts of a whole. It consists of two numbers and a fraction bar, and is written in the form $\frac{numerator}{denominator}$.

The denominator, the bottom part of the fraction, represents the whole. It can *never* equal zero. Suppose the whole is one yard. You could express the denominator in many ways: as 1 (the yard as a whole), 3 (the yard as 3 feet), or 36 (the yard as 36 inches).

The numerator, the top part of the fraction, represents parts of the whole. If you buy 2 feet of fabric out of a yard, you can express the numerator as 2 with the denominator as 3 (feet). The fraction $\frac{2}{3}$ represents how much of a yard of fabric you buy, or 2 of 3 feet. If you buy less fabric, say 9 inches, you can express the numerator as 9 with the denominator as 36 (inches). The fraction $\frac{9}{36}$ represents how much of a yard of fabric you buy, or 9 of 36 inches.

Suppose you are working with a medicine tablet that is scored (marked) for division in four equal parts, and you must administer one part of that tablet each day. The denominator represents the whole tablet, or all four parts. The numerator represents one part, the amount that you must administer each day. The fraction, or part, of the tablet that you must administer each day is written as:

$$\frac{numerator}{denominator} = \frac{1 \text{ part}}{4 \text{ parts}} = \frac{1}{4}.$$

This number is read "one-fourth" or "one-quarter." If you administer three parts of a tablet each day, the fraction of the whole tablet administered daily is $\frac{3}{4}$.

You may need to administer a tablet scored in two parts. Now the denominator is 2, since two parts make up the whole. If you administer one part each day, you administer $\frac{1}{2}$ of the tablet.

If you have trouble remembering which number is the numerator and which is the denominator, note that the words *denominator* and *down* begin with *d*. The <u>d</u>enominator is <u>d</u>own, under the fraction bar.

The fraction $\frac{2}{3}$, read as "two-thirds," means two parts out of the three parts that make up the whole. The fraction bar also means "divided by." Thus, $\frac{2}{3}$ can be read as "two divided by three," or $2 \div 3$. This definition is important when you change fractions to decimals.

Sometimes fractions show the relationship between part of a group and the whole group. For example, in a group of 15 patients with hyperthyroidism, 9 patients respond well to a medication. The other 6 patients show no change. The number of patients in the full group, 15, is the whole, or the denominator. You write the fraction of patients who respond well to the medication as

$$\frac{\text{part}}{\text{whole}} = \frac{\text{respond well}}{\text{whole group}} = \frac{9}{15}$$

Similarly, the fraction of patients who show no change is

$$\frac{\text{part}}{\text{whole}} = \frac{\text{show no change}}{\text{whole group}} = \frac{6}{15}$$

Proper and Improper Fractions. A proper fraction has a numerator that is smaller than the denominator. An improper fraction has a numerator that is equal to or greater than the denominator. Recall from past math classes that $<$ means "is less than" and $>$ means "is greater than." The open end of the symbols $<$ and $>$ is next to the larger value.

Rule 1-5

1. When the numerator is smaller than the denominator, the fraction is proper. Its value is *always* less than one. If numerator $<$ denominator, then $\frac{\text{numerator}}{\text{denominator}} < 1$.

2. When the numerator is larger than the denominator, the fraction is improper. Its value is *always* greater than one. If numerator $>$ denominator, then $\frac{\text{numerator}}{\text{denominator}} > 1$.

3. When the numerator is equal to the denominator, the fraction is improper. Its value is *always* exactly one. If numerator $=$ denominator, then $\frac{\text{numerator}}{\text{denominator}} = 1$.

EXAMPLE 1 Examples of proper fractions include $\frac{4}{5}, \frac{1}{17}, \frac{24}{25},$ and $\frac{107}{1000}$.

EXAMPLE 2 Examples of improper fractions include $\frac{5}{3}, \frac{25}{24},$ and $\frac{125}{10}$.

EXAMPLE 3 Examples of improper fractions that equal one are $\frac{5}{5}, \frac{12}{12},$ and $\frac{2}{2}$.

EXAMPLE 4 Insert $<$, $>$, or $=$ to make a true statement.

a. $\frac{7}{9}$ 1   a. Because $7 < 9$, $\frac{7}{9} < 1$.

b. $\frac{8}{8}$ 1   b. Because $8 = 8$, $\frac{8}{8} = 1$.

c. $\frac{20}{15}$ 1   c. Because $20 > 15$, $\frac{20}{15} > 1$.

The denominator of any fraction can never be zero. It can, however, equal 1.

When the denominator is 1, the fraction equals the number in the numerator.

EXAMPLE 1

$$\frac{4}{1} = 4; \frac{100}{1} = 100$$

Check these equations by treating each fraction as a division problem.

$$4 \div 1 = 4; 100 \div 1 = 100$$

Mixed numbers. A mixed number combines a whole number with a fraction. Examples include $2\frac{2}{3}$ (two and two-thirds), $1\frac{7}{8}$ (one and seven-eighths), and $12\frac{31}{32}$ (twelve and thirty-one thirty-seconds).

Rule 1-7

To convert an improper fraction to a mixed number,

1. Divide the numerator by the denominator. The result will be a whole number plus a remainder.

2. Write the remainder as the numerator over the original denominator.

3. Combine the whole number and the fractional remainder. This mixed number equals the original improper fraction.

EXAMPLE 1 Convert $\frac{11}{4}$ to a mixed number.

1. Divide the numerator by the denominator:

$$11 \div 4 = 2 \text{ R}3 \qquad (\text{R}3 \text{ means a remainder of 3.})$$

The result is the whole number 2 with a remainder of 3.

2. Write the remainder as the numerator over the original denominator of 4:

$$\frac{\text{remainder}}{\text{denominator}} = \frac{3}{4}$$

3. Combine the whole number and the fractional remainder:

$$2 + \frac{3}{4} = 2\frac{3}{4}$$

The mixed number $2\frac{3}{4}$ equals the original improper fraction $\frac{11}{4}$.

EXAMPLE 2 Convert $\frac{23}{7}$ to a mixed number.

1. $23 \div 7 = 3 \text{ R}2$

The result is the whole number 3 with a remainder of 2.

2. $\frac{\text{remainder}}{\text{denominator}} = \frac{2}{7}$

3. $3 + \frac{2}{7} = 3\frac{2}{7}$

The improper fraction $\frac{23}{7}$ equals the mixed number $3\frac{2}{7}$.

EXAMPLE 3 Convert $\frac{36}{12}$ to a mixed number.

1. $36 \div 12 = 3 \text{ R}0$

The result is the whole number 3 with a remainder of 0.

2. There is no remainder and, therefore, no fraction. Skip Step 2.

3. When there is no remainder, the answer is a whole number. In this example, $\frac{36}{12} = 3$.

You can also convert mixed numbers to improper fractions for those times that it is easier to work with improper fractions.

Rule 1-8

To convert a mixed number to an improper fraction,

1. Multiply the whole number by the denominator of the fraction.

2. Add the product from Step 1 to the numerator of the fraction.

3. Write the sum from Step 2 over the original denominator. This number is an improper fraction equal to the original mixed number.

EXAMPLE 1 Convert $5\frac{1}{3}$ to an improper fraction.

The whole number is 5. The denominator of the fraction is 3. The numerator of the fraction is 1.

1. Multiply the whole number by the denominator of the fraction.

$$5 \times 3 = 15$$

2. Add the product from Step 1 to the numerator of the fraction.

$$15 + 1 = 16$$

3. Write the sum from Step 2 over the original denominator.

$$\frac{16}{3}$$

Thus, $5\frac{1}{3} = \frac{16}{3}$

EXAMPLE 2 Convert $10\frac{7}{8}$ to an improper fraction.

The whole number is 10. The denominator is 8. The numerator is 7.

1. $10 \times 8 = 80$

2. $80 + 7 = 87$

3. $\frac{87}{8}$

Thus, $10\frac{7}{8} = \frac{87}{8}$

REVIEW and PRACTICE

WORKING WITH COMMON FRACTIONS

1. What is the numerator in $\frac{17}{100}$?

2. What is the numerator in $\frac{8}{3}$?

3. What is the denominator in $\frac{4}{100}$?

4. What is the denominator in $\frac{60}{1}$?

5. Which of the following fractions are proper fractions?

  a. $\frac{5}{24}$ **b.** $\frac{25}{10}$ **c.** $\frac{7}{7}$ **d.** $\frac{33}{50}$

6. Which of the following fractions are improper fractions?
   a. $\frac{150}{100}$ b. $\frac{9}{5}$ c. $\frac{1}{5}$ d. $\frac{12}{12}$

7. Twelve patients are in a hospital ward. Four have type A blood.
   a. What fraction of the patients have type A blood?
   b. What fraction of the patients do not have type A blood?

8. Twenty patients are in a hospital ward. Six have diabetes.
   a. What fraction of the patients have diabetes?
   b. What fraction of the patients do not have diabetes?

9. Write this expression as a fraction: $16 \div 3$

10. Write this expression as a fraction: $4 \div 15$

11. Insert $<$, $>$, or $=$ to make a true statement.
    a. $\frac{14}{14}$ 1   b. $\frac{24}{32}$ 1   c. $\frac{125}{100}$ 1

12. Insert $<$, $>$, or $=$ to make a true statement.
    a. $\frac{24}{3}$ 1   b. $\frac{75}{100}$ 1   c. $\frac{18}{18}$ 1

Convert the following improper fractions to mixed or whole numbers:

13. $\frac{43}{6}$ 14. $\frac{17}{3}$ 15. $\frac{100}{20}$ 16. $\frac{50}{50}$

17. $\frac{8}{5}$ 18. $\frac{167}{25}$

Convert the following mixed numbers to improper fractions:

19. $2\frac{16}{17}$ 20. $8\frac{8}{9}$ 21. $1\frac{1}{10}$ 22. $4\frac{1}{8}$

23. $103\frac{2}{3}$ 24. $6\frac{7}{8}$

To check your answers, see page 330.

Equivalent Fractions

Two or more fractions with the same value but written with different terms are equivalent fractions. They have different numerators and denominators, but they equal the same amount.

Suppose you and a friend are sharing a pizza equally, dividing it in half. If you cut the pizza into eight slices, you will each get four pieces, or $\frac{4}{8}$ of the whole pizza. If you cut the pizza into six slices, you will each get three pieces, or $\frac{3}{6}$. And if you cut the pizza into four slices, you will each get two slices, or $\frac{2}{4}$. Whether you get $\frac{4}{8}$, $\frac{3}{6}$, or $\frac{2}{4}$ of the pizza, you still have the same amount: half or $\frac{1}{2}$ of the pizza (see Figure 1-1). Thus, $\frac{4}{8} = \frac{3}{6} = \frac{2}{4} = \frac{1}{2}$. These four fractions are equivalent fractions.

Converting Fractions. Equivalent fractions help you compare measurements more easily. They also help you add and subtract fractions that have different denominators.

Figure 1-1

Equivalent fractions.

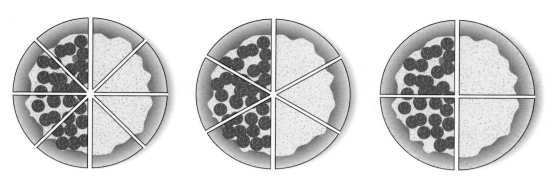

Rule 1-9

To find an equivalent fraction, multiply or divide both the numerator and denominator by the same number. *Exception:* The numerator and denominator cannot be multiplied or divided by zero.

EXAMPLE 1 Find equivalent fractions for $\frac{2}{4}$.

$$\frac{2 \times 2}{4 \times 2} = \frac{4}{8} \qquad \frac{2 \times 3}{4 \times 3} = \frac{6}{12} \qquad \frac{2 \div 2}{4 \div 2} = \frac{1}{2} \qquad \frac{2 \times 10}{4 \times 10} = \frac{20}{40}$$

Thus, $\frac{2}{4} = \frac{4}{8} = \frac{6}{12} = \frac{1}{2} = \frac{20}{40}$. These are equivalent fractions.

EXAMPLE 2 Find equivalent fractions for $\frac{4}{7}$.

$$\frac{4 \times 3}{7 \times 3} = \frac{12}{21} \qquad \frac{4 \times 5}{7 \times 5} = \frac{20}{35} \qquad \frac{4 \times 10}{7 \times 10} = \frac{40}{70} \qquad \frac{4 \times 100}{7 \times 100} = \frac{400}{700}$$

Thus, $\frac{4}{7} = \frac{12}{21} = \frac{20}{35} = \frac{40}{70} = \frac{400}{700}$. These are equivalent fractions.

EXAMPLE 3 Find equivalent fractions for 4.

To find equivalent fractions for a whole number, first write the whole number as a fraction. Then proceed as before.

$$4 = \frac{4}{1}$$

$$\frac{4 \times 2}{1 \times 2} = \frac{8}{2} \qquad \frac{4 \times 3}{1 \times 3} = \frac{12}{3} \qquad \frac{4 \times 4}{1 \times 4} = \frac{16}{4} \qquad \frac{4 \times 5}{1 \times 5} = \frac{20}{5}$$

Thus, $4 = \frac{4}{1} = \frac{8}{2} = \frac{12}{3} = \frac{16}{4} = \frac{20}{5}$. These are equivalent fractions.

EXAMPLE 4 Find equivalent fractions for $1\frac{4}{6}$.

To find equivalent fractions for a mixed number, first convert the mixed number to an improper fraction.

1. $1 \times 6 = 6$

2. $6 + 4 = 10$

3. $1\frac{4}{6} = \frac{10}{6}$

Now follow the same steps used in the previous examples.

$$\frac{10 \times 2}{6 \times 2} = \frac{20}{12} \qquad \frac{10 \times 3}{6 \times 3} = \frac{30}{18} \qquad \frac{10 \div 2}{6 \div 2} = \frac{5}{3} \qquad \frac{10 \times 10}{6 \times 10} = \frac{100}{60}$$

Thus, $1\frac{4}{6} = \frac{10}{6} = \frac{20}{12} = \frac{30}{18} = \frac{5}{3} = \frac{100}{60}$

A fraction equals 1 if its numerator equals its denominator.

$$\frac{2}{2} = 1 \qquad \frac{5}{5} = 1 \qquad \frac{21}{21} = 1 \qquad \frac{1000}{1000} = 1$$

These fractions have the same value, 1, and are equivalent:

$$\frac{2}{2} = \frac{5}{5} = \frac{21}{21} = \frac{1000}{1000}$$

Finding missing numerators. Suppose you want to convert a fraction into an equivalent one with a specific denominator. To convert $\frac{1}{5}$ to tenths, find the missing value in $\frac{1}{5} = \frac{?}{10}$. The ? stands for the number you want to find. This equation means, "One-fifth equals how many tenths?" In this case, compare the denominators. The new denominator, 10, is larger than the original denominator, 5. Therefore, 5 must be multiplied by some number to equal 10. To find this number, divide the larger denominator by the smaller one. Here, $10 \div 5 = 2$. Multiplying the numerator and denominator by 2 will lead to an equivalent fraction with 10 as the denominator.

$$\frac{1}{5} = \frac{1 \times 2}{5 \times 2} = \frac{2}{10} = \frac{?}{10} \text{ and } ? = 2$$

Rule 1-10

To find the missing numerator in an equivalent fraction,

1. If the denominator of the equivalent fraction is larger than the original denominator, then:
   a. Divide the larger denominator by the smaller one. (The answer to a division problem is the *quotient*.)
   b. Multiply the original numerator by the quotient from Step a.

2. If the denominator of the equivalent fraction is smaller than the original denominator, then:
   a. Divide the larger denominator by the smaller one.
   b. Divide the original numerator by the quotient from Step a.

EXAMPLE 1 $\frac{2}{3} = \frac{?}{12}$

a. Divide the larger denominator by the smaller one:

   $12 \div 3 = 4$

b. Multiply the original numerator by the quotient from Step a:

   $2 \times 4 = 8$

Thus, $\frac{2}{3} = \frac{2 \times 4}{3 \times 4} = \frac{8}{12}$ and ? = 8

EXAMPLE 2 $\frac{28}{60} = \frac{?}{15}$

a. Here the original denominator is the larger one. Divide the larger denominator by the smaller one:

   $60 \div 15 = 4$

b. Divide the original numerator by the quotient from Step a.

   $28 \div 4 = 7$

Thus, $\frac{28}{60} = \frac{28 \div 4}{60 \div 4} = \frac{7}{15}$ and ? = 7

EXAMPLE 3 $4 = \frac{?}{8}$

Convert 4 to an improper fraction. The equation is now $\frac{4}{1} = \frac{?}{8}$.

a. $8 \div 1 = 8$

b. $4 \times 8 = 32$

$$4 = \frac{4}{1} = \frac{4 \times 8}{1 \times 8} = \frac{32}{8} \text{ and ? } = 32$$

EXAMPLE 4 $\quad 2\frac{1}{2} = \frac{?}{6}$

First convert the mixed number into an improper fraction.

$$2\frac{1}{2} = \frac{(2 \times 2) + 1}{2} = \frac{5}{2}$$

The equation is now $\frac{5}{2} = \frac{?}{6}$

a. $6 \div 2 = 3$

b. $5 \times 3 = 15$

Thus, $2\frac{1}{2} = \frac{15}{6}$ and ? $= 15$

You can use a similar method to find a missing denominator in an equivalent fraction. In Chapter 2, you will learn another way to find the missing numerator by cross-multiplying.

REVIEW and PRACTICE

EQUIVALENT FRACTIONS

Find three equivalent fractions for each of the following:

1. $\frac{4}{5}$ **2.** $\frac{1}{10}$ **3.** $\frac{4}{2}$ **4.** $\frac{15}{9}$

5. 9 **6.** 24 **7.** $2\frac{1}{3}$ **8.** $3\frac{6}{9}$

Find the missing numerator in the following equations:

9. $\frac{3}{8} = \frac{?}{16}$ **10.** $\frac{1}{3} = \frac{?}{27}$ **11.** $\frac{16}{24} = \frac{?}{6}$ **12.** $\frac{18}{15} = \frac{?}{5}$

13. $3 = \frac{?}{4}$ **14.** $5 = \frac{?}{12}$ **15.** $1\frac{5}{16} = \frac{?}{160}$ **16.** $4\frac{2}{8} = \frac{?}{4}$

To check your answers, see page 330.

Simplifying Fractions to Lowest Terms

The last section showed how to find equivalent fractions by multiplying or dividing the numerator and denominator by the same number. When you divide, you simplify (or reduce) a fraction. By simplifying, you work with a smaller numerator and denominator, decreasing your chances of making an arithmetic mistake.

Rule 1-11

To reduce a fraction to its lowest terms, find the largest whole number that divides evenly into both the numerator and denominator. When no whole number except 1 divides evenly into them, the fraction is reduced to its lowest terms.

EXAMPLE 1 $\quad$ Reduce $\frac{10}{15}$ to its lowest terms.

Both 10 and 15 are divisible by 5.

$$\frac{10 \div 5}{15 \div 5} = \frac{2}{3}$$

No whole number other than 1 divides evenly into *both* 2 and 3. Thus, $\frac{10}{15}$ has been reduced to its lowest terms, $\frac{2}{3}$.

EXAMPLE 2

Reduce $\frac{24}{30}$ to its lowest terms.

Both 24 and 30 are divisible by 6.

$$\frac{24 \div 6}{30 \div 6} = \frac{4}{5}$$

No whole number other than 1 divides evenly into *both* 4 and 5. Thus, $\frac{24}{30}$ has been reduced to its lowest terms, $\frac{4}{5}$.

ERROR ALERT!

Reducing a fraction does not automatically mean you have simplified it to its lowest terms.

More than one number may divide evenly into both the numerator and the denominator. For example, both 18 and 42 are even numbers. To reduce $\frac{18}{42}$, you can divide by 2, so that

$$\frac{18 \div 2}{42 \div 2} = \frac{9}{21}$$

You are not done, though. Both 9 and 21 are divisible by 3, so that

$$\frac{18}{42} = \frac{9}{21} = \frac{9 \div 3}{21 \div 3} = \frac{3}{7}$$

Some fractions are easy to reduce. Looking at $\frac{2}{4}$, you can guess that 2 divides evenly into both the numerator and the denominator, so that $\frac{2 \div 2}{4 \div 2} = \frac{1}{2}$. In other cases, you may have to use several steps.

Table 1-2 Is a Number Divisible by 2, 3, 4, 5, 6, 8, 9, or 10?

Number	Hint	Example
2	Even numbers (numbers ending with 2, 4, 6, 8, or 0) are divisible by 2.	112, 734, 2936, 10,118, 365,920
3	If the sum of the digits of a number is divisible by 3, then the number is divisible by 3.	37,887 The sum of the digits is 3 + 7 + 8 + 8 + 7 = 33. 33 is divisible by 3.
4	If the last two digits of a number are divisible by 4, the entire number is divisible by 4.	126,936 The last two digits, 36, are divisible by 4.
5	Any number that ends with 5 or 0 is divisible by 5.	735 12,290
6	Combine the rules for 2 and 3. If a number is even *and* the sum of its digits is divisible by 3, then the number is divisible by 6.	582 The number is even. The sum of its digits, 5 + 8 + 2 = 15, is divisible by 3.
8	If the last three digits are divisible by 8, then the entire number is divisible by 8.	42,376 Here, 376 is divisible by 8.
9	If the sum of the digits is a multiple of 9, the number is divisible by 9.	42,705 4 + 2 + 7 + 0 + 5 = 18, which is divisible by 9.
10	If a number greater than 0 ends with 0, then the number is divisible by 10.	640

Prime numbers are numbers other than 1 that can be evenly divided only by themselves and 1. The first ten prime numbers are 2, 3, 5, 7, 11, 13, 17, 19, 23, and 29. If either the numerator or denominator is a prime number, and the other term is not divisible by that prime number, then the fraction is in lowest terms. For example, $\frac{17}{24}$ is in lowest terms. However, you can simplify $\frac{17}{34}$ to $\frac{1}{2}$, dividing both the numerator and denominator by 17.

REVIEW and PRACTICE

SIMPLIFYING FRACTIONS TO LOWEST TERMS

Reduce the following fractions to their lowest terms:

1. $\frac{10}{12}$　　　　2. $\frac{3}{6}$　　　　3. $\frac{27}{81}$　　　　4. $\frac{11}{22}$

5. $\frac{10}{100}$　　　6. $\frac{55}{100}$　　　7. $\frac{4}{5}$　　　　8. $\frac{6}{17}$

9. $\frac{21}{27}$　　　10. $\frac{35}{50}$　　　11. $\frac{48}{90}$　　　12. $\frac{49}{84}$

To check your answers, see page 330.

Finding Common Denominators

A common denominator is any number that is a common multiple of all the denominators in a group of numbers. The least common denominator (LCD) is the smallest of these numbers. Before you can add and subtract fractions with different denominators, you must first convert them to equivalent fractions with a common denominator. You must do the same to compare fractions with different denominators.

Rule 1-12

To find the least common denominator (LCD) of a group of fractions,

1. List the multiples of each denominator.

2. Compare the lists. Any numbers that appear on all lists are common denominators.

3. The smallest number that appears on all the lists is the LCD.

Once you have found the LCD, you can convert each fraction to an equivalent fraction with the LCD as the denominator.

EXAMPLE 1 Find the least common denominator of $\frac{1}{3}$ and $\frac{1}{2}$. Then convert each to an equivalent fraction with the LCD.

1. The number 3 divides evenly into 3, <u>6</u>, 9, <u>12</u>, 15, <u>18</u>, and 21. The number 2 divides evenly into 2, 4, <u>6</u>, 8, 10, <u>12</u>, 14, 16, and <u>18</u>.

2. The numbers 6, 12, and 18 are common denominators.

3. The smallest number that appears on both lists is 6. It is the least common denominator and is divisible by both 3 and 2.

Now convert $\frac{1}{3}$ and $\frac{1}{2}$ so that $\frac{1}{3} = \frac{?}{6}$, and $\frac{1}{2} = \frac{?}{6}$.

4. To convert $\frac{1}{3}$ to the equivalent fraction $\frac{?}{6}$,

a. $6 \div 3 = 2$

b. $\frac{1}{3} = \frac{1 \times 2}{3 \times 2} = \frac{2}{6}$

5. To convert $\frac{1}{2}$ to the equivalent fraction $\frac{?}{6}$,

    a. $6 \div 2 = 3$

    b. $\frac{1}{2} = \frac{1 \times 3}{2 \times 3} = \frac{3}{6}$

The least common denominator is 6. The equivalent fractions to $\frac{1}{3}$ and $\frac{1}{2}$ are $\frac{2}{6}$ and $\frac{3}{6}$.

EXAMPLE 2   Find the least common denominator of $\frac{1}{4}$, $\frac{1}{6}$, and $\frac{1}{8}$. Then convert each to an equivalent fraction with the LCD.

  1. The number 4 divides evenly into 4, 8, 12, 16, 20, and <u>24</u>.

     The number 6 divides evenly into 6, 12, 18, and <u>24</u>.

     The number 8 divides evenly into 8, 16, and <u>24</u>.

  2. The number 24 is a common denominator.

  3. In this case, 24 is the LCD.

  4. $\frac{1}{4} = \frac{?}{24}$

    a. $24 \div 4 = 6$

    b. $\frac{1}{4} = \frac{1 \times 6}{4 \times 6} = \frac{6}{24}$

  5. $\frac{1}{6} = \frac{?}{24}$

    a. $24 \div 6 = 4$

    b. $\frac{1}{6} = \frac{1 \times 4}{6 \times 4} = \frac{4}{24}$

  6. $\frac{1}{8} = \frac{?}{24}$

    a. $24 \div 8 = 3$

    b. $\frac{1}{8} = \frac{1 \times 3}{8 \times 3} = \frac{3}{24}$

The least common denominator is 24. The equivalent fractions to $\frac{1}{4}$, $\frac{1}{6}$, and $\frac{1}{8}$ are $\frac{6}{24}$, $\frac{4}{24}$, and $\frac{3}{24}$.

You may find it difficult to find common denominators of fractions with large denominators. However, you can simply multiply the individual denominators to find a common denominator.

Rule 1-13

To convert fractions with large denominators to equivalent fractions with a common denominator,

1. List the denominators of all the fractions.

2. Multiply the denominators. The product is a common denominator. Convert each fraction to an equivalent one with the common denominator.

EXAMPLE 1   Convert $\frac{1}{7}$ and $\frac{1}{19}$ to equivalent fractions with a common denominator.

1. The denominators are 7 and 19.

2. Multiply 7×19. The common denominator is 133.

$$\frac{1}{7} = \frac{1 \times 19}{7 \times 19} = \frac{19}{133} \text{ and } \frac{1}{19} = \frac{1 \times 7}{19 \times 7} = \frac{7}{133}$$

The equivalent fractions are $\frac{19}{133}$ and $\frac{7}{133}$.

EXAMPLE 2 Convert $\frac{2}{37}$ and $\frac{7}{90}$ to equivalent fractions with a common denominator.

1. The denominators are 37 and 90.

2. $37 \times 90 = 3330$

$$\frac{2 \times 90}{37 \times 90} = \frac{180}{3330} \text{ and } \frac{7 \times 37}{90 \times 37} = \frac{259}{3330}$$

The equivalent fractions are $\frac{180}{3330}$ and $\frac{259}{3330}$.

REVIEW and PRACTICE

FINDING COMMON DENOMINATORS

For each set of fractions, find the least common denominator. Then convert each fraction to an equivalent fraction with the LCD.

1. $\frac{1}{3}$ and $\frac{1}{7}$

2. $\frac{1}{5}$ and $\frac{1}{8}$

3. $\frac{1}{25}$ and $\frac{1}{40}$

4. $\frac{1}{24}$ and $\frac{1}{36}$

5. $\frac{1}{2}$ and $\frac{1}{12}$

6. $\frac{1}{6}$ and $\frac{1}{18}$

7. $\frac{5}{6}$ and $\frac{4}{7}$

8. $\frac{3}{4}$ and $\frac{5}{8}$

9. $\frac{11}{30}$ and $\frac{21}{80}$

10. $\frac{5}{48}$ and $\frac{7}{72}$

11. $\frac{1}{2}, \frac{1}{3}$, and $\frac{1}{4}$

12. $\frac{1}{6}, \frac{4}{9}$, and $\frac{13}{24}$

13. $\frac{2}{3}, \frac{4}{9}$, and $\frac{7}{15}$

14. $\frac{1}{4}, \frac{5}{6}$, and $\frac{7}{16}$

To check your answers, see page 330.

Comparing Fractions

Suppose a home patient is to take $\frac{3}{4}$ tablespoon of medication with lunch. You learn that the patient took $\frac{2}{3}$ tablespoon. Did the patient take too little, too much, or just the right amount? (You will answer this question in Exercise 19.) Now that you can convert fractions to equivalent fractions with a common denominator, you can also compare their sizes by comparing their numerators.

Rule 1-14

To compare fractions,

1. Write all fractions as equivalent fractions with a common denominator.

2. Write the fractions in order by the size of the numerator. The fraction with the largest numerator is the largest in the group.

3. Restate the comparisons with the original fractions.

EXAMPLE 1 Order from smallest to largest: $\frac{1}{5}, \frac{4}{5}$, and $\frac{3}{10}$.

1. Write the fractions as equivalent fractions with a common denominator. The least common denominator of $\frac{1}{5}, \frac{4}{5}$, and $\frac{3}{10}$ is 10.

$$\frac{1}{5} = \frac{?}{10} = \frac{1 \times 2}{5 \times 2} = \frac{2}{10}$$

$$\frac{4}{5} = \frac{?}{10} = \frac{4 \times 2}{5 \times 2} = \frac{8}{10}$$

$$\frac{3}{10} = \frac{3}{10}$$

Roman Numerals, Fractions, and Decimals **19**

If you have difficulty with this step, review "Equivalent Fractions" and "Finding Common Denominators" in this chapter.

2. Order the fractions by the size of their numerators, in this case, from smallest to largest:

$$\frac{2}{10} \quad \frac{3}{10} \quad \frac{8}{10}$$

Insert the proper comparison signs:

$$\frac{2}{10} < \frac{3}{10} < \frac{8}{10}$$

3. Restate with the original equivalent fractions:

$$\frac{1}{5} < \frac{3}{10} < \frac{4}{5}$$

EXAMPLE 2 ▷ Order from largest to smallest: $1\frac{7}{8}, \frac{6}{3}, 2, \frac{2}{8}$.

First, convert all whole and mixed numbers to improper fractions:

$$1\frac{7}{8} = \frac{15}{8}$$

$$2 = \frac{2}{1}$$

If you have difficulty with this step, review "Working With Common Fractions" in this chapter.

1. Write all fractions as equivalent fractions with a common denominator. The LCD for this set of fractions is 24:

$$1\frac{7}{8} = \frac{15}{8} = \frac{?}{24} = \frac{15 \times 3}{8 \times 3} = \frac{45}{24}$$

$$\frac{6}{3} = \frac{?}{24} = \frac{6 \times 8}{3 \times 8} = \frac{48}{24}$$

$$2 = \frac{2}{1} = \frac{?}{24} = \frac{2 \times 24}{1 \times 24} = \frac{48}{24}$$

$$\frac{2}{8} = \frac{?}{24} = \frac{2 \times 3}{8 \times 3} = \frac{6}{24}$$

2. Write the fractions in order by the size of their numerator:

$$\frac{48}{24}, \frac{48}{24}, \frac{45}{24}, \frac{6}{24}$$

Insert the proper comparison signs.

$$\frac{48}{24} = \frac{48}{24} > \frac{45}{24} > \frac{6}{24}$$

3. Restate with the original equivalent fractions:

$$2 = \frac{6}{3} > 1\frac{7}{8} > \frac{2}{8}$$

REVIEW and PRACTICE

COMPARING FRACTIONS

Insert $>$, $<$, or $=$ to make a true statement:

1. $\frac{1}{5}$ $\frac{3}{5}$ 2. $\frac{7}{9}$ $\frac{4}{9}$

3. $\frac{2}{8}$ $\frac{1}{4}$ 4. $\frac{7}{10}$ $\frac{7}{20}$

5. $\frac{3}{24}$ $\frac{1}{8}$ 6. $\frac{11}{3}$ $\frac{13}{9}$

7. 1 $\frac{2}{3}$ 8. $\frac{9}{4}$ 2

9. $1\frac{1}{12}$ $1\frac{5}{12}$

10. $3\frac{3}{5}$ $3\frac{2}{5}$

11. $1\frac{3}{4}$ $1\frac{7}{8}$

12. $2\frac{1}{10}$ $2\frac{1}{8}$

13. $3\frac{1}{5}$ $\frac{25}{8}$

14. $\frac{9}{5}$ $1\frac{8}{10}$

Place in order from largest to smallest:

15. $\frac{3}{4}, \frac{2}{5}, \frac{5}{6}, \frac{4}{7}$

16. $\frac{1}{3}, \frac{4}{7}, \frac{5}{9}, \frac{1}{2}$

17. $1\frac{3}{16}, \frac{9}{8}, \frac{5}{2}, 2\frac{1}{10}$

18. $2\frac{1}{2}, \frac{5}{3}, \frac{12}{9}, 1\frac{5}{6}$

19. A home patient is supposed to take $\frac{3}{4}$ tablespoon of medication with lunch. You learn that the patient took $\frac{2}{3}$ tablespoon. Did the patient take too little, too much, or just the right amount?

20. You want to prepare 150 units of a solution that consists of 25 units of medication mixed with 125 units of water. You find an already-prepared solution that has 1 unit of medication for every 5 units of water. Can you use 150 units of the already-prepared solution? Explain your answer.

21. Of 12 patients in the north wing, 8 have high blood pressure. Of 15 patients in the east wing, 9 have high blood pressure. Which wing has a larger portion of patients with high blood pressure?

22. You give George his medication once every 8 hours. You give Martha the same medication 4 times a day. Who receives medication more often? (In this problem, a day means 24 hours.)

To check your answers, see page 331.

Adding Fractions

Suppose you gave a patient $\frac{1}{2}$ tablespoon of medication with breakfast, $\frac{3}{8}$ tablespoon with lunch, $\frac{3}{4}$ tablespoon with dinner, and another $\frac{3}{8}$ tablespoon at bedtime. To determine the total amount of medication you have given the patient, you must add the fractions. (You will solve this problem in Exercise 21.)

Rule 1-15

To add fractions,

1. Write equivalent fractions with a common denominator.

2. Add the numerators. This number is the numerator of the sum of the fractions.

3. The common denominator is the denominator of the sum of the fractions.

4. Reduce the numerator and denominator to the lowest terms.

EXAMPLE 1   Add $\frac{2}{6} + \frac{3}{6}$

1. The fractions already have a common denominator.

2. Add the numerators: $2 + 3 = 5$

3. The denominator is 6.

4. The fraction $\frac{5}{6}$ is already reduced to lowest terms.

EXAMPLE 2 Add $\frac{3}{5} + \frac{4}{15}$

1. The least common denominator of $\frac{3}{5}$ and $\frac{4}{15}$ is 15.
$$\frac{3}{5} + \frac{4}{15} = \frac{9}{15} + \frac{4}{15}$$
2. Add the numerators: $9 + 4 = 13$

3. The common denominator is 15.

4. The fraction $\frac{13}{15}$ is already reduced to lowest terms.

EXAMPLE 3 Add $\frac{5}{6} + \frac{1}{4}$

1. The least common denominator is 12.
$$\frac{5}{6} + \frac{1}{4} = \frac{10}{12} + \frac{3}{12}$$
2. Add the numerators: $10 + 3 = 13$

3. $\frac{10}{12} + \frac{3}{12} = \frac{10 + 3}{12} = \frac{13}{12}$

4. Reduce the answer to lowest terms: $\frac{13}{12} = 1\frac{1}{12}$

You can add improper fractions the same way that you add proper fractions. You can also change improper fractions to mixed numbers first, and then add.

Rule 1-16

To add mixed numbers,

1. Add the whole numbers.

2. Add the fractional parts.

3. If the sum from Step 2 is an improper fraction, convert it to a mixed number.

4. Add the whole number and the fraction or mixed number. Reduce the answer to lowest terms.

EXAMPLE 1 Add $3\frac{1}{4} + 2\frac{1}{2}$

1. Add the whole numbers: $3 + 2 = 5$

2. Add the fractional parts: $\frac{1}{4} + \frac{1}{2}$

The least common denominator is 4.
$$\frac{1}{4} + \frac{1}{2} = \frac{1}{4} + \frac{2}{4} = \frac{1+2}{4} = \frac{3}{4}$$
3. $\frac{3}{4}$ is a proper fraction.

4. Add the whole number and the fraction: $5 + \frac{3}{4} = 5\frac{3}{4}$

EXAMPLE 2 Add $1\frac{7}{8} + 2\frac{1}{3}$

1. Add the whole numbers: $1 + 2 = 3$

2. Add the fractional parts: $\frac{7}{8} + \frac{1}{3}$

The least common denominator is 24.
$$\frac{7}{8} + \frac{1}{3} = \frac{21}{24} + \frac{8}{24} = \frac{29}{24}$$
3. Convert the improper fraction to a mixed number.
$$\frac{29}{24} = 1\frac{5}{24}$$

4. Add the whole number and the mixed number.

$$3 + 1\frac{5}{24} = 3 + 1 + \frac{5}{24} = 4 + \frac{5}{24} = 4\frac{5}{24}$$

Thus, $1\frac{7}{8} + 2\frac{1}{3} = 4\frac{5}{24}$

REVIEW and PRACTICE

ADDING FRACTIONS

Find the following sums. (Rewrite improper fractions as mixed numbers.)

1. $\frac{1}{8} + \frac{3}{8}$

2. $\frac{1}{7} + \frac{3}{7}$

3. $\frac{1}{7} + \frac{2}{14}$

4. $\frac{2}{5} + \frac{4}{15}$

5. $\frac{1}{6} + \frac{3}{8}$

6. $\frac{4}{10} + \frac{2}{25}$

7. $\frac{5}{8} + \frac{7}{12}$

8. $\frac{5}{6} + \frac{7}{9}$

9. $2 + \frac{4}{5}$

10. $\frac{8}{11} + 3$

11. $1\frac{1}{2} + \frac{1}{3}$

12. $2\frac{3}{8} + \frac{1}{5}$

13. $1\frac{2}{5} + 4\frac{3}{7}$

14. $2\frac{1}{8} + 1\frac{1}{2}$

15. $\frac{1}{2} + \frac{1}{5} + \frac{1}{8}$

16. $\frac{1}{3} + \frac{1}{4} + \frac{1}{5}$

17. $\frac{3}{4} + \frac{3}{8} + \frac{7}{12}$

18. $\frac{1}{2} + \frac{2}{3} + \frac{3}{5}$

19. The patient's chart indicates that he weighed 158 pounds at the end of April. He then gained $\frac{3}{4}$ pound in May and $1\frac{1}{2}$ pounds in June. What did he weigh at the end of June?

20. Since breakfast, Kelly drank $1\frac{1}{4}$ cups of water, $\frac{2}{3}$ cup of juice, and $\frac{3}{4}$ cup of milk. How much liquid has Kelly had since breakfast?

21. During the day, you gave one of your patients $\frac{1}{2}$ tablespoon of medication with breakfast, $\frac{3}{8}$ tablespoon with lunch, $\frac{3}{4}$ tablespoon with dinner, and $\frac{3}{8}$ tablespoon at bedtime. What is the total amount of medication you gave your patient?

22. You are observing your patient's sleep pattern over the past 24 hours. She slept $7\frac{1}{2}$ hours at night, $1\frac{3}{4}$ hours after breakfast, and $2\frac{1}{4}$ hours after lunch. She also had a $\frac{1}{4}$ hour nap before lunch and a $\frac{1}{4}$ hour nap after dinner. How many hours did she sleep?

To check your answers, see page 331.

Subtracting Fractions

Subtracting fractions is similar to adding fractions.

Rule 1-17

To subtract fractions,

1. Write equivalent fractions with a common denominator.

2. Subtract the numerators. (The difference is the new numerator.)

3. Keep the common denominator.

4. Reduce your answer to its lowest terms.

Subtract: $\frac{2}{6} - \frac{3}{12}$

EXAMPLE 1

1. Write equivalent fractions with a common denominator. Here, 12 is the lowest common denominator: $\dfrac{2}{6} - \dfrac{3}{12} = \dfrac{4}{12} - \dfrac{3}{12}$

2. Subtract the numerators: $4 - 3 = 1$

3. Keep the common denominator: $\dfrac{4}{12} - \dfrac{3}{12} = \dfrac{4 - 3}{12} = \dfrac{1}{12}$

4. $\dfrac{1}{12}$ is already reduced to lowest terms.

Rule 1-18

To subtract from a whole or mixed number,

1. Write the fractional parts as equivalent fractions with a common denominator.

2. If necessary, borrow one unit from the whole number. Add it to the fractional part, creating an improper fraction.

3. Complete the subtraction. Subtract whole numbers first. Then subtract the fractional parts and reduce to lowest terms.

4. State the answer.

EXAMPLE 1 Subtract: $14\dfrac{1}{2} - \dfrac{7}{8}$

1. Write the fractional parts as equivalent fractions with a common denominator. The least common denominator is 8.

$$14\dfrac{1}{2} - \dfrac{7}{8} = 14\dfrac{4}{8} - \dfrac{7}{8}$$

2. Borrow one unit from the whole number 14. Add it to the fractional part.

$$14\dfrac{4}{8} = 13 + 1 + \dfrac{4}{8} = 13 + \dfrac{8}{8} + \dfrac{4}{8} = 13 + \dfrac{8 + 4}{8} = 13 + \dfrac{12}{8} = 13\dfrac{12}{8}$$

3. Complete the subtraction.

Subtract the whole numbers first: $13 - 0 = 13$

Subtract the fractional parts: $\dfrac{12}{8} - \dfrac{7}{8} = \dfrac{12 - 7}{8} = \dfrac{5}{8}$

Thus, $14\dfrac{1}{2} - \dfrac{7}{8} = 13\dfrac{12}{8} - \dfrac{7}{8} = 13\dfrac{5}{8}$

4. The answer is $13\dfrac{5}{8}$.

EXAMPLE 2 Subtract: $9\dfrac{2}{3} - 3\dfrac{11}{12}$

1. Write the fractional portions as equivalent fractions with a common denominator. The least common denominator is 12.

The problem is now: $9\dfrac{8}{12} - 3\dfrac{11}{12}$

2. Borrow one unit from the whole number 9.

$$9\dfrac{8}{12} = 8 + 1 + \dfrac{8}{12} = 8 + \dfrac{12}{12} + \dfrac{8}{12} = 8 + \dfrac{12 + 8}{12} = 8 + \dfrac{20}{12} = 8\dfrac{20}{12}$$

3. The problem is now: $8\dfrac{20}{12} - 3\dfrac{11}{12}$

Subtract the whole numbers first: $8 - 3 = 5$

Subtract the fractional parts: $\dfrac{20}{12} - \dfrac{11}{12} = \dfrac{9}{12} = \dfrac{3}{4}$

4. The answer is $5\dfrac{3}{4}$.

EXAMPLE 3 Subtract: $6 - 3\dfrac{1}{4}$

Here you can combine the first two steps. Rewrite 6 as follows:

$$6 = 5 + 1 = 5 + \dfrac{4}{4} = 5\dfrac{4}{4}$$

Now complete the subtraction.

$$6 - 3\frac{1}{4} = 5\frac{4}{4} - 3\frac{1}{4}$$

$$5 - 3 = 2 \text{ and } \frac{4}{4} - \frac{1}{4} = \frac{3}{4}$$

The answer is $2\frac{3}{4}$.

REVIEW and PRACTICE

SUBTRACTING FRACTIONS

Find the following differences.

1. $7\frac{7}{15} - 4\frac{4}{15}$ 2. $\frac{7}{25} - \frac{2}{25}$ 3. $\frac{11}{3} - \frac{2}{6}$ 4. $\frac{4}{7} - \frac{3}{21}$

5. $\frac{5}{6} - \frac{4}{9}$ 6. $\frac{3}{4} - \frac{1}{6}$ 7. $1\frac{7}{8} - \frac{1}{4}$ 8. $2\frac{5}{8} - \frac{1}{2}$

9. $6\frac{1}{3} - \frac{5}{6}$ 10. $4\frac{1}{2} - \frac{3}{4}$ 11. $14\frac{9}{10} - 3\frac{1}{3}$ 12. $6\frac{6}{7} - 2\frac{3}{5}$

13. $24\frac{1}{8} - 3\frac{3}{16}$ 14. $8\frac{7}{10} - 3\frac{3}{4}$ 15. $6 - \frac{2}{3}$ 16. $7 - \frac{3}{7}$

17. You give a patient $\frac{3}{4}$ cup of juice, but he only drinks $\frac{3}{8}$ cup. How much juice remains?

18. You give a patient $1\frac{1}{4}$ cups of water to drink before supper. When you bring in the meal, you see that $\frac{5}{8}$ cup remains in the glass. How much water did the patient drink?

19. At the beginning of the day, you have $6\frac{1}{2}$ bottles of a medication on hand. At the end of the day, $2\frac{3}{4}$ bottles remain. How much of the medication was used during the day?

20. Brenda weighed $153\frac{1}{2}$ pounds when she began a diet. The first month she lost $2\frac{3}{4}$ pounds. The second month she lost $4\frac{1}{2}$ pounds. The third month she lost $2\frac{1}{2}$ pounds. What does she weigh now? (Hint: You can subtract each month separately, or you can calculate her total weight loss first.)

To check your answers, see page 331.

Multiplying Fractions

Unlike adding and subtracting fractions, you do not need a common denominator to multiply fractions. Think about what $\frac{2}{3} \times \frac{1}{2}$ means. This problem could be read as "two-thirds times one-half" or "two-thirds of one-half." In Figure 1-2a, a pizza is divided into six slices. Half of the pizza (three slices) has pepperoni. When you look for $\frac{2}{3}$ of $\frac{1}{2}$ of the pizza, you are looking for two-thirds of the pepperoni half.

In Figure 1-2b, two-thirds of the pepperoni half also has mushrooms. The mushroom slices represent $\frac{2}{3}$ of $\frac{1}{2}$ of the pizza, or $\frac{2}{3} \times \frac{1}{2}$. They also represent $\frac{2}{6}$ of the entire pizza. Thus, $\frac{2}{3} \times \frac{1}{2} = \frac{2}{6} = \frac{1}{3}$

Figure 1-2

Multiplying fractions.

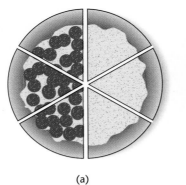 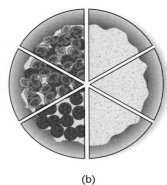

(a)   (b)

Rule 1-19

To multiply fractions,

1. Convert any mixed or whole numbers to improper fractions.

2. Multiply the numerators. Then multiply the denominators.

3. Reduce the product to its lowest terms.

EXAMPLE 1 Multiply $\frac{1}{6} \times \frac{3}{4}$

1. There are no mixed or whole numbers.

2. The product of the numerators is $1 \times 3 = 3$. The product of the denominators is $6 \times 4 = 24$. Thus, $\frac{1}{6} \times \frac{3}{4} = \frac{3}{24}$

3. $\frac{3}{24}$ reduces to $\frac{1}{8}$.

EXAMPLE 2 Multiply $\frac{1}{2} \times \frac{7}{3} \times \frac{4}{9}$

The only difference from the previous example is that now you are multiplying three numerators and three denominators.

$$\frac{1}{2} \times \frac{7}{3} \times \frac{4}{9} = \frac{1 \times 7 \times 4}{2 \times 3 \times 9} = \frac{28}{54}$$

$\frac{28}{54}$ reduces to $\frac{14}{27}$.

EXAMPLE 3 Multiply $1\frac{4}{7} \times 2\frac{3}{5}$

1. First convert the mixed numbers to improper fractions.

$$1\frac{4}{7} = \frac{11}{7} \text{ and } 2\frac{3}{5} = \frac{13}{5}$$

2. Now multiply the numerators and denominators.

$$1\frac{4}{7} \times 2\frac{3}{5} = \frac{11}{7} \times \frac{13}{5} = \frac{11 \times 13}{7 \times 5} = \frac{143}{35}$$

3. $\frac{143}{35}$ converts to $4\frac{3}{35}$.

EXAMPLE 4 Multiply $3 \times \frac{2}{3}$

First convert 3 to the improper fraction $\frac{3}{1}$. Now solve.

$$3 \times \frac{2}{3} = \frac{3}{1} \times \frac{2}{3} = \frac{3 \times 2}{1 \times 3} = \frac{6}{3}$$

$\frac{6}{3}$ reduces to 2.

Canceling terms provides a short cut that makes multiplying large fractions easier. It lets you work with smaller numbers, reducing the potential for arithmetic errors. If you divide both the numerator and the denominator of a fraction by the same number, you have not changed the fraction's value. You already use this rule to reduce a fraction. Canceling applies the rule to two or more fractions.

To find the product of $\frac{8}{21} \times \frac{7}{16}$, you could multiply the numerators and multiply the denominators.

$$\frac{8}{21} \times \frac{7}{16} = \frac{8 \times 7}{21 \times 16} = \frac{56}{336}$$

$\frac{56}{336}$ reduces to $\frac{1}{6}$, although that may not be immediately clear to you. By canceling terms, however, you work with smaller numbers.

Rule 1-20

To cancel terms in a product of fractions, divide both a numerator and a denominator by the same number. You may only cancel terms if a numerator and denominator can both be divided evenly.

EXAMPLE 1 Cancel terms to solve $\frac{8}{21} \times \frac{7}{16}$.

Both the numerator 8 and the denominator 16 can be divided evenly by 8. You can now write the problem as

$\frac{\overset{1}{8}}{21} \times \frac{7}{\underset{2}{16}}$, which is equivalent to $\frac{1}{21} \times \frac{7}{2}$

The slash marks indicate that 8 and 16 were canceled. In this case, they were divided by 8, reducing 8 and 16 to 1 and 2. Both the numerator 7 and the denominator 21 are divisible by 7. After you cancel again, you can rewrite the problem as

$\frac{\overset{1}{8}}{\underset{3}{21}} \times \frac{\overset{1}{7}}{\underset{2}{16}}$ which is equivalent to $\frac{1}{3} \times \frac{1}{2}$

Now when you solve, the product will already be in lowest terms:

$$\frac{8}{21} \times \frac{7}{16} = \frac{\overset{1}{8}}{\underset{3}{21}} \times \frac{\overset{1}{7}}{\underset{2}{16}} = \frac{1}{3} \times \frac{1}{2} = \frac{1}{6}$$

EXAMPLE 2 $\frac{27}{36} \times \frac{4}{5}$

In this problem, one of the fractions has not been reduced to lowest terms. Both 27 and 36 are divisible by 9.

$\frac{\overset{3}{27}}{\underset{4}{36}} \times \frac{4}{5}$ becomes $\frac{3}{4} \times \frac{4}{5}$

You can also cancel 4 from the numerator 4 and what had begun as the denominator 36. The problem now becomes:

$$\frac{\overset{3}{27}}{\underset{4}{\underset{1}{36}}} \times \frac{\overset{1}{4}}{5} = \frac{3}{\overset{}{\underset{1}{4}}} \times \frac{\overset{1}{4}}{5} = \frac{3}{1} \times \frac{1}{5} = \frac{3}{5}$$

The product $\frac{3}{5}$ is already reduced to lowest terms.

EXAMPLE 3 $2\frac{1}{2} \times \frac{8}{15} \times \frac{45}{4}$

First convert the mixed number $2\frac{1}{2}$ to the improper fraction $\frac{5}{2}$. Now the problem becomes

$$\frac{5}{2} \times \frac{8}{15} \times \frac{45}{4}$$

Both the numerator 45 and the denominator 15 are divisible by 15. Both the numerator 8 and the denominator 2 are divisible by 2.

$$\frac{5}{\underset{1}{\cancel{2}}} \times \frac{\overset{4}{\cancel{8}}}{\underset{1}{\cancel{15}}} \times \frac{\overset{3}{\cancel{45}}}{4} = \frac{5}{1} \times \frac{4}{1} \times \frac{3}{4}$$

You have another opportunity to cancel 4 from both a numerator and denominator. The problem now becomes:

$$\frac{5}{\underset{1}{\cancel{2}}} \times \frac{\overset{4}{\cancel{8}}}{\underset{1}{\cancel{15}}} \times \frac{\overset{3}{\cancel{45}}}{4} = \frac{5}{1} \times \frac{\overset{1}{\cancel{4}}}{1} \times \frac{3}{\underset{1}{\cancel{4}}} = \frac{5}{1} \times \frac{1}{1} \times \frac{3}{1} = \frac{15}{1} = 15$$

If you are not sure what numbers will divide evenly into both the numerator and denominator, review Table 1-2.

ERROR ALERT!

Avoid canceling too many terms.

A term that you plan to cancel may be a factor in more than one numerator or more than one denominator. Each time you cancel a term, you must cancel it from *one* numerator **and** one denominator.

Suppose you are multiplying $\frac{7}{12} \times \frac{8}{20}$. You can cancel 4 from the numerator 8. You can also cancel 4 from either of the denominators 12 or 20, but not from both. Either of the following is correct.

$$\frac{7}{\underset{3}{\cancel{12}}} \times \frac{\overset{2}{\cancel{8}}}{20} \text{ or } \frac{7}{12} \times \frac{\overset{2}{\cancel{8}}}{\underset{5}{\cancel{20}}}$$

However, *you cannot cancel 4 as follows* in this problem:

$$\frac{7}{\underset{3}{\cancel{12}}} \times \frac{\overset{2}{\cancel{8}}}{\underset{5}{\cancel{20}}}$$

If the problem were $\frac{5}{12} \times \frac{9}{24}$, where 3 can be canceled twice from the numerator 9, then you can cancel 3 twice in the denominators. Thus,

$$\frac{5}{12} \times \frac{9}{24} = \frac{5}{\underset{4}{\cancel{12}}} \times \frac{\overset{1}{\overset{3}{\cancel{9}}}}{\underset{8}{\cancel{24}}} = \frac{5}{4} \times \frac{1}{8} = \frac{5}{32}$$

REVIEW and PRACTICE

MULTIPLYING FRACTIONS

Find the following products. (Rewrite improper fractions as mixed numbers.)

1. $\frac{1}{6} \times \frac{1}{8}$ 2. $\frac{2}{7} \times \frac{3}{5}$ 3. $\frac{1}{2} \times \frac{6}{8}$ 4. $\frac{6}{9} \times \frac{1}{6}$

5. $\frac{3}{8} \times \frac{4}{9}$ 6. $\frac{5}{12} \times \frac{6}{15}$ 7. $\frac{10}{14} \times \frac{7}{5}$ 8. $\frac{5}{3} \times \frac{9}{10}$

9. $\frac{9}{8} \times \frac{8}{2}$ 10. $\frac{4}{3} \times \frac{15}{8}$ 11. $1\frac{7}{8} \times \frac{4}{5}$ 12. $3\frac{1}{3} \times \frac{9}{15}$

13. $3\frac{6}{8} \times 5\frac{2}{9}$ 14. $1\frac{5}{6} \times 7\frac{4}{5}$

15. $\frac{7}{16} \times \frac{4}{3} \times \frac{1}{2}$ 16. $\frac{5}{7} \times \frac{3}{10} \times \frac{3}{4}$

17. $\frac{11}{32} \times \frac{4}{22} \times 12$ 18. $5 \times \frac{7}{15} \times \frac{3}{14}$

19. $\frac{12}{25} \times \frac{8}{9} \times \frac{15}{16}$ 20. $\frac{49}{20} \times \frac{12}{7} \times \frac{5}{21}$

21. A bottle of liquid medication contains 24 doses. If the hospital has a supply of $9\frac{3}{4}$ bottles of the medication, how many doses are available?

22. A tablet contains $\frac{1}{4}$ grain of a medication. If you give a patient $1\frac{1}{2}$ tablets three times per day, how many grains of the medication are you giving to the patient each day?

23. A patient is supposed to take $\frac{1}{3}$ tablespoon of medicine four times per day. However, the patient misunderstood the directions and took $\frac{1}{4}$ tablespoon of medicine three times per day.
   a. How much medicine should the patient have taken per day?
   b. How much medicine did the patient take per day?
   c. What is the difference per day between the two amounts?

24. For four days, you give a patient $1\frac{1}{2}$ ounces of a medication five times per day. How much medication did you give the patient over the four days?

To check your answers, see page 332.

Dividing Fractions

You have now learned most of the steps needed to divide fractions. Suppose you have $\frac{3}{4}$ bottle of liquid medication available. The regular dose you would give a patient is $\frac{1}{16}$ bottle, and you want to know how many doses remain in the bottle. You solve this problem by dividing fractions.

You want to solve $\frac{3}{4} \div \frac{1}{16}$, where $\frac{3}{4}$ is the dividend, $\frac{1}{16}$ is the divisor, and your answer is the quotient. The problem is read "three-quarters divided by one-sixteenth," where you are finding out how many times $\frac{1}{16}$ goes into $\frac{3}{4}$.

To solve this problem, multiply the dividend $\frac{3}{4}$ by the reciprocal of the divisor $\frac{1}{16}$. You find the reciprocal of a fraction by inverting it—flipping it so that the numerator becomes the denominator and the denominator becomes the numerator. The reciprocal of $\frac{1}{16}$ is $\frac{16}{1}$. Thus,

$$\frac{3}{4} \div \frac{1}{16} = \frac{3}{4} \times \frac{16}{1}$$

You now solve this as a multiplication problem:

$$\frac{3}{\cancel{4}_1} \times \frac{\cancel{16}^{4}}{1} = \frac{3}{1} \times \frac{4}{1} = \frac{12}{1} = 12$$

The bottle has 12 doses remaining.

Rule 1-21

To divide fractions,
   1. Convert any mixed or whole numbers to improper fractions.
   2. Invert (flip) the divisor to find its reciprocal.
   3. Multiply the dividend by the reciprocal of the divisor and reduce.

EXAMPLE 1 Divide $\frac{1}{2} \div \frac{1}{4}$
   1. The problem has no mixed or whole numbers.
   2. Invert (flip) the divisor $\frac{1}{4}$ to find its reciprocal $\frac{4}{1}$.

3. Multiply the dividend by the reciprocal of the divisor:

$$\frac{1}{2} \div \frac{1}{4} = \frac{1}{2} \times \frac{4}{1} = \frac{1}{\underset{1}{2}} \times \frac{\overset{2}{4}}{1} = \frac{2}{1} = 2$$

EXAMPLE 2 Divide $1\frac{1}{2} \div \frac{1}{4}$

1. Convert the mixed number to an improper fraction.

$$1\frac{1}{2} = \frac{3}{2}$$

2. Invert (flip) the divisor $\frac{1}{4}$ to find its reciprocal $\frac{4}{1}$.

3. Multiply the dividend by the reciprocal of the divisor:

$$1\frac{1}{2} \div \frac{1}{4} = \frac{3}{2} \div \frac{1}{4} = \frac{3}{\underset{1}{2}} \times \frac{\overset{2}{4}}{1} = \frac{3}{1} \times \frac{2}{1} = \frac{6}{1} = 6$$

You may have to solve a *complex fraction,* in which the numerator and the denominator are themselves fractions. The main fraction bar will often be wider and darker than the fraction bars within the numerator and the denominator. You can simply rewrite a complex fraction as an ordinary division problem and proceed.

EXAMPLE 3 Simplify $\dfrac{\frac{7}{10}}{\frac{3}{5}}$

Here, $\frac{7}{10}$ is the numerator and $\frac{3}{5}$ is the denominator. Rewrite the complex fraction as a regular division problem, then solve.

$$\frac{\frac{7}{10}}{\frac{3}{5}} = \frac{7}{10} \div \frac{3}{5} = \frac{7}{10} \times \frac{5}{3} = \frac{7}{\underset{2}{10}} \times \frac{\overset{1}{5}}{3} = \frac{7}{2} \times \frac{1}{3} = \frac{7}{6} = 1\frac{1}{6}$$

ERROR ALERT!
Write division problems carefully to avoid mistakes.

1. Convert whole numbers to fractions, especially if you use complex fractions.

You cannot tell if $\dfrac{\frac{3}{8}}{4}$ is $3 \div \frac{8}{4}$ or $\frac{3}{8} \div 4$

2. Be sure to find the reciprocal of the correct fraction. You want the reciprocal of the *divisor* when you convert the problem from division to multiplication.

$$\frac{2}{3} \div \frac{4}{5} = \frac{2}{3} \times \frac{5}{4}, \textbf{ not } \frac{3}{2} \times \frac{4}{5}$$

REVIEW and PRACTICE

DIVIDING FRACTIONS

Find the following quotients. (Rewrite improper fractions as mixed numbers.)

1. $\dfrac{4}{9} \div \dfrac{5}{7}$ 2. $\dfrac{3}{11} \div \dfrac{4}{5}$ 3. $\dfrac{3}{8} \div \dfrac{1}{2}$ 4. $\dfrac{1}{6} \div \dfrac{3}{4}$

5. $\dfrac{3}{5} \div \dfrac{2}{8}$ 6. $\dfrac{6}{9} \div \dfrac{5}{11}$ 7. $\dfrac{9}{10} \div \dfrac{3}{5}$ 8. $\dfrac{7}{12} \div \dfrac{21}{36}$

9. $1\frac{3}{4} \div \frac{2}{3}$ 10. $\frac{7}{8} \div 1\frac{3}{4}$ 11. $4\frac{2}{9} \div 2\frac{3}{8}$ 12. $3\frac{1}{2} \div 1\frac{1}{4}$

13. $1\frac{7}{8} \div 9$ 14. $6 \div \frac{5}{8}$ 15. $\dfrac{\frac{9}{12}}{\frac{4}{6}}$ 16. $\dfrac{\frac{2}{9}}{\frac{1}{8}}$

17. A bottle of pills has 40 tablets scored so that each tablet can be divided into four pieces. If a typical dose is $\frac{1}{4}$ tablet, how many doses does the bottle contain?

18. A nurse administered doses of $2\frac{1}{2}$ milliliters (mL) of medication from a bottle that contained 150 mL. How many $2\frac{1}{2}$ mL doses was the nurse able to give from the bottle?

19. A patient is told to drink the equivalent of 8 glasses of water each day. How many times must the patient drink $\frac{1}{2}$ glass of water to reach the daily goal?

20. A pharmacy technician opens a case that has a total of 84 ounces of medication. If each vial in the case holds $1\frac{3}{4}$ ounces, how many vials are in the case?

To check your answers, see page 332.

Decimals

The decimal system provides another way to represent whole numbers and their fractional parts. Health care practitioners use decimals in their daily work. The metric system, which is decimal-based, is used in dosage calculations, instrument calibrations, and general charting work. You must be able to work with decimals and convert fractions and mixed numbers into decimals.

Working With Decimals

In the decimal system, the location of a digit relative to the decimal point determines its value. The decimal point separates the whole number from the decimal fraction.

Writing Decimals.   Each position in a decimal number has a place value. You already know values to the left of a decimal point. The places to the right of a decimal point represent fractions.

Table 1-3 Decimal Place Values

The number 1,542.567 can be represented as follows:

Whole Number				Decimal Point	Decimal Fraction		
Thousands	Hundreds	Tens	Ones	.	Tenths	Hundredths	Thousandths
1,	5	4	2	.	5	6	7

The number 1,542.567 is read "one thousand five hundred forty-two *and* five hundred sixty-seven thousandths."

Rule 1-22

When you write a decimal number,

1. Write the whole number part to the left of the decimal point.

2. Write the decimal fraction part to the right of the decimal point. Decimal fractions are equivalent to fractions that have denominators of 10, 100, 1,000, and so forth.

3. Use zero as a placeholder to the right of the decimal point just as you use zero for whole numbers. The decimal number 0.203 represents 0 ones, 2 tenths, 0 hundredths, and 3 thousandths.

EXAMPLE 1

Decimal	Description	Mixed Number
12.5	twelve and five tenths	$12\frac{5}{10}$
206.34	two hundred six and thirty-four hundredths	$206\frac{34}{100}$
0.33	thirty-three hundredths	$\frac{33}{100}$
1.125	one and one-hundred-twenty-five thousandths	$1\frac{125}{1000}$

EXAMPLE 2 Write $3\frac{4}{10}$ in decimal form.

$3\frac{4}{10}$ is 3 ones and 4 tenths. In decimal form, $3\frac{4}{10} = 3.4$

EXAMPLE 3 Write $20\frac{7}{100}$ in decimal form.

$20\frac{7}{100}$ is 2 tens, 0 ones, 0 tenths, and 7 hundredths. In decimal form, $20\frac{7}{100} = 20.07$

Rule 1-23

Always write a zero to the left of the decimal point when the decimal number has no whole number part. Using the zero makes the decimal point more noticeable. It helps to prevent errors caused by illegible handwriting.

EXAMPLE 1 Write the following fractions in decimal form:

(a) $\frac{4}{10}$ (b) $\frac{25}{1000}$

(a) $\frac{4}{10} = 0.4$ Do *not* write .4

(b) $\frac{25}{1000} = 0.025$ Do *not* write .025

Comparing Decimals. The more places a number is to the right of the decimal point, the smaller its value. For example, 0.3 is $\frac{3}{10}$, or three tenths; 0.03 is $\frac{3}{100}$, or three hundredths; and 0.003 is $\frac{3}{1000}$, or three thousandths.

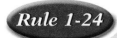

Rule 1-24

To compare the values of a group of decimal numbers,

1. Look first at the whole number part. The decimal number with the greatest whole number is the greatest decimal number.

2. If the whole numbers of two decimals are equal, compare the digits in the tenths place. The tenths place is the first place to the right of the decimal point.

3. If the tenths are equal, move to the right and compare the hundredths place digits.

4. Continue moving to the right, comparing digits until one is greater than the other. This will be the larger number. Zeros added to the right of the last nonzero digit after the decimal point do not change the value of the number.

EXAMPLE 1 Which is larger: 2.1 or 2.3?

The whole number 2 is the same in both numbers. Move one space to the right of the decimal. Compare the tenths digits. Because 3 > 1,

$$2.3 > 2.1$$

EXAMPLE 2 Which is larger: 0.3 or 0.05?

There is no whole number. Move one space to the right of the decimal. Compare the tenths digits. Because 3 > 0,

$$0.3 > 0.05$$

EXAMPLE 3 Which is larger: 0.121 or 0.13?

There is no whole number. Move one space to the right of the decimal. Compare the tenths. These digits are equal. Move one space to the right and compare the hundredths digits. Because 3 > 2,

$$0.13 > 0.121$$

REVIEW and PRACTICE

WORKING WITH DECIMALS

Write the following fractions in decimal form:

1. $\dfrac{2}{10}$ 2. $\dfrac{17}{100}$ 3. $6\dfrac{5}{10}$ 4. $7\dfrac{19}{100}$

5. $\dfrac{3}{1000}$ 6. $\dfrac{23}{1000}$

Place > or < between each pair of decimals to make a true statement:

7. 4.27   4.02   8. 12.25   12.18

9. 0.4   0.6   10. 2.22   2.20

11. 0.0170   0.0172   12. 0.3001   0.2998

To check your answers, see page 332.

Rounding Decimals

In health care settings, you will usually round decimals to the nearest tenth or hundredth, especially if you use a calculator. The answer you get may contain many more decimal places than you need, and you must round the answer. For example, $10 \div 3 = 3.333333. \ldots$ You can round this number to the nearest tenth: 3.3

Rule 1-25

To round decimals,

1. Underline the place value to which you want to round.

2. Look at the digit to the right of this target place value. If this digit is 0, 1, 2, 3, or 4, do not change the digit in the target place value. If this digit is 5, 6, 7, 8, or 9, round the digit in the target place value up one unit.

3. Drop all digits to the right of the target place value.

EXAMPLE 1 Round 2.42 to the nearest tenth.

1. Underline the tenths place (the target place value): 2.<u>4</u>2

2. The digit to the right of the tenths place is 2. Do not change the digit in the tenths place.

3. Drop the digits to the right of the tenths place. 2.42 rounded to the nearest tenth equals 2.4

EXAMPLE 2 Round 0.035 to the nearest hundredth.

1. 0.0<u>3</u>5

2. The digit to the right of the hundredths place is 5. Round the digit in the hundredths place up one unit: 0.0<u>4</u>

3. 0.035 rounded to the nearest hundredth equals 0.04

EXAMPLE 3 Round 3.99 to the nearest tenth.

1. 3.<u>9</u>9

2. The digit to the right of the tenths place is 9. Round the digit in the tenths place up one unit. When 9 is rounded up, it becomes 10. Place the 0 in the tenths place and carry the 1 to the ones place. When 1 is added to the ones place, 3 becomes 4. The rounded number becomes 4.<u>00</u>

3. 3.99 rounded to the nearest tenth equals 4.0

CRITICAL THINKING ON THE JOB

Rounding Errors With 9

A medical assistant is calculating how much medication to inject. The patient should receive 4.95 milliliters, but the syringe being used is calibrated (marked) in tenths. He must round the calculation to the nearest tenth.

The medical assistant looks at the 5 in the hundredths place and rounds the tenths place up from 9 to 0. However, the medical assistant neglects to carry the unit to the ones place and draws 4.0 milliliters of medication into the syringe.

Think Before You Act

Because the medical assistant forgets to carry a unit from the tenths place into the ones place, an error results. The patient does not receive a full dose of medication. With correct rounding, the patient should receive 5.0 milliliters, not 4.0 milliliters.

ROUNDING DECIMALS

Round to the nearest tenth:

1. 14.34	**2.** 3.45	**3.** 0.86
4. 0.19	**5.** 1.007	**6.** 0.2083

Round to the nearest hundredth:

7. 9.293	**8.** 55.168	**9.** 4.0060
10. 2.2081	**11.** 5.5195	**12.** 11.999

Round to the nearest whole number:

13. 11.493	**14.** 19.98
15. 2.099	**16.** 50.505

17. You are preparing a syringe to inject 3.75 milliliters of medication. The syringe is calibrated in tenths. How much medication should you draw into the syringe?

18. A nurse is preparing a syringe for injection. The calculations indicate that 0.38 milliliters should be given to the patient. The syringe is calibrated in hundredths. How much medication should the nurse draw into the syringe?

To check your answers, see page 332.

Converting Fractions Into Decimals

Conversions between fractions and decimals is important in health care settings. For example, you may receive a drug order in fractions, but the equipment is measured in decimals. When you convert proper fractions to decimals, the equivalent decimals are less than one. When you convert improper fractions, the equivalent decimals are greater than one. When you convert fractions to decimals, think of the fractions as division problems. You can write $\frac{1}{4}$ as $1 \div 4$. Reducing fractions first (if possible) makes the division easier.

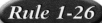
Rule 1-26

To convert a fraction to a decimal, divide the numerator by the denominator.

EXAMPLE 1 Convert $\frac{3}{4}$ to a decimal.

Divide the numerator by the denominator:

$$
\begin{array}{r}
0.75 \\
4\overline{)3.00} \\
\underline{2\ 8} \\
20 \\
\underline{20} \\
\end{array}
$$

$$\frac{3}{4} = 0.75$$

EXAMPLE 2   Convert $\frac{2}{3}$ to a decimal.

$$
\begin{array}{r}
0.666 \\
3\overline{)2.000} \\
\underline{1\ 8} \\
20 \\
\underline{18} \\
20 \\
\underline{18} \\
2\ \ldots
\end{array}
$$

Sometimes the decimal repeats rather than terminates, as with $\frac{2}{3}$. In such cases, you round, for example, to the nearest hundredth:

$$\frac{2}{3} = 0.67$$

EXAMPLE 3   Convert $\frac{8}{5}$ to a decimal.

$$
\begin{array}{r}
1.6 \\
5\overline{)8.0} \\
\underline{5} \\
3.0 \\
\underline{3.0}
\end{array}
\qquad \frac{8}{5} = 1.6
$$

EXAMPLE 4   Convert $1\frac{7}{8}$ to a decimal.

$$
\begin{array}{r}
0.875 \\
8\overline{)7.000} \\
\underline{6\ 4} \\
60 \\
\underline{56} \\
40 \\
\underline{40}
\end{array}
\qquad 1\frac{7}{8} = 1 + \frac{7}{8} = 1 + 0.875 = 1.875
$$

REVIEW and PRACTICE

CONVERTING FRACTIONS INTO DECIMALS

Convert the following numbers into decimals. Where necessary, round to the nearest thousandth:

1. $\frac{2}{5}$ 2. $\frac{7}{20}$ 3. $\frac{9}{12}$ 4. $\frac{12}{24}$

5. $\frac{1}{3}$ 6. $\frac{4}{9}$ 7. $\frac{15}{27}$ 8. $\frac{21}{36}$

9. $\frac{12}{8}$ 10. $\frac{11}{5}$ 11. $\frac{7}{3}$ 12. $\frac{9}{8}$

13. $1\frac{4}{5}$ 14. $2\frac{1}{10}$ 15. $6\frac{3}{4}$ 16. $3\frac{1}{2}$

To check your answers, see page 333.

Converting Decimals Into Fractions

Sometimes you need to convert a decimal to a fraction, especially when you use a calculator that provides decimals, but you need a fraction. When you work with decimals, treat the number to the left of the decimal point as a whole number and the number to the right of the decimal point as a fraction. For example, 12.5 is twelve and five tenths, or $12\frac{5}{10}$. The place value of the digit farthest to the right of the decimal point is the denominator. For 12.5, this place value is the tenths place. The denominator is 10. The numerator is 5, the number to the right of the decimal point.

Rule 1-27

To convert a decimal to a fraction or mixed number,
1. Write the number to the left of the decimal point as the whole number.
2. Write the number to the right of the decimal point as the numerator of the fraction.
3. Use the place value of the digit farthest to the right of the decimal point as the denominator.
4. Reduce the fraction part to its lowest terms.

EXAMPLE 1 Convert 3.75 to a mixed number.
1. Write the number to the left of the decimal point, 3, as the whole number.
2. Write the number to the right of the decimal point, 75, as the numerator of the fraction.
3. The digit farthest to the right of the decimal point, 5, is in the hundredths place. Thus, the denominator is 100. The mixed number is $3\frac{75}{100}$.
4. Reduce to lowest terms: $3\frac{75}{100} = 3\frac{3}{4}$

EXAMPLE 2 Convert 0.010 to a fraction.
1. The number to the left of the decimal point is 0, so 0.010 has no whole number.
2. The number 010 is to the right of the decimal point. Because 010 = 10, write 10 as the numerator of the fraction.
3. The digit farthest to the right of the decimal point is 0, in the thousandths place. The denominator is 1000. The fraction is
$$\frac{10}{1000}$$
4. $\frac{10}{1000} = \frac{1}{100}$

REVIEW and PRACTICE

CONVERTING DECIMALS INTO FRACTIONS

Convert the following decimals to fractions or mixed numbers. Reduce the answer to its lowest terms.

1. 1.2	**2.** 98.6	**3.** 0.3	**4.** 0.442
5. 5.03	**6.** 0.301	**7.** 100.04	**8.** 206.070

To check your answers, see page 333.

Adding and Subtracting Decimals

When you add or subtract decimals, you align them by their place value, just as you do to add or subtract whole numbers.

Rule 1-28

To add or subtract decimals,

1. Write the problem vertically, as you would with whole numbers. Align the decimal points.

2. Perform the operation, starting from the right. Include the decimal point in your answer.

EXAMPLE 1 Add 2.47 + 0.39

1. Write the problem vertically.
   Align the decimal points.

$$\begin{array}{r} 2.47 \\ +\ 0.39 \end{array}$$

2. Perform the operation.

$$\begin{array}{r} 2.47 \\ +\ 0.39 \\ \hline 2.86 \end{array}$$

EXAMPLE 2 Subtract 52.04 − 14.31

Align the decimal points.

$$\begin{array}{r} 52.04 \\ -\ 14.31 \\ \hline 37.73 \end{array}$$

When the decimals have an unequal number of places, add zeros to the end of the decimal fraction so that all numbers are the same length past the decimal point. Writing zeros after the last digit to the right of the decimal point does not change the number's value. Including these zeros helps prevent errors in calculations.

EXAMPLE 3 Add 14.3 + 1.56 + 9 + 0.352

Align the numbers. (Rewrite 9 as 9.0 to help you align it properly.) Fill in zeros so that all decimal fractions are of equal length. Then add.

$$\begin{array}{r} 14.3 \\ 1.56 \\ 9.0 \\ 0.352 \end{array} \qquad \begin{array}{r} 14.300 \\ 1.560 \\ 9.000 \\ 0.352 \\ \hline 25.212 \end{array}$$

EXAMPLE 4 Subtract 7.3 − 1.005

Align the numbers. Fill in zeros so that all decimal fractions are of equal length. Then subtract.

$$\begin{array}{r} -\ 7.3 \\ -\ 1.005 \end{array} \qquad \begin{array}{r} -\ 7.300 \\ -\ 1.005 \\ \hline 6.295 \end{array}$$

EXAMPLE 5 Subtract 10 − 0.75

$$\begin{array}{r} 10.00 \\ -\ 0.75 \\ \hline 9.25 \end{array}$$

ADDING AND SUBTRACTING DECIMALS

Add or subtract the following pairs of numbers.

1. 7.58 + 3.24

2. 143.05 + 22.07

3. 13.561 + 0.099

4. 24.102 + 2.410

5. 2.01 + 0.5

6. 2.30 + 0.005

7. 0.075 + 0.73

8. 4 + 0.025

9. 31.64 − 17.39

10. 16.250 − 1.625

11. 5.66 − 0.09

12. 14.7 − 0.9

13. 1.22 − 0.4

14. 12.2 − 0.972

15. 8 − 0.076

16. 12 − 0.02

17. Steve's temperature on Wednesday morning was 101.4 degrees Fahrenheit. By Thursday afternoon, it was 99.5 degrees. By how many degrees had his temperature changed?

18. While waiting to see her father, Helene ate at the hospital cafeteria, where she spent $1.30 for a soda, $2.65 for a bowl of soup, and $3.50 for a garden salad. How much did Helene spend?

19. You are supposed to administer 9 grains of a medication. You give the patient one tablet with 4.5 grains and a second tablet with 2.25 grains. How much more medication should you administer?

20. A bottle of liquid medication contains 50 milliliters (mL). The following amounts are given to patients from the bottle: 2.5 mL, 3.1 mL, 1.75 mL, 3 mL, and 2.25 mL. How much medication remains in the bottle?

To check your answers, see page 333.

Multiplying Decimals

Multiplying decimals is similar to multiplying whole numbers, except you must determine where to place the decimal point.

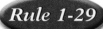

Rule 1-29

To multiply decimals,

1. First multiply without considering the decimal points, as if the numbers were whole numbers.

2. Count the total number of places to the right of the decimal points in *both* factors.

3. To place the decimal point in the product, start at its right end. Move the decimal point to the left the same number of places as the sum from Step 2.

EXAMPLE 1 Multiply 3.42 × 2.5

When multiplying, the decimal points *do not* need to line up as they do for adding and subtracting.

1. First multiply without considering the decimal points.

$$
\begin{array}{r}
3.42 \\
\times\ 2.5 \\
\hline
1710 \\
684 \\
\hline
8550
\end{array}
$$

2. Count the total number of decimal places (to the right of the decimal point) in the factors. 3.42 has 2 decimal places; 2.5 has 1 decimal place. The factors have a total of 3 decimal places.

3. Place the decimal point in the product. Start at the right of the product 8550. Move the decimal point three places to the left: 8.550 *After* placing the decimal point, you can drop the final zero so that the product is 8.55

EXAMPLE 2 Multiply 0.001 × 0.02

1. Multiply

$$
\begin{array}{r}
0.001 \\
\times\ 0.02 \\
\hline
2
\end{array}
$$

2. 0.001 has 3 decimal places, and 0.02 has 2 decimal places. The factors have a total of 5 decimal places.

3. Start to the right of the product 2. Move the decimal point five places to the left. Insert zeros to the left of 2 in order to correctly place the decimal point. The correct answer is 0.00002

REVIEW and PRACTICE

MULTIPLYING DECIMALS

Multiply the following numbers.

1. 7.4 × 8.2

2. 8.21 × 1.1

3. 4.2 × 0.3

4. 3.04 × 0.04

5. 0.55 × 0.5

6. 0.027 × 0.4

7. 0.003 × 0.02

8. 0.25 × 0.75

9. 1.03 × 14

10. 12 × 0.09

11. 0.004 × 15.5

12. 0.004 × 40.01

13. A patient is given 7.5 milliliters of liquid medication 5 times per day. How many milliliters does she receive per day?

14. A small syringe is used to give a patient 0.28 milliliter of medication 4 times per day for 4 days. How much medication does he receive over the 4 days?

15. A tablet has a strength of 0.25 milligram of medication. You give the patient $1\frac{1}{2}$ tablets 3 times per day. How many milligrams of medication do you give the patient each day? (Hint: Convert $1\frac{1}{2}$ to decimal form first.)

16. A tablet has a strength of 0.4 milligram of medication. If you give the patient $\frac{1}{4}$ tablet twice a day, how many milligrams of medication does the patient receive per day?

To check your answers, see page 333.

Dividing Decimals

The key to dividing decimals correctly is to place the decimal point properly. Recall that the dividend is the number that will be divided. If the divisor is a decimal, you want to convert the problem to one in which the divisor is a whole number.

Rule 1-30

To divide decimals,

1. Write the problem as a fraction. (The dividend is the numerator and the divisor is the denominator.)

2. Move the decimal point to the right the *same* number of places in both the numerator and denominator until the denominator is a whole number. Insert zeros to the numerator as necessary.

3. Complete the division as you would with whole numbers. Align the decimal point of the quotient with the decimal point of the numerator, if needed.

EXAMPLE 1 Divide $0.8 \div 0.02$

1. Write the problem as a fraction: $\dfrac{0.8}{0.02}$

2. Move the decimal point two places to the right in both the numerator and the denominator. The denominator is now a whole number.

$$\frac{0.8}{0.02} = \frac{8}{0.2} = \frac{80}{2}$$

(This step is equivalent to multiplying $\dfrac{0.8}{0.02} \times \dfrac{100}{100}$.)

3. Complete the division:

$$2\overline{)80} \quad \begin{array}{r} 40 \\ \hline 80 \end{array} \quad \text{so that } 0.8 \div 0.02 = 40$$

EXAMPLE 2 Divide $0.066 \div 0.11$

1. $\dfrac{0.066}{0.11}$

2. $\dfrac{0.066}{0.11} = \dfrac{6.6}{11}$ Move the decimal point two places to the right so that the denominator (divisor) is a whole number.

3. $\quad\quad\quad 11\overline{)6.6} \quad \begin{array}{r} 0.6 \\ \hline 6.6 \end{array}$

Align the decimal point of the quotient with the decimal point of the numerator (dividend). Here, $0.066 \div 0.11 = 0.6$

CRITICAL THINKING ON THE JOB

Placing Decimals Correctly

A medical assistant was instructed to give 0.25 gram of medication for every 1.0 kilogram of body weight. A baby she was treating weighed 6.25 kilograms. She set up this calculation:

```
    6.25
  × .25
  3125
  1250
156.25
```

Think Before You Act

The practitioner got confused when placing the decimal in the answer. She followed the rule for addition rather than for multiplication of decimals. The result, had the error not been caught, would have been a disastrous overdose. The baby should have received 1.5625 grams of medication, which rounds to 1.56 grams.

REVIEW and PRACTICE

DIVIDING DECIMALS

Divide the following numbers.

1. $3.2 \div 1.6$

2. $48.6 \div 1.8$

3. $24.5 \div 0.2$

4. $0.004 \div 0.002$

5. $1.25 \div 0.5$

6. $0.32 \div 0.8$

7. $0.05 \div 4$

8. $12.6 \div 4$

9. $40 \div 0.8$

10. $0.44 \div 4.4$

11. $29.05 \div 100$

12. $3.48 \div 1000$

13. $39.666 \div 0.03$

14. $54.54 \div 0.009$

15. A bottle holds 60 milliliters of medication. If the average dose is 0.75 milliliters, how many doses does the bottle hold?

16. A bottle contains 32 ounces of medication. If the average dose is 0.4 ounces, how many doses does the bottle contain?

17. A patient received a total of 2.25 grains of a medication. If the patient received the total over a 3-day period and was given 3 doses per day, what was the strength of each dose?

18. A patient weighs 197.5 pounds. The patient's goal is to weigh 152.5 pounds a year from now. How much weight should the patient lose per month to be successful?

To check your answers, see page 333.

CHAPTER 1 REVIEW

CHECK UP

Write the following Roman numerals as Arabic numbers:

1. XXIV   **2.** IX   **3.** xviii   **4.** xxix

Convert the following mixed numbers to improper fractions:

5. $2\frac{3}{8}$ **6.** $1\frac{2}{7}$ **7.** $9\frac{9}{10}$ **8.** $12\frac{11}{12}$

Reduce the following fractions to their lowest terms:

9. $\frac{12}{36}$ **10.** $\frac{39}{48}$ **11.** $\frac{45}{9}$ **12.** $\frac{58}{8}$

Find the least common denominator. Then write an equivalent fraction for each.

13. $\frac{3}{10}$ and $\frac{4}{5}$ **14.** $\frac{5}{6}$ and $\frac{4}{9}$

15. $\frac{3}{8}, \frac{3}{4},$ and $\frac{1}{6}$ **16.** $\frac{7}{10}, \frac{1}{4},$ and $\frac{2}{3}$

Place $>$, $<$, or $=$ between the following pairs of fractions to make a true statement:

17. $\frac{3}{10}$ $\frac{3}{16}$ **18.** $\frac{3}{2}$ $\frac{8}{5}$

19. $1\frac{2}{3}$ $1\frac{16}{24}$ **20.** $\frac{4}{25}$ $\frac{16}{75}$

Perform the following calculations. Give the answer in lowest terms.

21. $\frac{9}{4} + \frac{2}{3}$ **22.** $\frac{3}{5} + 1\frac{2}{5}$

23. $\frac{2}{10} + \frac{1}{100} + \frac{4}{50}$ **24.** $6 + \frac{5}{8} + \frac{1}{3} + \frac{5}{12}$

25. $\frac{11}{9} - \frac{1}{3}$ **26.** $\frac{4}{5} - \frac{3}{4}$

27. $3\frac{1}{4} - 1\frac{7}{8}$ **28.** $3 - \frac{2}{7}$

29. $\frac{5}{6} \times \frac{2}{3}$ **30.** $\frac{7}{9} \times \frac{3}{14}$

31. $2\frac{2}{5} \times \frac{10}{3}$ **32.** $\frac{3}{8} \times 11$

33. $\frac{1}{7} \div \frac{3}{4}$ **34.** $\frac{12}{13} \div \frac{3}{52}$

35. $2\frac{5}{8} \div \frac{1}{6}$ **36.** $\frac{1}{3} \div 1\frac{1}{4}$

Place $>$, $<$, or $=$ between the following pairs of decimals to make a true statement:

37. 5.7   5.09   **38.** 0.04   0.004

39. 6.3   6.300   **40.** 9.033   9.303

Round to the nearest hundredth:

41. 0.229   **42.** 7.091   **43.** 46.001   **44.** 9.885

Round to the nearest tenth:

45. 4.34   **46.** 3.65   **47.** 6.991   **48.** 0.073

Round to the nearest whole number:

49. 8.96   **50.** 20.6   **51.** 0.931   **52.** 12.449

Convert the following fractions to decimals:

53. $\dfrac{7}{14}$ **54.** $\dfrac{5}{8}$ **55.** $2\dfrac{3}{5}$ **56.** $\dfrac{32}{4}$

Convert the following decimals to fractions. Reduce the answers to lowest terms.

57. 0.82   **58.** 0.65   **59.** 3.5   **60.** 1.001

Perform the following calculations:

61. 7.23 + 12.38   **62.** 4.59 + 0.2

63. 0.031 + 0.99   **64.** 12 + 0.004 + 1.7

65. 7.49 − 0.38   **66.** 4.28 − 3.39

67. 0.852 − 0.61   **68.** 14.01 − 0.788

69. 2.3 × 4.9   **70.** 0.33 × 0.002

71. 5 × 0.999   **72.** 12.01 × 1.005

73. 38.85 ÷ 2.1   **74.** 4.875 ÷ 3.25

75. 2.2 ÷ 0.11   **76.** 1.4 ÷ 0.07

77. A medical unit has 18 patients. Eight have Type O blood. Five have Type A blood. Two have Type AB blood. Three have Type B blood. Write the fractions that describe the portions of the medical unit patients that have each blood type.

78. A patient is supposed to receive $\dfrac{1}{2}$ cup of medication three times per day. Instead, the patient receives $\dfrac{1}{3}$ cup twice per day. During the day, how much medicine does the patient receive? How does that amount compare with the amount ordered?

79. During the day, Brian drank $\dfrac{3}{4}$ cup of water seven times, 1 cup of milk two times, and $\dfrac{1}{2}$ cup of juice three times. How much liquid did Brian consume?

80. A bottle contains 48 milliliters of liquid medication.
  a. If the average dose is $\dfrac{3}{4}$ milliliter, how many doses does the bottle contain?
  b. If the average dose is 1.2 milliliters, how many doses does the bottle contain?

CRITICAL THINKING

A medical assistant is asked to arrange a set of instruments on a tray in order from smallest to largest on the basis of the instruments' diameters. The diameters are marked $\dfrac{1}{4}$, $\dfrac{7}{16}$, $\dfrac{1}{2}$, $\dfrac{1}{8}$, $\dfrac{1}{16}$, $\dfrac{3}{16}$, and $\dfrac{5}{16}$. How should the medical assistant arrange the instruments? Look at the pattern of increase in these measurements. Are any instruments missing in the sequence? If so, which ones?

CASE STUDY

A nurse is tracking the weight of a patient who is retaining fluids because of congestive heart failure. On day 3, the patient is given a diuretic. Here is a summary of the weight changes that occurred. In the column marked Change, write the amount of weight change since the previous measurement. Write + before weight gained, and − before weight lost.

Time	Weight	Change
Day 1 8:00 a.m.	$142\frac{1}{2}$	n/a
Day 2 8:00 a.m.	144	
Day 3 8:00 a.m.	$145\frac{3}{4}$	
Day 3 8:00 a.m.	Patient receives diuretic Lasix (furosemide) 40 milligrams.	
Day 3 2:00 p.m.	$144\frac{3}{4}$	
Day 3 4:00 p.m.	Lasix 40 milligrams	
Day 4 8:00 a.m.	$142\frac{3}{4}$	
Day 4 8:00 a.m.	Lasix 20 milligrams	
Day 4 4:00 p.m.	$140\frac{1}{2}$	

To check your answers see page 334.

INTERNET ACTIVITY

When you use the Internet, you must critically evaluate any information you find for accuracy and reliability. Understanding basic web site addresses, in the form *www.name.ending*, can help.

Basic addresses ending in *.gov* are official federal, state, and local government sites. Information from known government organizations such as the National Institutes of Health (*www.nih.gov*) is considered to be reliable.

Addresses ending in *.edu* originate at educational institutions. Be aware that individual pages at an educational site are often written and supported by students and faculty members. The content of these pages is not necessarily reviewed by the institution.

Sites ending in *.org* are primarily for nonprofit organizations. The credibility of the information depends on the credibility of the organization. Well-known groups such as the American Medical Association (*www.ama-assn.org*) or the American Cancer Society (*www.cancer.org*) usually have reliable, useful information. In general, though, be wary. Any nonprofit group, regardless of its interests or agenda, can create a Web site.

Sites ending in *.com* are sites maintained by commercial organizations. (The ending *.net* is also used by a variety of organizations.) Some provide detailed, accurate information of general interest. Others contain slanted statistics designed to promote their products.

Commercial organizations also sponsor Web sites maintained by millions of individuals throughout the world. These sites can be written by anyone from an elementary school child to a Nobel Prize winner. Be cautious when using information from private sites.

If you have doubts about the information from an Internet site, confirm it with a textbook, reference book, or other traditional information source before you use it.

Assignment: Search for sites that contain information on dosage calculation or medication math. If you find a site you like and trust, bookmark it (save it in a listing on your computer) so that you can easily find the site again. (Suggested key words: "dosage + calculations," "medication + math," "algebra," and "student + nursing.")

PERCENTS, RATIOS, and PROPORTIONS

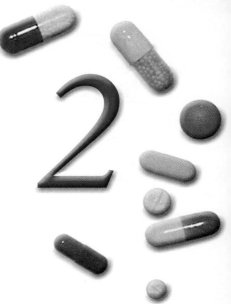

2

Objectives

When you have completed Chapter 2, you will be able to:

- Describe the relationship among percents, ratios, decimals, and fractions.
- Calculate equivalent measurements using percents, ratios, decimals, and fractions.
- Indicate solution strengths by using percents and ratios.
- Explain the concept of proportion.
- Calculate missing values in proportions by using ratios (means and extremes) and fractions (cross-multiplying).

Percents

Percents, like decimals and fractions, provide a way to express the relationship of parts to a whole. Indicated by the symbol %, *percent* literally means "per 100" or "divided by 100." The whole is always 100 units. Table 2-1 shows the same number expressed as a decimal, a fraction, and a percent. A number less than one is expressed as less than 100 percent. A number greater than one is expressed as greater than 100 percent. Any expression of one (for instance, 1.0 or $\frac{5}{5}$) equals 100 percent.

Table 2-1 Comparing Decimals, Fractions, and Percents

Words	Decimal	Fraction	Percent
eight hundredths	0.08	$\frac{8}{100}$	8%
twenty-three hundredths	0.23	$\frac{23}{100}$	23%
seven-tenths	0.7	$\frac{7}{10}$	70%
one	1.0	$\frac{1}{1}$	100%
one and five-tenths or one and one half	1.5	$1\frac{5}{10}$ or $1\frac{1}{2}$	150%

Working With Percents

Converting between percents and decimals requires little more than dividing and multiplying by 100.

Rule 2-1

> To convert a percent to a decimal, remove the percent symbol. Then divide the remaining number by 100.

Converting a percent to a decimal is similar to dividing a number by 100—you move the decimal point two places to the left. If the percent is a fraction or a mixed number, first convert it to a decimal (see Chapter 1 for review). Then divide by 100, moving the decimal point two places to the left.

EXAMPLE 1 Convert 42% to a decimal.

$$42\% = 42.\% = .42. = 0.42$$

Insert the zero before the decimal point for clarity.

EXAMPLE 2 Convert 175% to a decimal.

$$175\% = 175.\% = 1.75. = 1.75$$

EXAMPLE 3 When you move the decimal point to the left, you may need to insert zeros.
Convert 0.3% to a decimal.

$$0.3\% = 000.3\% = 0.00.3 = 0.003$$

EXAMPLE 4 Convert $25\frac{1}{2}\%$ to a decimal.

$$25\frac{1}{2}\% = 25\frac{5}{10}\% = 25.5\% = 025.5\% = 0.25.5 = 0.255$$

EXAMPLE 5 Convert $\frac{3}{4}\%$ to a decimal.
First convert $\frac{3}{4}$ to a decimal.

$$\frac{3}{4} = 4\overline{)3.00}^{\,0.75} = 0.75$$

$$\frac{3}{4}\% = 0.75\% = 000.75\% = 0.00.75 = 0.0075$$

Rule 2-2

> To change a decimal into a percent, multiply the decimal by 100. Then add the percent symbol.

Converting a decimal to a percent is similar to multiplying a number by 100—you move the decimal point two places to the right. Because 100% = 1.00, multiplying a number by 100% does not change its value.

EXAMPLE 1 Convert 1.42 to a percent.

$$1.42 \times 100\% = 142.00\% = 142\%$$

You can write this as $1.42 = 1.42\% = 142\%$

EXAMPLE 2 Convert 0.02 to a percent.

$$0.02 \times 100\% = 2.00\% = 2\%$$

You can write this as $0.02 = 0.02\% = 2\%$

When you move the decimal point to the right, you may need to insert zeros.

EXAMPLE 3 Convert 0.8 to a percent.

$$0.8 \times 100\% = 80.0\% = 80\%$$

You can write this as $0.8 = 0.80 = 0.80\% = 80\%$

Because percent means "per 100" or "divided by 100," you can easily convert percents to equivalent fractions.

Rule 2-3

To convert a percent to an equivalent fraction, write the value of the percent as the numerator and 100 as the denominator. Then reduce the fraction to its lowest terms.

EXAMPLE 1 Convert 8% into an equivalent fraction.

$$8\% = \frac{8}{100} = \frac{\overset{2}{\cancel{8}}}{\underset{25}{\cancel{100}}} = \frac{2}{25}$$

EXAMPLE 2 Convert 130% to an equivalent mixed number.

$$130\% = \frac{130}{100} = \frac{\overset{13}{\cancel{130}}}{\underset{10}{\cancel{100}}} = \frac{13}{10} = 1\frac{3}{10}$$

EXAMPLE 3 Change 0.6% to an equivalent fraction.

$$0.6\% = \frac{0.6}{100} = \frac{6}{1000} = \frac{\overset{3}{\cancel{6}}}{\underset{500}{\cancel{1000}}} = \frac{3}{500}$$

Here, $\frac{0.6}{100}$ was multiplied by $\frac{10}{10}$ in order to eliminate the decimal from the fraction.

EXAMPLE 4 Change $\frac{3}{4}$% to an equivalent fraction.

$$\frac{3}{4}\% = \frac{3}{4} \div 100 = \frac{3}{4} \times \frac{1}{100} = \frac{3}{400}$$

For a review of division with fractions, see Chapter 1.

Rule 2-4

To convert a fraction to a percent, first convert the fraction to a decimal. Round the decimal to the nearest hundredth. Then follow the rule for converting a decimal to a percent.

EXAMPLE 1 Convert $\frac{1}{2}$ to a percent.

First convert $\frac{1}{2}$ to a decimal.

$$\frac{1}{2} = 1 \div 2 = 0.5$$

Now convert the decimal to a percent.

$$\frac{1}{2} = 0.5 = 0.5 \times 100\% = 50\%$$

You can write this as $0.5 = 0.50 = 0.50.\% = 50\%$

EXAMPLE 2 Convert $\frac{2}{3}$ to a percent.

Convert $\frac{2}{3}$ to a decimal. Round to the nearest hundredth.

$$\frac{2}{3} = 2 \div 3 = 0.666 = 0.67$$

Now convert to a percent.

$$\frac{2}{3} = 0.67 = 0.67 \times 100\% = 67\%$$

You can write this as $0.67 = 0.67.\% = 67\%$

EXAMPLE 3 Convert $1\frac{3}{4}$ to a percent.

$$1\frac{3}{4} = \frac{7}{4} = 1.75 = 1.75 \times 100\% = 175\%$$

You can write this as $1\frac{3}{4} = 1.75.\% = 175\%$

REVIEW and PRACTICE

WORKING WITH PERCENTS

Convert the following percents to decimals:

1. 14%   2. 30%   3. 2%

4. 9%   5. 103%   6. 300%

7. 0.021%   8. 0.4%   9. $42\frac{1}{2}\%$

10. $3\frac{4}{5}\%$ 11. 4.5%   12. 250.75%

Convert the following decimals to percents:

13. 4.04   **14.** 2.3   **15.** 0.7

16. 0.33   **17.** 0.06   **18.** 0.013

19. 15   **20.** 32

Convert the following percents to fractions. Reduce the answers to their lowest terms:

21. 22%   **22.** 4%   **23.** 158%

24. 300%   **25.** 0.1%   **26.** 0.8%

27. $\frac{9}{10}$%   **28.** $1\frac{2}{5}$%

Convert the following fractions to percents:

29. $\frac{6}{8}$ **30.** $\frac{4}{5}$ **31.** $\frac{1}{6}$ **32.** $\frac{5}{9}$

33. $1\frac{1}{10}$ **34.** $2\frac{1}{4}$ **35.** $\frac{175}{100}$ **36.** $\frac{40}{100}$

To check your answers, see page 335.

Solution Strengths

Percents are commonly used to indicate the strength of intravenous (IV) solutions. They are sometimes used to designate the strength of medications such as ointments.

These terms are important to understanding solutions: solute, solvent or diluent, and solution.

- The *solute* is the drug or substance being dissolved.
- The *solvent* or *diluent* is the liquid with which the solute is combined.
- The *solution* is the combined mixture.

Suppose you dissolve one teaspoon of salt into eight ounces of fresh water. The salt is the solute. The fresh water is the solvent or diluent. The resulting salt water is the solution.

Rule 2-5

If the drug is a dry drug, then the percent strength of a solution represents the amount of dry drug, measured in grams, that is in 100 milliliters (mL) of solution.

Note that the 100 mL of solution is a mixture of dry drug (solute) and solvent.

EXAMPLE 1 Determine how many grams of dry drug are in 100 mL of a 1% solution.

Each percent strength of a 100 mL solution represents 1 gram of dry drug. Therefore, the 1% solution contains 1 gram of dry drug.

EXAMPLE 2 Determine how many grams of dry drug are in 200 mL of a 2% solution.

A 2% solution contains 2 grams of dry drug in 100 mL of solution. Since 200 mL is twice the amount of solution as 100 mL, it will contain twice the amount of dry drug, or 4 grams. The percent has not changed, just the total volume.

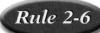

Rule 2-6

If the drug is a liquid, then the percent strength of a solution represents the amount of liquid drug, measured in milliliters (mL), that is in 100 mL of solution.

EXAMPLE 1 If 100 mL of solution contains 15 mL of liquid drug, what is the solution's strength?

When measuring liquid drugs, each mL of drug in 100 mL of solution represents 1% strength. Since this solution has 15 mL, its strength is 15%.

EXAMPLE 2 How much liquid medication is in 50 mL of an 8% solution?

100 mL of an 8% solution has 8 mL of liquid medication. 50 mL is half of 100 mL. It would have half the amount of liquid medication, or 4 mL.

Since percent means "per 100," the percent strength of a solution is *always* calculated on the amount of drug *per 100* mL. Solutions with higher percent strengths contain more drug in each 100 mL and, therefore, are stronger solutions. A 10% solution has twice as much drug as a 5% solution.

Table 2-2 Comparing Solution Strengths

Amount of Solution	Solution Strength	Grams of Dry Drug	mL of Liquid Drug
50 mL	1%	0.5 grams	0.5 mL
100 mL	1%	1.0 grams	1.0 mL
200 mL	1%	2.0 grams	2.0 mL
50 mL	2%	1.0 grams	1.0 mL
100 mL	2%	2.0 grams	2.0 mL
200 mL	2%	4.0 grams	4.0 mL
100 mL	5%	5.0 grams	5.0 mL
50 mL	10%	5.0 grams	5.0 mL
100 mL	10%	10.0 grams	10.0 mL
200 mL	10%	20.0 grams	20.0 mL

CRITICAL THINKING ON THE JOB

Confusing Percent Strength With Percent Conversions

A pharmacy technician is asked to make a 2% drug solution using a dry drug. Before mixing the solution, the technician converts 2% to a decimal. Since 2% = 0.02, the technician adds 0.02 grams of drug to 100 mL of solution.

Think Before You Act

The technician confused percent strength with percent conversion. The definition of percent strength is the amount of the drug, in grams, that is dissolved in 100 mL. In this case, the technician did not need to convert 2% to a decimal. Instead, the technician should have asked, "How many grams of drug dissolved in 100 mL will equal 2%?" The answer is 2 grams.

SOLUTION STRENGTHS

Note: 100 mL = 100 cc. The abbreviation *cc* represents cubic centimeters. Measurements and abbreviations such as mL and cc will be discussed in Chapter 3.

1. How many grams of drug are in 100 mL of a 5% solution?

2. How many grams of drug are in 100 mL of a 6% solution?

3. An IV bag contains 200 cc of dextrose 5% (a 5% drug solution). How many grams of dextrose are in the bag?

4. How many grams of dextrose will a patient receive from a 100 mL bag of dextrose 10% (a 10% solution of dextrose)?

5. A full 1000-cc bag of a 10% drug solution contains how many grams of the drug?

6. A 1000-cc bag of a 5% drug solution is now half empty. How many grams of the drug remain in the bag?

To check your answers, see page 335.

Ratios

Ratios also express the relationship of a part to the whole. They may relate a quantity of liquid drug to a quantity of solution, as with intravenous drugs. Ratios can also be used to calculate dosages of dry medication such as tablets.

A ratio is usually written in the form A:B. The colon tells you to compare A to B. A:B is read "A to B." For example, a 1:100 drug solution ("one to one hundred") describes a solution that has 1 part drug to every 100 parts of solution. The ratio 1:100 is equivalent to the fraction $\frac{1}{100}$, the decimal 0.01, and the percent 1%.

When ratios describe dry medications, the whole unit is often 1, as in 1 tablet. Thus, 25 milligrams (mg) of drug to one tablet would be written as the ratio 25:1. This concept of a ratio is important when you calculate dosage.

Working With Ratios

You may use only whole numbers when you write a ratio. Correct ratios include 8:1, 2:5, and 1:100. Incorrect ratios include 2.5:10, 1:4.5, and $3\frac{1}{2}$:100.

Ratios should almost always be expressed in lowest terms. Just as $\frac{4}{100}$ reduces to $\frac{1}{25}$, the ratio 4:100 should be written 1:25. Similarly, you would reduce 2:10 to 1:5 and 10:12 to 5:6.

Rule 2-7

Reduce a ratio as you would a fraction. Find the largest whole number that divides evenly into both values A and B.

EXAMPLE 1   Reduce 2:12 to its lowest terms.

Both values 2 and 12 are divisible by 2.

$$2 \div 2 = 1 \qquad 12 \div 2 = 6$$

Thus, 2:12 is written 1:6.

EXAMPLE 2 Reduce 10:15 to its lowest terms.

Both values 10 and 15 are divisible by 5.

$$10 \div 5 = 2 \qquad 15 \div 5 = 3$$

$$10:15 = 2:3$$

Because a ratio relates two quantities, value A and value B, you can convert a ratio to a fraction.

Rule 2-8

To convert a ratio to a fraction, write value A (the first number) as the numerator and value B (the second number) as the denominator, so that $A:B = \dfrac{A}{B}$.

EXAMPLE 1 Convert the following ratios to fractions.

a. 1:2

b. 4:5

c. 1:100

d. 7:3

e. 8:5

a. $1:2 = \dfrac{1}{2}$

b. $4:5 = \dfrac{4}{5}$

c. $1:100 = \dfrac{1}{100}$

d. $7:3 = \dfrac{7}{3}$

e. $8:5 = \dfrac{8}{5}$

If the first number in the ratio is smaller than the second number, the equivalent fraction is a proper fraction. If the first number in the ratio is larger than the second number, the fraction is an improper fraction. If the first number equals the second number, then the fraction has a value of one.

Rule 2-9

To convert a fraction to a ratio, write the numerator as the first value A and the denominator as the second value B.

$$\dfrac{A}{B} = A:B$$

Convert a mixed number to a ratio by first writing the mixed number as an improper fraction.

EXAMPLE 1 Convert the following to ratios.

a. $\dfrac{7}{12}$

b. $\dfrac{3}{10}$

c. $\dfrac{3}{2}$

d. $\dfrac{47}{12}$

a. $\dfrac{7}{12} = 7:12$

b. $\dfrac{3}{10} = 3:10$

c. $\dfrac{3}{2} = 3:2$

d. $\dfrac{47}{12} = 47:12$

e. $3\frac{1}{3}$ **e.** $3\frac{1}{3} = \frac{10}{3} = 10{:}3$

f. $2\frac{1}{2}$ **f.** $2\frac{1}{2} = \frac{5}{2} = 5{:}2$

When you convert between ratios and fractions, you do not have to perform any calculations. You simply rearrange the presentation of the numbers.

Rule 2-10

To convert a ratio to a decimal,

1. Write the ratio as a fraction.

2. Convert the fraction to a decimal. (See Chapter 1.)

EXAMPLE 1 Convert 1:10 to a decimal.

1. Write the ratio as a fraction.

$$1{:}10 = \frac{1}{10}$$

2. Convert the fraction to a decimal.

$$\frac{1}{10} = 1 \div 10 = 0.1$$

Thus, $1{:}10 = \frac{1}{10} = 0.1$

EXAMPLE 2 Convert 3:2 to a decimal.

1. $3{:}2 = \frac{3}{2}$

2. $\frac{3}{2} = 3 \div 2 = 1.5$

Thus, $3{:}2 = \frac{3}{2} = 1.5$

Rule 2-11

To convert a decimal to a ratio,

1. Write the decimal as a fraction. (See Chapter 1.)

2. Reduce the fraction to lowest terms.

3. Restate the fraction as a ratio by writing the numerator as value A and the denominator as value B.

EXAMPLE 1 Convert 0.8 to a ratio.

1. Write the decimal as a fraction.

$$0.8 = \frac{8}{10}$$

2. Reduce the fraction to lowest terms.

$$\frac{8}{10} = \frac{\overset{4}{\cancel{8}}}{\underset{5}{\cancel{10}}} = \frac{4}{5}$$

3. Restate the number as a ratio.

$$\frac{4}{5} = 4{:}5$$

Thus, $0.8 = \frac{8}{10} = \frac{4}{5} = 4{:}5$

EXAMPLE 2 Convert 0.05 to a ratio.

1. $0.05 = \dfrac{5}{100}$

2. $\dfrac{5}{100} = \dfrac{\overset{1}{\cancel{5}}}{\underset{20}{\cancel{100}}} = \dfrac{1}{20}$

3. $\dfrac{1}{20} = 1{:}20$

Thus, $0.05 = \dfrac{1}{20} = 1{:}20$

EXAMPLE 3 Convert 2.5 to a ratio.

1. $2.5 = 2\dfrac{5}{10} = \dfrac{25}{10}$

2. $\dfrac{25}{10} = \dfrac{\overset{5}{\cancel{25}}}{\underset{2}{\cancel{10}}} = \dfrac{5}{2}$

3. $\dfrac{5}{2} = 5{:}2$

Thus, $2.5 = \dfrac{5}{2} = 5{:}2$

Recall that you can write a percent as a fraction with the denominator of 100. This step helps you to convert a ratio to a percent and a percent to a ratio.

Rule 2-12

To convert a ratio to a percent,

1. Convert the ratio to a decimal.

2. Write the decimal as a percent by multiplying the decimal by 100 and adding the % symbol.

EXAMPLE 1 Convert 1:50 to a percent.

1. Convert the ratio to a decimal.

$1{:}50 = \dfrac{1}{50} = 0.02$

2. Multiply 0.02 by 100 and add the % symbol.

$0.02 \times 100\% = 2\%$

$1{:}50 = \dfrac{1}{50} = 0.02 = 2\%$

EXAMPLE 2 Convert 2:3 to a percent.

1. $2{:}3 = \dfrac{2}{3} = 0.67$

2. $0.67 \times 100\% = 67\%$

$2{:}3 = \dfrac{2}{3} = 0.67 = 67\%$

EXAMPLE 3 Convert 5:2 to a percent.

1. $5{:}2 = \dfrac{5}{2} = 2.5 = 2.50$

2. $2.50 \times 100\% = 250\%$

$5{:}2 = \dfrac{5}{2} = 2.50 = 250\%$

Rule 2-13

To convert a percent to a ratio,

1. Write the percent as a fraction.

2. Reduce the fraction to lowest terms.

3. Write the fraction as a ratio by writing the numerator as value A and the denominator as value B, in the form A:B.

EXAMPLE 1 Convert 25% to a ratio.

1. Write the percent as a fraction.
$$25\% = \frac{25}{100}$$

2. Reduce the fraction.
$$\frac{25}{100} = \frac{1}{4}$$

3. Restate the fraction as a ratio. Write the numerator as value A and the denominator as value B.
$$\frac{1}{4} = 1{:}4$$

Thus, $25\% = \frac{1}{4} = 1{:}4$

EXAMPLE 2 Convert 450% to a ratio.

1. $450\% = \frac{450}{100}$

2. $\frac{450}{100} = \frac{45}{10} = \frac{9}{2}$

3. $\frac{9}{2} = 9{:}2$

Thus, $450\% = \frac{9}{2} = 9{:}2$

EXAMPLE 3 Convert 0.3% to a ratio.

1. Write the percent as a fraction. In this case, rewrite the fraction without decimal points.
$$0.3\% = \frac{0.3}{100} = \frac{3}{1000}$$

2. $\frac{3}{1000}$ is reduced to its lowest terms.

3. $\frac{3}{1000} = 3{:}1000$

Thus, $0.3\% = \frac{3}{1000} = 3{:}1000$

REVIEW and PRACTICE

WORKING WITH RATIOS

Convert the following ratios to fractions or mixed numbers:

1. 3:4   2. 4:9   3. 5:3

4. 10:1   5. 1:20   6. 1:250

Convert the following fractions to ratios:

7. $\frac{2}{3}$ **8.** $\frac{6}{7}$ **9.** $\frac{5}{4}$ **10.** $\frac{7}{3}$

11. $1\frac{7}{8}$ **12.** $3\frac{1}{3}$ **13.** $\frac{6}{10}$ **14.** $\frac{18}{27}$

15. $\frac{1}{50}$ **16.** $\frac{1}{75}$

Convert the following ratios to decimals. Round to the nearest hundredth, if necessary.

17. 1:4   **18.** 1:8   **19.** 3:4   **20.** 2:5

21. 50:1   **22.** 25:2   **23.** 8:3   **24.** 5:6

Convert the following decimals to ratios:

25. 0.9   **26.** 0.3   **27.** 0.01   **28.** 0.45

29. 6   **30.** 2.4

Convert the following ratios to percents. If necessary, round to the nearest percent.

31. 1:4   **32.** 1:25   **33.** 2:9   **34.** 7:17

35. 20:1   **36.** 15:2

Convert the following percents to ratios:

37. 14%   **38.** 65%   **39.** 400%

40. 175%   **41.** 0.6%   **42.** 0.18%

To check your answers, see page 335.

Ratio Strengths

Ratios can describe liquid and solid medication strengths.

Ratio Strengths and Solutions

The ratio strength of a solution relates the amount of drug to the amount of solution. This relationship is the *dosage strength* of the medication. The first number represents the amount of drug. The second number represents the amount of solution. For example, a 1:10 solution strength represents 1 part drug for every 10 parts solution. A 10:1 solution strength represents 10 parts drug for every 1 part solution.

When the amount of solution in which a fixed amount of drug is dissolved decreases, its overall strength increases. For example, a 1:50 drug solution is stronger than a 1:100 solution but weaker than a 1:10 drug solution.

 Write a ratio to describe 50 mL of solution containing 3 grams of a drug.

The first number represents the amount of drug, 3 grams. The second number represents the amount of solution, 50 mL. The ratio is 3:50.

EXAMPLE 2 Write a ratio to describe 25 milligrams (mg) of a drug dissolved in 150 mL of solution.

The amount of the drug is 25 milligrams. The amount of the solution is 150 mL. The ratio is 25:150, which can be reduced.

$$25:150 = 1:6$$

The ratio is 1:6.

ERROR ALERT! *Do not assume the units of measurement.*

The last two examples had ratios of 3:50 and 1:6. While both the 50 and 6 represent milliliters (mL) in these ratios, the 3 and 1 represent different units of measure. The first ratio measures grams (g) per mL, the second ratio measures milligrams (mg) per mL. In other cases, the first value could represent micrograms (mcg), units (U), or even mL. The second value could represent not only mL, but also ounces (oz) or liters (L). Always check the units of measurement before you begin your calculations.

CRITICAL THINKING ON THE JOB

Reversing Terms in a Ratio Strength

A pharmacy technician who is preparing 1000 mL of a 1:10 solution of dextrose mistakenly mixes 10,000 grams of dextrose in 1000 mL of solution. The ratio 1:10 means 1 gram of dextrose in every 10 mL of solution. The technician reversed the terms, adding 10 grams of dextrose for every 1 mL of solution. The technician has prepared a 10:1 solution.

Think Before You Act

The technician should have used 100 grams of dextrose in 1000 mL of solution. Note that 100:1000 = 1:10. Thinking critically about the task, the technician should consider whether 10,000 grams is an unreasonably large amount of dextrose to dissolve in 1000 mL of solution. Furthermore, the technician should realize that in a 1:10 solution, the quantity of grams should be smaller than the quantity of milliliters. The fact that 10,000 is larger, not smaller, than 1000 should alert the technician to the error.

Ratio Strengths and Solid Medications

You can use ratios to express the strength of medication in tablet or capsule form, as well as for solutions. The first value in the ratio represents the amount of drug. The second value represents the number of tablets or capsules.

If a medication has 50 milligrams (mg) in one tablet, the ratio of medication to tablets is 50:1. For two tablets, each with 50 mg of drug, the ratio 100 mg:2 tablets is still 50:1. As you increase the number of tablets, the total quantity of medication increases. However, the dosage strength (the amount of drug per tablet) remains the same.

EXAMPLE 1 Write a ratio to describe a tablet with 15 mg of a drug.

The unit for a tablet is the tablet itself. An individual tablet has a measure of 1. Here 15 mg of a drug are contained in 1 tablet. The corresponding ratio is 15 mg:1 tablet.

EXAMPLE 2 Write a ratio to describe 3 tablets containing a total of 36 mg of medication.

The first value, the amount of drug, is 36. The second value, the number of tablets, is 3. The ratio is 36 mg:3 tablets, which reduces to 12 mg:1 tablet. Each tablet has 12 mg of medication.

RATIO STRENGTHS

Write a ratio to describe each of the following. Reduce the ratio to its lowest terms.

1. 100 mL of solution contain 5 grams of drug.

2. 500 mL of solution contain 25 grams of dextrose.

3. Each capsule contains 5 mg of drug.

4. 40 mg of drug are in every tablet.

5. 20 mg of drug are in 100 mL of solution.

6. 150 mg of drug are in 1500 mL of solution.

7. Three tablets contain 90 mg of drug.

8. Two tablets contain 20 mg of drug.

9. 75 mL of solution contain 15 mL of drug.

10. Each 500 mL of solution contains 250 mL of drug.

11. 10 grains of drug are in 2 tablets.

12. 4 tablets contain a total of 1 gram of drug.

To check your answers, see page 336.

Proportion

A proportion is a mathematical statement that two ratios are equal. Because ratios are often written as fractions, a proportion is also a statement that two fractions are equal.

Writing Proportions

You have learned that 2:3 is read "two to three." A double colon in a proportion means "as." The proportion 2:3::4:6 reads "two is to three as four is to six." This proportion states that the relationship of 2 to 3 is the same as the relationship of 4 to 6. By now, you know that 2 divided by 3 is the same as 4 divided by 6. *When you write proportions, do not reduce the ratios to their lowest terms.*

You can write proportions by replacing the double colon with an equal sign. Thus, 2:3::4:6 is the same as 2:3 = 4:6. You can also write a proportion with fractions. For example, 2:3::4:6 can be written

$$\frac{2}{3} = \frac{4}{6}$$

This format is referred to later as a *fraction proportion*.

Rule 2-14

To write a ratio proportion as a fraction proportion,

1. Change the double colon to an equal sign.

2. Convert both ratios to fractions.

EXAMPLE 1 Write 3:4::9:12 as a fraction proportion.

1. Change the double colon to an equal sign.

$$3{:}4{::}9{:}12 \rightarrow 3{:}4 = 9{:}12$$

2. Convert both ratios to fractions. Here, 3:4 becomes $\frac{3}{4}$ and 9:12 becomes $\frac{9}{12}$, so that

$$3{:}4{::}9{:}12 \rightarrow \frac{3}{4} = \frac{9}{12}$$

EXAMPLE 2 Write 5:10::50:100 as a fraction proportion.

1. $5{:}10{::}50{:}100 \rightarrow 5{:}10 = 50{:}100$

2. $5{:}10{::}50{:}100 \rightarrow \frac{5}{10} = \frac{50}{100}$

EXAMPLE 3 Write 8:6::4:3 as a fraction proportion.

1. $8{:}6{::}4{:}3 \rightarrow 8{:}6 = 4{:}3$

2. $8{:}6{::}4{:}3 \rightarrow \frac{8}{6} = \frac{4}{3}$

Rule 2-15

To write a fraction proportion as a ratio proportion,

1. Convert each fraction to a ratio.

2. Change the equal sign to a double colon.

EXAMPLE 1 Write $\frac{5}{6} = \frac{10}{12}$ as a ratio proportion.

1. Convert each fraction to a ratio.

$$\frac{5}{6} = 5{:}6 \text{ and } \frac{10}{12} = 10{:}12 \text{ so that } 5{:}6 = 10{:}12$$

2. Change the equal sign to a double colon.

$$5{:}6 = 10{:}12 \rightarrow 5{:}6{::}10{:}12$$

EXAMPLE 2 Write $\frac{3}{8} = \frac{9}{24}$ as a ratio proportion.

1. $\frac{3}{8} = 3{:}8 \text{ and } \frac{9}{24} = 9{:}24 \text{ so that } 3{:}8 = 9{:}24$

2. $3{:}8 = 9{:}24 \rightarrow 3{:}8{::}9{:}24$

EXAMPLE 3 Write $\frac{10}{2} = \frac{5}{1}$ as a ratio proportion.

1. $\frac{10}{2} = 10{:}2 \text{ and } \frac{5}{1} = 5{:}1 \text{ so that } 10{:}2 = 5{:}1$

2. $10{:}2 = 5{:}1 \rightarrow 10{:}2{::}5{:}1$

WRITING PROPORTIONS

Write the following ratio proportions as fraction proportions:

1. 4:5::8:10   **2.** 5:12::10:24   **3.** 1:10::100:1000

4. 2:3::20:30   **5.** 50:25::10:5   **6.** 6:4::18:12

Write the following fraction proportions as ratio proportions:

7. $\frac{3}{4} = \frac{75}{100}$ **8.** $\frac{1}{5} = \frac{3}{15}$ **9.** $\frac{8}{4} = \frac{2}{1}$

10. $\frac{8}{7} = \frac{24}{21}$ **11.** $\frac{18}{16} = \frac{9}{8}$ **12.** $\frac{10}{1} = \frac{40}{4}$

Means and Extremes

You often work with proportions to calculate dosages. When you know three of four values of a proportion, you will find the missing value. In this section, you will learn to find the missing value in a ratio proportion. Then, you will learn to find the missing value in a fraction proportion. Both methods lead to the same answer. Which method you select is a matter of personal preference.

It is not enough to learn to find the missing value. You must also learn to set up the proportion correctly. If you set up the proportion incorrectly, you could give the wrong amount of medication, with serious consequences for the patient. Use critical thinking skills to select the appropriate information and set up the proportion. In later chapters, you will learn to read physician's orders and drug labels, the sources for the information that goes into the proportion. The remainder of this chapter focuses on finding missing values.

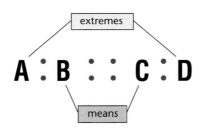

When you set up a ratio proportion in the form A:B::C:D, the values A and D are the *extremes*. The values B and C are the *means*. If you have trouble remembering which is which, think "Extremes are on the Ends. Means are in the Middle."

In any true ratio proportion, the product of the means always equals the product of the extremes.

Rule 2-16

To determine if a ratio proportion is true,

1. Multiply the means.

2. Multiply the extremes.

3. Compare the product of the means and the product of the extremes. If the products are equal, the proportion is true.

EXAMPLE 1 ▷ Determine if 1:2::3:6 is a true proportion.

1. Multiply the means: $2 \times 3 = 6$

2. Multiply the extremes: $1 \times 6 = 6$

3. Compare the products of the means and the extremes.
   $6 = 6$
The statement 1:2::3:6 is a true proportion.

EXAMPLE 2 Determine if 100:40::50:20 is a true proportion.

1. $40 \times 50 = 2000$

2. $100 \times 20 = 2000$

3. $2000 = 2000$

The proportion 100:40:50:20 is true.

EXAMPLE 3 Determine if 100:20::5:4 is a true proportion.

1. $20 \times 5 = 100$

2. $100 \times 4 = 400$

3. $400 \neq 100$

The proportion 10:20::5:4 is not true.

By definition, both sides of an equation are equal. If you perform the same calculation on both sides of an equation, they will still be equal. For instance, consider the equation

$$4 \times 2 = 8$$

You can add 3 to both sides or subtract 5 from both sides of the equation and the resulting equations are still true.

$$(4 \times 2) + 3 = 8 + 3 \qquad\qquad (4 \times 2) - 5 = 8 - 5$$
$$11 = 11 \qquad\qquad\qquad\qquad 3 = 3$$

You can also multiply or divide both sides by the same non-zero number.

$$(4 \times 2) \times 6 = 8 \times 6 \qquad\qquad (4 \times 2) \div 4 = 8 \div 4$$
$$48 = 48 \qquad\qquad\qquad\qquad 2 = 2$$

Now you can use the means and extremes to help you find a missing value in a proportion. Suppose you have the proportion

$$2:4::?:12$$

where ? represents the missing value. The product of the means equals the product of the extremes.

$$4 \times ? = 2 \times 12$$
$$4 \times ? = 24$$

To find the value of ?, you must write the equation so that ? stands alone on one side of the equal sign. Here you simply divide both sides by the number before ?, or 4.

$$4 \times ? = 24$$
$$\frac{4 \times ?}{4} = \frac{24}{4}$$
$$? = 6$$

Check that the proportion is now true:

$$2:4::6:12$$
$$4 \times 6 = 24 \text{ and } 2 \times 12 = 24$$

Because $4 \times 6 = 2 \times 12$, the proportion is true. Remember: taking the time to check your work will help you avoid errors.

Rule 2-17

To find the missing value in a ratio proportion,

1. Write an equation setting the product of the means equal to the product of the extremes.

2. Solve the equation for the missing value.

3. Restate the proportion, inserting the missing value.

4. Check your work. Determine if the ratio proportion is true.

EXAMPLE 1 Find the missing value in 25:5::50:?

1. Write an equation setting the product of the means equal to the product of the extremes.

$$5 \times 50 = 25 \times ?$$
$$250 = 25 \times ?$$

2. Solve the equation. Here, divide both sides by 25.

$$\frac{250}{25} = \frac{25 \times ?}{25}$$
$$10 = ?$$

3. Restate the proportion, inserting the missing value.

25:5::50:10

4. Check your work.

$$5 \times 50 = 25 \times 10$$
$$250 = 250$$

The missing value is 10.

EXAMPLE 2 If 100 mL of solution contains 20 mg of drug, how many milligrams of drug will be in 500 mL of solution?

Start by setting up the ratios. The ratio strength of the first solution is 20 mg to 100 mL, or 20:100. Remember not to reduce ratios used for proportions. The missing value, ?, is the amount of drug in the second solution. The ratio strength of the second solution is ? mg to 500 mL, or ?:500. The proportion sets the first ratio equal to the second ratio.

20:100::?:500

Now solve for ?, the missing value.

1. $100 \times ? = 20 \times 500$

$100 \times ? = 10,000$

2. $\dfrac{100 \times ?}{100} = \dfrac{10,000}{100}$

$? = 100$

3. 20:100::100:500

4. $100 \times 100 = 20 \times 500$

$10,000 = 10,000$

The second solution will contain 100 mg of drug in 500 mL of solution.

EXAMPLE 3 15 grams (g) of drug are dissolved in 300 mL of solution. If you want 45 g in the same strength solution, how much solution do you need?

First write the ratios. The first solution has 15 g of drug to 300 mL of solution. Its ratio strength is 15:300. The second solution has 45 g of drug to an unknown amount of solution, or 45:? Now set up the proportion and solve.

15:300::45:?

1. $300 \times 45 = 15 \times ?$

$13,500 = 15 \times ?$

2. $\dfrac{13,500}{15} = \dfrac{15 \times ?}{15}$

$900 = ?$

3. 15:300::45:900

4. $300 \times 45 = 15 \times 900$

$13{,}500 = 13{,}500$

You will need 900 mL of solution to have 45 g of drug with the same strength solution.

REVIEW and PRACTICE

MEANS AND EXTREMES

Determine whether the following proportions are true:

1. 6:12::12:24

2. 3:8::9:32

3. 5:75::15:250

4. 8:100::20:250

Use the means and extremes to find the missing values.

5. 10:?::5:8

6. 10:4::20:?

7. 4:25::16:?

8. ?:15::100:75

9. 21:27::?:45

10. 100:?::50:2

11. 3:12::?:36

12. 33:39::55:?

13. If one tablet contains 30 mg of drug, how many milligrams of drug do 5 tablets contain?

14. If 10 grams of drug are in 250 mL of solution, how many grams of drug are in 1000 mL of solution?

15. If 3 tablets contain 45 mg of drug, how many milligrams of drug are in 1 tablet?

16. If 60 mg of drug are in 500 mL of solution, how many milliliters of solution contain 36 mg of drug?

To check your answers, see page 336.

Cross-Multiplying

Earlier in this chapter, you learned that a proportion can be written with ratios or with fractions. For example, the proportion 2:4::5:10 can be written as $\frac{2}{4} = \frac{5}{10}$. More generally, A:B::C:D can be written $\frac{A}{B} = \frac{C}{D}$

To determine whether a proportion is true, compare the products of the extremes (A and D) with the product of the means (B and C). When a proportion is written with fractions, use a similar method, *cross-multiplying*, to determine if it is true. The numerator of the first fraction, A, and the denominator of the second fraction, D, are the extremes of the ratio proportion. The denominator of the first fraction, B, and the numerator of the second fraction, C, are the means.

multiply the extremes

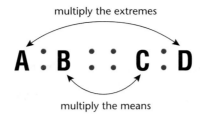

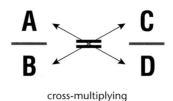

multiply the means

cross-multiplying

Rule 2-18

To determine if a fraction proportion is true,

1. Cross-multiply. Multiply the numerator of the first fraction with the denominator of the second fraction. Then multiply the denominator of the first fraction with the numerator of the second fraction.

2. Compare the products. The products must be equal.

EXAMPLE 1 Determine if $\frac{2}{5} = \frac{10}{25}$ is a true proportion.

1. Cross-multiply.

$$\frac{2}{5} \bowtie \frac{10}{25} \rightarrow 2 \times 25 = 5 \times 10$$

2. Compare the products on both sides of the equal sign.

$$50 = 50$$

$\frac{2}{5} = \frac{10}{25}$ is a true proportion.

EXAMPLE 2 Determine if $\frac{100}{1000} = \frac{500}{5000}$ is a true proportion.

1. $\frac{100}{1000} \bowtie \frac{500}{5000} \rightarrow 100 \times 5000 = 1000 \times 500$

2. $500{,}000 = 500{,}000$

$\frac{100}{1000} = \frac{500}{5000}$ is a true proportion.

EXAMPLE 3 Determine if $\frac{5}{8} = \frac{40}{72}$ is a true proportion.

1. $\frac{5}{8} \bowtie \frac{40}{72} \rightarrow 5 \times 72 = 8 \times 40$

2. $360 \neq 320$

The proportion $\frac{5}{8} = \frac{40}{72}$ is not true.

In the previous section, you learned to use means and extremes to find a missing value in a ratio proportion. As you might expect, you can cross-multiply to find the missing value in a fraction proportion.

Rule 2-19

To find the missing value in a fraction proportion,

1. Cross-multiply. Write an equation setting the products equal to each other.

2. Solve the equation to find the missing value.

3. Restate the proportion, inserting the missing value.

4. Check your work. Determine if the fraction proportion is true.

EXAMPLE 1 Find the missing value in $\frac{3}{5} = \frac{6}{?}$

1. Cross-multiply.

$$\frac{3}{5} \bowtie \frac{6}{?} \rightarrow 3 \times ? = 5 \times 6$$

$$3 \times ? = 30$$

2. Solve the equation. Here, divide both sides by 3.

$$\frac{3 \times ?}{3} = \frac{30}{3}$$

$$? = 10$$

3. Restate the proportion, inserting the missing value.

$$\frac{3}{5} = \frac{6}{10}$$

4. Check your work by cross-multiplying.

$$3 \times 10 = 5 \times 6$$

$$30 = 30$$

The missing value is 10.

EXAMPLE 2 Find the missing value in $\frac{25}{5} = \frac{50}{?}$

1. $\frac{25}{5} \bowtie \frac{50}{?} \rightarrow 25 \times ? = 5 \times 50$

$$25 \times ? = 250$$

2. $\frac{25 \times ?}{25} = \frac{250}{25}$

$$? = 10$$

3. $\frac{25}{5} = \frac{50}{10}$

4. $25 \times 10 = 5 \times 50$

$$250 = 250$$

The missing value is 10.

EXAMPLE 3 If 100 mL of solution contains 20 mg of drug, how many milligrams of drug will be in 500 mL of solution?

Set up the fraction. The ratio strength of the first solution is 20 mg to 100 mL, or $\frac{20}{100}$. The missing value, ?, is the amount of drug in the second solution. The ratio strength of the second solution is ? to 500 mL, or $\frac{?}{500}$. The proportion sets the first fraction equal to the second fraction.

$$\frac{20}{100} = \frac{?}{500}$$

Now solve for ?, the missing value.

1. $\frac{20}{100} \bowtie \frac{?}{500} \rightarrow 20 \times 500 = 100 \times ?$

$$10,000 = 100 \times ?$$

2. $\frac{10,000}{100} = \frac{100 \times ?}{100}$

$$100 = ?$$

3. $\frac{20}{100} = \frac{100}{500}$

4. $20 \times 500 = 100 \times 100$

$$10,000 = 10,000$$

The second solution will contain 100 mg of drug in 500 mL of solution.

EXAMPLE 4 15 g of drug are dissolved in 300 mL of solution. If you want 45 g in the same strength solution, how much solution do you need?

Write the ratios. The first solution has 15 g of drug to 300 mL of solution. Its ratio strength is $\frac{15}{300}$. The second solution has 45 g of drug to an unknown amount of solution, or $\frac{45}{?}$. Now set up the proportion and solve.

$$\frac{15}{300} = \frac{45}{?}$$

1. $\frac{15}{300} \diagup\!\!\!\!\diagup \frac{45}{?} \rightarrow 15 \times ? = 300 \times 45$

$$15 \times ? = 13,500$$

2. $\frac{15 \times ?}{15} = \frac{13,500}{15}$

$$? = 900$$

3. $\frac{15}{300} = \frac{45}{900}$

4. $15 \times 900 = 300 \times 5$

$$13,500 = 13,500$$

You will need 900 mL of solution to have 45 g of drug with the same strength solution.

These last three examples are the same examples from the previous section. Before, you used ratios and the means-extreme method; here, you used fractions and cross-multiplying. Once you have tried both methods to find missing values, you can decide which method works best for you.

When you set up proportions using fractions, the units in the two numerators must be the same and the units in the two denominators must be the same. For example, in Example 4, the proportion including units of measurement is

$$\frac{15 \text{ grams}}{300 \text{ mL}} = \frac{45 \text{ grams}}{900 \text{ mL}}$$

Both the numerators are grams, and both the denominators are milliliters. When you solve problems such as these, include the units.

CRITICAL THINKING ON THE JOB

Confusing Multiplying Fractions With Cross-Multiplying

A pharmacy technician is preparing a 5% solution of dextrose in batches of 500 cubic centimeters (cc). She sets up the calculation as follows: $\frac{5 \text{ g}}{100 \text{ cc}} = \frac{?}{500 \text{ cc}}$. Distracted by a call, she returns to the calculation and computes

$$5 \times ? = 100 \times 500 = 50,000$$

This calculation leads to

$$? = 10,000$$

Think Before You Act

The technician realizes that mixing 10,000 g for a solution with 500 cc is not reasonable. Looking at her work, she realizes she has treated the problem as if she was multiplying fractions rather than solving a proportion problem. She has mistakenly multiplied the two numerators and set their product equal to the product of the two denominators.

To calculate correctly, the technician should cross-multiply $100 \times ?$ and 5×500. In turn,

$$100 \times ? = 2500$$
$$? = 25$$

The technician will need 25 g, *not* 10,000 g, of dextrose.

The technician was distracted in the middle of the calculation. Distractions cause a lot of calculation errors. *If you are interrupted in the middle of a calculation, go back and start the calculation again from the beginning.*

CROSS-MULTIPLYING

Determine if the following proportions are true:

1. $\dfrac{7}{16} = \dfrac{28}{48}$

2. $\dfrac{6}{9} = \dfrac{24}{36}$

3. $\dfrac{100}{250} = \dfrac{150}{375}$

4. $\dfrac{50}{125} = \dfrac{125}{300}$

Cross-multiply to find the missing value.

5. $\dfrac{3}{15} = \dfrac{?}{5}$

6. $\dfrac{2}{?} = \dfrac{8}{100}$

7. $\dfrac{?}{20} = \dfrac{120}{100}$

8. $\dfrac{50}{75} = \dfrac{100}{?}$

9. $\dfrac{10}{3} = \dfrac{?}{60}$

10. $\dfrac{?}{4} = \dfrac{4}{16}$

11. $\dfrac{25}{?} = \dfrac{75}{3}$

12. $\dfrac{2}{3} = \dfrac{6}{?}$

13. A patient must take 3 tablets per day for 14 days. How many tablets should the pharmacy supply to fill this order?

14. If 15 mL of solution contains 75 mg of drug, how many milligrams of drug are in 60 mL of solution?

15. A nurse is instructed to administer 600 mL of a solution every 8 hours. How many hours will be needed to administer 1800 mL of the solution?

16. Two tablets contain a total of 50 mg of drug. How many milligrams of drug are in 10 tablets?

To check your answers, see page 337.

CRITICAL THINKING ON THE JOB

Setting Up Correct Proportions

A physician's order calls for a patient to receive 250 mg of amoxicillin oral suspension t.i.d. (three times a day). Amoxicillin oral suspension is a dry medication that is mixed with a solvent before it is given to a patient. Each 5 mL of solution contains 125 mg of drug.

The nurse sets up the calculation as $\dfrac{5}{125} = \dfrac{250}{?}$. His answer tells him to administer 6250 mL of the solution.

Think Before You Act

Fortunately, the nurse thinks critically about the answer. He realizes that 6250 mL is an unreasonably large amount of medication to give to the patient three times a day. He reworks the problem, this time including the units of measurement. He sets up the proportion as

$$\dfrac{5 \text{ mL}}{125 \text{ mg}} = \dfrac{? \text{ mL}}{250 \text{ mg}}$$

Now the nurse calculates correctly, concluding that ? = 10 mL of solution.

Thinking critically is a necessary part of dosage calculations. For each calculation, you must ask, "Is this answer reasonable?" Even if the arithmetic of the calculation is correct, the problem may be set up incorrectly.

Critical thinking is especially necessary when you use a calculator. Sometimes the proportion is not set up correctly. Sometimes the proportion is correct, but you press the wrong buttons on the calculator. If you have any doubts about the reasonableness of an answer, recalculate the problem. If necessary, ask the physician or another licensed health care worker to check your work.

CHAPTER 2 REVIEW

CHECK UP

In each row of the table below, use the information to calculate the equivalent values. For instance, in Row 1, convert the ratio 2:3 to a fraction, a decimal, and a percent. Where necessary, round decimals to the nearest hundredth. Round percents to the nearest percent. Do not reduce ratios and fractions.

	Fraction	Decimal	Ratio	Percent
1.			2:3	
2.	$\frac{5}{4}$			
3.				28%
4.		0.03		
5.	$\frac{40}{8}$			
6.			4:12	
7.	$\frac{9}{27}$			
8.		1.4		
9.				0.5%
10.			3:50	
11.				25%
12.		6		
13.	$\frac{1}{9}$			
14.				150%
15.			6:97	
16.		12.8		

Find the missing value:

17. 1:10::4:?

18. 3:27::?:9

19. ?:6::8:12

20. 5:?::10:50

21. $\dfrac{4}{8} = \dfrac{24}{?}$

22. $\dfrac{?}{14} = \dfrac{5}{70}$

23. $\dfrac{3}{?} = \dfrac{30}{20}$

24. $\dfrac{1}{25} = \dfrac{?}{125}$

25. If one tablet contains 25 mg of drug, how many milligrams of drug are in three tablets?

26. If 100 mL of drug are in 600 mL of solution, how many milliliters of drug are in 1800 mL of solution?

27. A solution is 5% dextrose. How many grams (g) of dextrose are in 500 cc of solution?

28. A solution contains 1 gram (g) of drug for every 50 mL of solution. How much solution would you need to give a patient to administer 3 g of drug?

29. 10 mL of a liquid medication contain 250 mg of drug. How many milliliters contain 50 mg of drug?

30. If 30 grams of drug are in 100 mL of solution, what is the ratio strength of the solution?

CRITICAL THINKING

A pharmacy technician has just finished preparing 250 mL of a 6% solution (using a dry drug) when he learns that the physician wants an 8% solution, not a 6% solution. How many additional grams of dry drug should the technician add to the 6% solution he has just prepared?

CASE STUDY

A physician's order calls for Ceclor oral suspension 750 mg to be given daily for 14 days. The daily dosage is to be divided into three equal doses per day. Ceclor oral suspension is a drug that is mixed with solvent before it is administered.

a. How many milligrams of drug should be given in each dose?

b. If 5 mL of solution contain 125 mg of drug, how many milliliters should be given in each dose?

To check your answers, see page 337.

INTERNET ACTIVITY

Note: The Internet is a research tool from which to get basic information. Validate the accuracy of all Internet information.

A classmate is feeling uncertain about his ability to work with ratios and proportions.

Assignment: Look for a Web site that will help your classmate review these concepts. (Hint: Search for the specific topic that is giving your classmate difficulty, rather than a general topic such as mathematics.)

SYSTEMS of WEIGHTS and MEASURES

3

Objectives

When you have completed Chapter 3, you will be able to:

- List the fundamental units of the metric system for length, weight, and volume.
- Summarize metric notation.
- Calculate equivalent measurements within the metric system.
- Identify the most frequently used equivalent measurements among metric, household, and apothecaries' measurements.
- Recognize the symbols for dram, ounce, grain, and drop.
- Convert measurements within and among the metric, household, and apothecaries' systems of measurement.
- Calculate temperature and time conversions.

Metric System

The metric system is the most widely used system of measurement in the world today. The system, which was defined in 1792, gets its name from the meter, the basic unit of length. A meter is approximately three inches longer than a yard.

Units of measurement in the metric system are sometimes referred to as SI units, an abbreviation for International System of Units. This system was established in 1960 to make units of measurement for the metric system standard throughout the world. Table 3-1 lists the basic metric units for length, weight, and volume.

Table 3-1 Basic Units of Metric Measurement

Type of Measure	Basic Unit	Abbreviation
Length	meter	m
Weight (or Mass)	gram	g (or gm)
Volume	liter	L

Notice that meter and gram are abbreviated with lowercase letters, but liter is abbreviated with an uppercase L. Using the uppercase L minimizes the chance of confusing the lowercase letter L (l) with the digit 1. You will use length mostly when expressing measurements such as patient height, infant head circumference, and lesion or wound size. However, you will use weight and volume frequently when you calculate dosages. Most dosages and drug strengths are expressed using the metric system.

Understanding Metric Notation

Like the decimal system, the metric system is based on multiples of 10. The more confidence you have working with decimals, the more comfortable you will be working with metric units. (To review decimals, see Chapter 1.)

A prefix before the basic unit indicates relative size. For example, *kilo-* indicates that you multiply the basic unit by 1000. A kilometer is 1000 meters, a kilogram is 1000 grams, and a kiloliter is 1000 liters. When you divide a meter into 1000 equal lengths, each length is one millimeter. The prefix *milli-* means one-thousandth. A millimeter is one-thousandth of a meter, a milliliter is one-thousandth of a liter, and a milligram is one-thousandth of a gram. Table 3-2 lists several common prefixes, their abbreviations, and their value relative to the basic unit.

Table 3-2 Common Metric System Prefixes

Prefix	Length	Value
kilo- (k)	kilometer (km)	1 km = 1000 m
(basic unit)	meter (m)	1 m
centi- (c)	centimeter (cm)	$1 \text{ cm} = \frac{1}{100} \text{ m} = 0.01 \text{ m}$
milli- (m)	millimeter (mm)	$1 \text{ mm} = \frac{1}{1000} \text{ m} = 0.001 \text{ m}$
micro- (mc or μ)	micrometer (mcm)	$1 \text{ mcm} = \frac{1}{1,000,000} \text{ m} = 0.000001 \text{ m}$

As a health care provider, you will most often use the metric prefixes *kilo-*, *centi-*, *milli-*, and *micro-*. (Micro- is often abbreviated with μ, the Greek letter mu. Table 3-3 shows the most commonly used combinations of prefixes and basic units.

Table 3-3 Combining Prefixes and Units

Prefix	Length (meter)	Weight (Mass) (gram)	Volume (liter)
kilo- (× 1000)	kilometer km	kilogram kg	kiloliter kL
centi- (÷ 100)	centimeter cm	centigram cg	centiliter cL
milli- (÷ 1000)	millimeter mm	milligram mg	milliliter mL
micro- (÷ 1,000,000)	micrometer mcm	microgram mcg	microliter mcL

Rule 3-1

Use Arabic numerals, with decimals to represent any fractions.

EXAMPLE 1 Write 1.25 g to represent $1\frac{1}{4}$ g.

Rule 3-2

If the quantity is less than 1, include a 0 before the decimal point. Delete any other zeros that are not necessary.

EXAMPLE 1 Do not write .750; instead, write 0.75, adding a zero before the decimal point and deleting the unnecessary zero at the end.

Rule 3-3

Write the quantity before, not after, the unit.

EXAMPLE 1 Write 30 mg, not mg 30.

Rule 3-4

Write the prefix before the basic unit of measurement.

EXAMPLE 1 To represent micrograms, write mcg, not gmc or micro g.

Rule 3-5

Use lowercase letters for metric abbreviations. However, use uppercase L to represent liter.

EXAMPLE 1 Write mg, not MG. Write mL, not ml. While *ml* is technically correct, you will avoid errors if you use an uppercase L.

Rule 3-6

Insert a space between the quantity and the unit.

EXAMPLE 1 Write 35 kg, not 35kg.

EXAMPLE 2 Select the correct metric notation for six and two-eighths milliliters from the following choices:

a. 6.28mL　　　　**b.** ml 6.25　　　　**c.** $6\frac{1}{4}$ mcL　　　　**d.** 6.25 mL

The correct choice is *d*, 6.25 mL. Two-eighths is 0.25 in decimal form. Answer *a* confuses two-eighths with twenty-eight hundredths and does not include a space between the quantity and the unit. In answer *b*, the quantity should appear before the unit. The abbreviation should be mL, not ml, to avoid confusing the letter l with the digit 1. In answer *c*, two-eighths reduces to one-fourth, but the number should be written in decimal form. In addition, milliliters is written mL, not mcL.

EXAMPLE 3 ▷ Select the correct metric notation for one-half milligram from the following choices:

a. 0.5 mg **b.** .5 mg **c.** 0.50 mG **d.** mg 0.5

The correct choice is *a*, 0.5 mg. In answer *b*, a zero should precede the decimal point when the decimal is less than 1. In answer *c*, the zero at the end of 0.50 is unnecessary. Also, the appropriate abbreviation for milligram should be mg, not mG. Answer *d* incorrectly places the unit before the quantity.

REVIEW and PRACTICE

UNDERSTANDING METRIC NOTATION

In Exercises 1–6, select the correct metric notation.

1. two and one-half kilograms
   a. 2.5 Kg   **b.** 2.05 kg   **c.** $2\frac{1}{2}$ kg   **d.** 2.5 kg

2. seven-tenths of a milliliter
   a. $\frac{7}{10}$ mL   **b.** .7mL   **c.** ml 0.7   **d.** 0.7 mL

3. four-hundredths of a gram
   a. 400 G   **b.** 0.4g   **c.** 0.04 g   **d.** .04 g

4. thirty-one millimeters
   a. 31mm   **b.** 0.031 mm   **c.** 31.0 mlm   **d.** 31 mm

5. eight liters
   a. 8.0 l   **b.** 8 L   **c.** 8.0L   **d.** 0.8 l

6. one hundred twenty-five micrograms
   a. 125 mg   **b.** 0.125 mcg   **c.** 125 mcg   **d.** 125mg

In Exercises 7–12, write the indicated amounts.

7. four and one-half milliliters

8. sixty-two hundredths of a gram

9. three-quarters of a milliliter

10. seven-tenths of a meter

11. twelve liters

12. nine-twelfths of a kilogram

To check your answers, see page 338.

Converting Within the Metric System

Recall from Chapters 1 and 2 that when you multiply a decimal number by 100, you move the decimal point two places to the right and get a larger number. When you divide a decimal number by 100, you move the decimal point two places to the left and get a smaller number.

Converting one metric unit of measurement to another is similar to multiplying and dividing decimal numbers. For example, if you travel 1 kilometer, you travel 1000 meters. When you convert from the larger unit of measurement (kilometer) to the smaller unit (meter), the quantity of units increases. Therefore, you multiply, moving the decimal point to the right.

If you convert from meters to kilometers, the quantity of units decreases. If you travel 1000 meters, you travel 1 kilometer. When you convert from a smaller unit (meter) to a larger unit (kilometer), the quantity of units decreases. Therefore, you divide, moving the decimal point to the left.

Rule 3-7

When you convert a quantity from one unit of metric measurement to another,

1. Move the decimal point to the right if you convert from a larger to a smaller unit.

2. Move the decimal point to the left if you convert from a smaller to a larger unit.

3. Determine how many places to move the decimal point.

Figure 3-1 will help you determine both the direction and the number of places to move the decimal point when you convert between units of metric measurement. For example, milliliter is three places to the right of liter, the basic unit. To convert a quantity from liters (larger) to milliliters (smaller), move the decimal point three places to the right. Similarly, to convert a quantity from grams (smaller) to kilograms (larger), move the decimal point three places to the left.

Figure 3-1

Metric system place values.

kilo-		hecto-	deka-	base unit	deci-	centi-	milli-		decimilli-	centimilli-	micro-
km kg kL				meter gram liter			mm mg mL				mcm mcg mcL
1 km = 1000 m 1 kg = 1000 g 1 kL = 1000 L				1.0 m 1.0 g 1.0 L			1 mm = 0.001 m 1 mg = 0.001 g 1 mL = 0.001 L				1 mcm = 0.000001 m 1 mcg = 0.000001 g 1 mcL = 0.000001 L

EXAMPLE 1 Convert 4 L to mL

A milliliter (mL) is smaller than a liter (L); a quantity will have more milliliters than liters. Using Figure 3-1, you can see that milliliter is three places to the right of liter. Move the decimal point for 4 (or 4.0) three places to the right to find the number of milliliters. Add zeros as necessary to help you with your calculation.

$$4 \text{ L} = 4.000 \text{ L} = 4000 \text{ mL}$$

EXAMPLE 2 How many m are in 75 mm?

A meter (m) is larger than a millimeter (mm); a quantity will have fewer meters than millimeters. Using Figure 3-1, you can see that meter is three places to the left of millimeter. Write 75 as 75.0, and move the decimal point in 75 three places to the left. Add zeros as necessary.

$$75 \text{ mm} = 75.0 \text{ mm} = 0.075 \text{ m}$$

Rule 3-7 covers all metric conversions. When you calculate dosages, you will work most often with four metric units of weight and three metric units of volume. The four units of weight are kg, g, mg, and mcg. Two of the units of volume are L and mL. The third is cc (cubic centimeter), which is equivalent to mL.

The four units of weight, or mass, are related to each other by a factor of 1000. A kilogram is 1000 times larger than a gram. Thus, 1 kg = 1000 g. In turn, a gram is 1000 times larger than a milligram, which is 1000 times larger than a microgram. The same relationship is true for liters and milliliters; a liter is 1000 times larger than a milliliter. Table 3-4 lists four of the most commonly used equivalent measurements. Because they are so important to dosage calculations, you should memorize them.

Table 3-4 Equivalent Metric Measurements

1 kg = 1000 g	1 mg = 1000 mcg
1 g = 1000 mg	1 L = 1000 mL

Rule 3-8

To convert quantities between kilograms and grams, grams and milligrams, milligrams and micrograms, or liters and milliliters,

1. Move the decimal point three places to the right if you are converting from the larger unit to the smaller unit.

2. Move the decimal point three places to the left if you are converting from the smaller unit to the larger unit.

Note that this rule applies when you convert between the pairs of measurements listed above.

Convert 8.5 L to mL

You are converting from a larger to a smaller unit. Multiply 8.5 by 1000, moving the decimal point three places to the right.

$$8.5 \text{ L} \times 1000 = 8.500 \text{ L} \times 1000 = 8500 \text{ mL}$$

Convert 4.5 mcg to mg

You are converting from a smaller unit to a larger one. Divide 4.5 by 1000, moving the decimal point three places to the left.

$$4.5 \text{ mcg} \div 1000 = 0004.5 \text{ mcg} \div 1000 = 0.0045 \text{ mg}$$

Convert 62 kg to g

You are converting from a larger unit to a smaller one. Multiply 62 by 1000, moving the decimal point three places to the right.

$$62 \text{ kg} \times 1000 = 62.000 \text{ kg} \times 1000 = 62{,}000 \text{ g}$$

Convert 300 mg to g

You are converting from a smaller unit to a larger one. Divide 300 by 1000, moving the decimal point three places to the left.

$$300 \text{ mg} \div 1000 = 0300.0 \text{ mg} \div 1000 = 0.3 \text{ g}$$

Remember: The larger the unit, the smaller the quantity. The smaller the unit, the larger the quantity.

You may be tempted to multiply when you convert from a smaller unit to a larger unit, thinking that you are increasing in size. If you find yourself confused, think about conversions you have made all your life.

For example, a dollar bill is a larger unit of money than a quarter, which is a larger unit of money than a penny. When you write their relationship, look at how the quantity changes:

1 dollar bill = 4 quarters = 100 pennies

When you convert from the larger unit to the smaller one, the quantity increases. Writing the money relationship as

100 pennies = 4 quarters = 1 dollar bill

shows you that as the unit increases in size, the quantity decreases. You see the same relationship with units of time and in the metric system:

1 hour = 60 minutes = 3600 seconds

1 g = 1000 mg = 1,000,000 mcg

CRITICAL THINKING ON THE JOB

Placing the Decimal Point Correctly

A child suffering from congestive heart failure is rushed into an emergency room. The physician orders 0.05 mg of Lanoxin for the child. The attending nurse quickly calculates that 0.05 mg = 500 mcg. Lanoxin is available for injection in quantities of 500 mcg. The nurse hands the syringe to the doctor.

Fortunately, the doctor catches the error before the Lanoxin is administered. The child should be given 50 mcg, not 500 mcg of Lanoxin. As it turns out, Lanoxin is available as an elixir in doses of 50 mcg. This quantity should be administered. The larger dose of 500 mcg could be fatal to the child.

Think Before You Act

When you convert quantities from one unit of measure to another, pay close attention to the decimal point. In going from mg to mcg, the quantity should be multiplied by 1000; the decimal should move three places to the right.

$0.05 \text{ mg} \times 1000 = 0.050 \text{ mg} \times 1000 = 50 \text{ mcg}$

Be even more careful when the patient is a child. Dosages that are perfectly safe for adults may be life-threatening for children. As you will learn in Chapter 6, you must carefully read the labels on all drugs. In the case of Lanoxin, both the elixir and the injection have labels marked in both mcg and mg. A careful look at the labels would help prevent this error.

REVIEW and PRACTICE

CONVERTING WITHIN THE METRIC SYSTEM

In Exercises 1–18, complete the conversions.

1. 7 g = _____ mg

2. 1200 mg = _____ g

3. 23 g = _____ kg

4. 8 kg = _____ g

5. 8.01 L = _____ mL

6. 100 mL = _____ L

7. 3.6 m = _____ mm

8. 5233 mm = _____ m

9. 500 m = _____ km

10. 3.25 km = _____ m

11. 0.25 mg = _____ mcg

12. 462 mg = _____ mcg

13. 250 mcg = _____ mg

14. 75 mcg = _____ mg

15. 0.06 g = _____ mcg

16. 0.5 g = _____ mcg

17. 8000 mcg = _____ g

18. 20,000 mcg = _____ g

To check your answers, see page 338.

Other Systems of Measurement

The trend in health care is clearly toward using the metric system of measurement. However, two older systems, the apothecary and household systems, are still in use. Two other measures, milliequivalents and units, are also used for some medications.

Apothecary System

The apothecary system is an old system of measurement. Used first by apothecaries (early pharmacists), it traveled across Europe from Greece and Rome to France and England. Eventually, it crossed the Atlantic to colonial America. The household system familiar to most Americans evolved from the apothecary system. Although this system is not widely used today, you must still be familiar with it. Certain medications, especially older ones such as aspirin and morphine, are still measured in apothecary units.

Units of Measure. The basic unit of weight in the apothecary system is the grain (gr). Originally, the grain was defined as the weight of a single grain of wheat, hence its name.

ERROR ALERT!

Do not confuse grains and grams.

Because they have names and abbreviations that are similar, grains (gr) and grams (g) are easily confused. A grain is a measure in the apothecary system; a gram is a measure in the metric system. If you are not sure whether an order refers to grains or grams, check with the physician or pharmacist. For most conversions, one grain equals either 60 or 65 milligrams (mg), which means

1 gr = 60 mg = 0.06 g *or*

1 gr = 65 mg = 0.065 g

In either case, 1 grain is significantly smaller than 1 gram. Medications that are measured in grains do not all use the same conversion. However, their labels list the metric units as well.

The three common units of volume in the apothecary system are the minim ($\mathfrak{m}$), the dram ($\mathfrak{z}$), and the ounce ($\mathfrak{z}$). As you will see in Chapter 4, many syringes continue to have marks that indicate minims, and most measuring cups have marks for drams and ounces. While ounces continue to be used, minims and drams are rarely used today. Still, you should be familiar with them.

ERROR ALERT!

Do not confuse the symbols for drams and ounces.

The symbols for drams and ounces appear similar. When they are typed, the symbol for dram $\mathfrak{z}$ looks similar to the numeral 3; the symbol for ounce $\mathfrak{z}$ has an extra line at the top. When they are handwritten, the symbol for dram $\mathfrak{z}$ can look like the written letter z. Again, the symbol for ounce $\mathfrak{z}$ has an extra line at the top. Because 1 ounce = 8 drams, if you confuse one for the other, you could give a patient a much different amount of medication than was ordered. As always, if you are in doubt about which symbol is used, check with the physician who wrote the order.

Apothecary notation. The system of apothecary notation has special rules that combine fractions, Roman and Arabic numerals, symbols, and abbreviations. Even the order in which information is written differs from the order most familiar to you. Recall that Roman numbers may be written with a bar above them.

Rule 3-9

When writing a value in the apothecary system,

1. If a value is less than 1, write it as a fraction. However, if the value is one-half, write it as the abbreviation *ss*.

2. Write the values 1–10, 20, and 30 with lowercase Roman numerals. Write other whole numbers, such as 12 and 15, with Arabic numerals.

3. Use the abbreviation gr to represent grain. Use the symbols m, ℥, and ℥ to represent minim, dram, and ounce.

4. Write the abbreviation, symbol, or unit before the quantity.

EXAMPLE 1 Write *four grains* using apothecary notation.

Use lowercase Roman numerals to represent four as iv. Abbreviate grains as gr and place it before the quantity: gr iv or gr īv

EXAMPLE 2 Write *twelve ounces* using apothecary notation.

Use the Arabic numeral 12. Use the symbol for ounces and place it before the quantity: ℥ 12

EXAMPLE 3 Write *two and one-half grains* using apothecary notation.

Use lowercase Roman numerals to represent two as ii. Abbreviate one-half as ss, writing two and one-half as iiss. The abbreviation for grain precedes this quantity: gr iiss.

Household System

The household system of measurement is still commonly used today. Patients who take medication at home are more likely to use everyday household measures than metric ones. Many over-the-counter medications provide instructions for patients relying on household measures. For instance, a patient will be told to take two teaspoons of a cough syrup.

While the household system is the most familiar one to patients, in practice it is the least accurate. For instance, patients who take a teaspoon of a syrup will often use everyday spoons that vary in size, rather than baking or other calibrated spoons. Instructions for over-the-counter medications can even invite inaccuracies. A patient may be told to mix a rounded teaspoon of powder with a quantity of water. The interpretation of *rounded* will vary from patient to patient.

Units of Measure. Basic units of volume in the household system, in increasing size, include drop, teaspoon, tablespoon, ounce, cup, pint, quart, and gallon. Of these, the four smallest measures are most commonly used for medications.

When specifically discussing medications, the word *ounce* generally implies volume; it represents fluid ounce. In other contexts, *ounce* may represent a unit of weight, as does *pound*.

Household Notation. As with the metric system, household notation places the quantity in Arabic numerals before the abbreviation for the unit. Table 3-5 summarizes the standard abbreviations.

Table 3-5 Abbreviations for Household Measures

Unit of Measurement	Abbreviation
drop	gtt
teaspoon	tsp or t
tablespoon	tbs or T
ounce	oz or ℥
cup	cup or c
pint	pt
quart	qt
gallon	gal

EXAMPLE 1 Write *six drops* using household notation.

Write the quantity with Arabic numerals before the abbreviation for the unit: 6 gtt

EXAMPLE 2 Write *twelve ounces* using household notation.

Write the quantity with Arabic numerals before the abbreviation for the unit: 12 oz

Apothecary and Household Equivalents

Units of measurement found in both the apothecary and the household systems are equal: an apothecary ounce equals a household ounce. Unlike the metric system, neither the apothecary system nor the household system is based on multiples of 10. You must become familiar with their equivalent measures (see Table 3-6). In practice, the size of a drop depends on the dropper and the liquid. A drop by itself is not a reliably accurate form of measurement.

Table 3-6 Apothecary and Household Equivalent Measures

drop	1 drop	=	1 minim
teaspoon	1 teaspoon	=	60 drops
tablespoon	1 tablespoon	=	3 teaspoons
ounce	1 ounce	=	2 tablespoons
cup	1 cup	=	8 ounces

EXAMPLE 1 How many teaspoons of solution are contained in 1 ounce of solution?

From Table 3-6, you can see that 1 ounce contains 2 tablespoons. In turn, each tablespoon contains 3 teaspoons. Therefore,

$$1 \text{ oz} = 2 \times 1 \text{ tbs} = 2 \times 3 \text{ tsp} = 6 \text{ tsp}$$

One ounce of solution contains six teaspoons of solution.

EXAMPLE 2 How many tablespoons are in $\frac{1}{2}$ cup of solution?

Convert 1 cup to ounces, then ounces to tablespoons. From Table 3-6, you know that 1 cup = 8 oz and 1 oz = 2 tbs:

$$\frac{1}{2} \text{ cup} = \frac{1}{2} \times 1 \text{ cup} = \frac{1}{2} \times 8 \text{ oz} = 4 \text{ oz}$$
$$= 4 \times 1 \text{ oz} = 4 \times 2 \text{ tbs} = 8 \text{ tbs}$$

One-half cup of solution contains eight tablespoons of solution.

Milliequivalents and Units

Some drugs are measured in *milliequivalents* (mEq). A unit of measure based on the chemical combining power of the substance, the mEq is defined as $\frac{1}{1000}$ of an equivalent weight of a chemical. Electrolytes, such as sodium and potassium, are often measured in mEq. Sodium bicarbonate and potassium chloride are examples of drugs that are prescribed in mEq. You do not need to learn to convert from mEq to another system of measurement.

Medications such as insulin, heparin, and penicillin are measured in *USP Units* (U). (See Chapter 6 to learn more about USP.) A Unit is the amount of a medication required to produce a certain effect. *The size of a Unit varies for each drug.* Some medications, such as vitamins, are measured in standardized units called International Units (IU). These IUs represent the amount of medication needed to produce a certain effect, but they are standardized by international agreement. As with mEq, you do not need to convert from Units to other measures. Medications that are ordered in Units will also be labeled in Units.

REVIEW and PRACTICE

OTHER SYSTEMS OF MEASUREMENT

In Exercises 1–10, write the symbols or abbreviations.

1. minim

2. dram

3. grain

4. ounce

5. drop

6. teaspoon

7. tablespoon

8. pint

9. milliequivalent

10. Unit

In Exercises 11–24, write the amounts using either apothecary or household notation, as appropriate. (Some exercises may require you to write the amount using both notations.)

11. seven grains

12. five drams

13. three ounces

14. eight ounces

15. fourteen grains

16. seventeen grains

17. one-half teaspoon

18. one-half tablespoon

19. one-half grain

20. one-half ounce

21. two and one-half ounces

22. five and one-half ounces

23. two thousand Units

24. forty milliequivalents

To check your answers, see page 339.

Converting Among Metric, Apothecary, and Household Systems

When you calculate dosages, you must often convert among the metric, apothecary, and household systems of measurement. To do so, you will need to know how the measure of a quantity in one system compares with its measure in another system. For example, you learned the relationships between mL and L and between tsp and tbs. To convert between systems, you may also need to know the relationship between mL and tsp. When you convert between systems, you lose a certain amount of exactness, especially when you round numbers. Thus, two measures are often approximately the same, though not exactly the same.

Equivalent Volume Measurements

A standard equivalent measure is that 1 tsp = 5 mL. In Chapter 2, you learned 1 mL = 1 cubic centimeter (cc). Thus,

$$1 \text{ tsp} = 5 \text{ mL} = 5 \text{ cc}$$

You can now determine most relationships between household or apothecary systems and metric systems. For instance, because 1 tbs = 3 tsp,

$$1 \text{ tbs} = 3 \text{ tsp} = 3 \times 1 \text{ tsp} = 3 \times 5 \text{ mL} = 15 \text{ mL}$$

Therefore, 1 tbs = 15 mL. Furthermore, because 1 oz = 2 tbs,

$$1 \text{ oz} = 2 \text{ tbs} = 2 \times 1 \text{ tbs} = 2 \times 15 \text{ mL} = 30 \text{ mL}$$

Therefore, 1 oz = 30 mL.

$$1 \text{ oz} = 30 \text{ mL}$$

Earlier you learned that 1 oz = 8 dr. Therefore,

$$1 \text{ oz} = 8 \text{ dr} = 2 \text{ tbs} = 30 \text{ mL}$$

The importance of this relationship will be clear in Chapter 4, when you learn about medicine cups.

Table 3-7 summarizes several important volume relationships.

Table 3-7 Approximate Equivalent Measures for Volume

Metric	Household	Apothecary
5 mL	1 tsp	1 dr
15 mL	1 tbs	3 or 4 dr*
30 mL	2 tbs = 1 oz	1 oz
240 mL	8 oz = 1 c	8 oz
480 mL	2 c = 1 pt	16 oz
960 mL	2 pt = 1 qt	32 oz

*see the following paragraph

This table indicates that 1 qt is approximately 960 mL. However, a commonly used equivalent measure is 1 qt = 1 L, even though 1 L = 1000 mL, not 960 mL. You might notice another discrepancy. If 4 dr = 15 mL, then dividing each side by 3, 1.33 dr = 5 mL. However, the table lists 1 dr = 5 mL. These discrepancies are a result of the approximate nature of the equivalent measures.

Equivalent Weight Measurements

Earlier you learned that 1 grain is equivalent to either 60 or 65 milligrams:

gr i = 60 mg *or* gr i = 65 mg

The relationship between grains and milligrams or grams is actually more complex. The conversion varies from 60 mg to 66.7 mg per gr. You will need to use information from the drug label or a drug reference to help you determine which equivalent measure to use for a given drug.

Figure 3-2

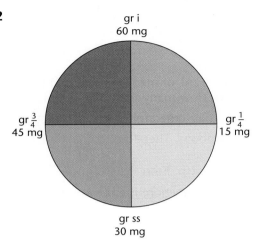

In cases where you use 60 mg as the equivalent measure, one way to remember the relationship between grains and milligrams is to think of a clock (see Figure 3-2). If each "minute" is one milligram, then an entire hour is one grain. This image of the clock may help you when you need to find the equivalent of $\frac{1}{2}$ grain (gr ss) or $\frac{1}{4}$ grain (gr $\frac{1}{4}$). Each half of an "hour" or grain is 30 "minutes" or milligrams. Similarly, each quarter of an "hour" or grain is 15 "minutes" or milligrams.

Table 3-8 summarizes important weight equivalent measures, including the relationship between kilograms and pounds (lb).

Table 3-8 Approximate Equivalent Measures for Weight

Metric	Apothecary
60 mg	gr i (1 grain)
30 mg	gr ss ($\frac{1}{2}$ grain)
15 mg	gr $\frac{1}{4}$
1 mg	gr $\frac{1}{60}$
1 g (1000 mg)	gr xv (15 grains)
0.5 g	gr viiss ($7\frac{1}{2}$ grains)
1 kg	2.2 lb

Converting Using Conversion Factors

A conversion factor expresses an equivalent measure. It helps you switch from one unit of measure to an equivalent one. Its numerator and denominator are equivalent. Both the factor and its reciprocal equal 1. For example, $\frac{1 \text{ mg}}{1000 \text{ mcg}}$ and $\frac{1000 \text{ mcg}}{1 \text{ mg}}$ are conversion factors that relate mg and mcg. Both factors equal 1. Similarly, $\frac{\text{gr i}}{60 \text{ mg}}$ and $\frac{60 \text{ mg}}{\text{gr i}}$ relate gr and mg.

You can use fraction proportions with conversion factors to convert a quantity from one unit of measure to another. (Recall from Chapter 2 that you cross-multiply to find a missing value in a fraction proportion.)

Rule 3-10

To convert a quantity from one unit of measure to another,

1. Write the first fraction so that the numerator is the quantity that you know and the denominator is the quantity you want (the missing value).

2. For the second fraction, use a conversion factor with the same respective units of measurement in the numerator and denominator.

3. Write a proportion. Set the two fractions equal to each other.

4. Cross-multiply to find the missing value, the denominator of the first fraction.

EXAMPLE 1 You are instructing a patient to take 10 mL of medication at home, using a calibrated teaspoon to measure the medication. How many teaspoons should the patient use?

1. The quantity you know is 10 mL, the numerator of the first fraction. The quantity you want to find is the number of teaspoons. Therefore, the first fraction is $\frac{10 \text{ mL}}{? \text{ tsp}}$.

2. From Table 3-7, you know 5 mL = 1 tsp. Both $\frac{5 \text{ mL}}{1 \text{ tsp}}$ and $\frac{1 \text{ tsp}}{5 \text{ mL}}$ are conversion factors equal to 1. Select $\frac{5 \text{ mL}}{1 \text{ tsp}}$ as the second fraction; it has mL in the numerator and tsp in the denominator.

3. Write a proportion. Set the two fractions equal to each other.

$$\frac{10 \text{ mL}}{? \text{ tsp}} = \frac{5 \text{ mL}}{1 \text{ tsp}}$$

4. Cross-multiply to solve.

$$10 \times 1 = ? \times 5$$
$$10 = 5 \times ?$$
$$2 = ?$$

Thus, $\frac{10 \text{ mL}}{2 \text{ tsp}} = \frac{5 \text{ mL}}{1 \text{ tsp}}$. The patient should take 2 tsp of medication to get the equivalent of 10 mL.

EXAMPLE 2 How many kg does a 62-pound child weigh?

1. The quantity you know is 62 lb. The quantity you want to find is the number of kg. Write your first fraction as $\frac{62 \text{ lb}}{? \text{ kg}}$.

2. From Table 3-8, you know 1 kg = 2.2 lb. Write the second fraction so that the numerator is lb and the denominator is kg, to match the first fraction. The second fraction is $\frac{2.2 \text{ lb}}{1 \text{ kg}}$.

3. Write the proportion.

$$\frac{62 \text{ lb}}{? \text{ kg}} = \frac{2.2 \text{ lb}}{1 \text{ kg}}$$

4. Cross-multiply to solve.

$$62 \times 1 = ? \times 2.2$$
$$62 = 2.2 \times ?$$
$$28.18 = ?$$

The child weighs 28.18 kg. Sometimes the amount of medication you give to a child is dependent on the child's body weight. Knowing how to convert between pounds and kilograms is important.

EXAMPLE 3 — A physician orders morphine gr $\frac{1}{8}$ for a patient. How many milligrams of morphine will the patient receive?

1. The first fraction is $\dfrac{\text{gr } \frac{1}{8}}{? \text{ mg}}$.

2. From Table 3-7, you find that 60 mg = gr i. You write the conversion factor with gr in the numerator and mg in the denominator, matching the first fraction: $\dfrac{\text{gr i}}{60 \text{ mg}}$

3. $\dfrac{\text{gr } \frac{1}{8}}{? \text{ mg}} = \dfrac{\text{gr i}}{60 \text{ mg}}$

4. $\dfrac{1}{8} \times 60 = ? \times 1$

   $7.5 = ?$

The patient will receive 7.5 mg of morphine.

Converting Using Ratio-Proportion Method

In Chapter 2, you learned to use means and extremes to find a missing value in a ratio proportion. By writing the conversion factor as a ratio, you can use those same steps to convert a quantity from one unit of measure to another.

Rule 3-11

To convert a quantity from one unit of measure to another using the ratio-proportion method,

1. Write the first ratio as A:B so that A is the quantity you know and B is the quantity you want (the missing value).

2. Write a conversion factor as a ratio C:D so that C and D have the same units of measure as A and B, respectively.

3. Write a ratio proportion in the form A:B::C:D

4. Find the missing value B by using means and extremes.

EXAMPLE 1 — You are instructing a patient to take 10 mL of medication at home, using a calibrated teaspoon to measure the medication. How many teaspoons should the patient use?

1. Write the first ratio with the quantity you know, 10 mL, as A and the quantity you want, ? tsp, as B. Thus,

   10 mL:? tsp

2. From Table 3-7, you know that 5 mL = 1 tsp. Write this relationship as a ratio C:D, where the unit of C matches the unit of A (mL) and the unit of D matches the unit of B (tsp). Thus,

   5 mL:1 tsp

3. Write a proportion in the form A:B::C:D

   10 mL:? tsp::5 mL:1 tsp

4. Find the missing value, using the means and extremes. The means are ? and 5 and the extremes are 10 and 1. Thus,

   $? \times 5 = 10 \times 1$

   $5 \times ? = 10$

   $? = 2$

The patient should take 2 tsp of medication to get the equivalent of 10 mL. This example is the same as Example 1 in the previous section. Here, the ratio-proportion method is used to find the missing value. Previously, the conversion factor method was used. Both methods lead you to the same solution. Which method you use is a matter of personal choice.

CRITICAL THINKING ON THE JOB

Selecting the Correct Conversion Factor

Greg is teaching a patient how much liquid medication to take. The physician has ordered 30 mL of Milk of Magnesia, but the patient will be using teaspoons to measure her medication. Using a conversion chart, Greg confuses 1 tbs with 1 tsp, and reads 1 tsp = 15 mL. Using this incorrect information, he calculates the dose as follows:

$$\frac{30 \text{ mL}}{? \text{ tsp}} = \frac{15 \text{ mL}}{1 \text{ tsp}}$$
$$30 \times 1 = ? \times 15$$
$$2 = ?$$

Greg tells the patient to take 2 tsp of Milk of Magnesia. This amount is only one-third of the amount that the patient should take; the patient does not get the relief desired.

Think Before You Act

Even though Greg set up the proportion correctly, he used the wrong conversion factor. Certain equivalent measures, such as 1 tsp = 5 mL, are so commonly used that you should memorize them. However, when you use a conversion chart, always check that you use the correct unit of measure. Be sure that you read across the same line. Do not match the first half of a conversion with the second half from a different line.

Had Greg used the correct conversion, 1 tsp = 5 mL, he would have calculated as follows:

$$\frac{30 \text{ mL}}{? \text{ tsp}} = \frac{5 \text{ mL}}{1 \text{ tsp}}$$
$$30 \times 1 = ? \times 5$$
$$6 = ?$$

The patient would be told to take 6 tsp of medication, not 2 tsp.

REVIEW and PRACTICE

CONVERTING AMONG METRIC, APOTHECARY, AND HOUSEHOLD SYSTEMS

In Exercises 1–10, convert the measures from one system of measurement to another.

1. 4 dr = _____ tsp

2. 125 mL = _____ cc

3. 120 mL = _____ tsp

4. 240 cc = _____ oz

5. 15 mg = gr_____

6. gr 15 = _____ mg

7. 10 mg = gr_____

8. 2.5 g = gr _____

9. 42 kg = _____ lb

10. 42 lb = _____ kg

11. During the total course of his treatment, a patient will receive 720 mL of medication. How many pints will he receive?

12. If an order calls for the patient to receive 2 tsp of cough syrup, how many mL of syrup should the patient receive?

13. A patient weighs 65 kg. How many pounds does she weigh?

14. A patient weighs 187 lb. How many kg does he weigh?

15. A physician orders 8 dr of liquid medication. How many tbs should the patient take?

16. A patient drinks 4 c of liquid during the morning. How many mL did the patient drink?

17. An order is for gr iii of medication. How many g should the patient be given?

18. A physician orders that a patient be given 10 mg of medication three times per day. How many gr of medication should the patient be given per day?

To check your answers, see page 339.

Temperature

Both the Fahrenheit (F) and Celsius (C) temperature scales are used in health care settings. The Fahrenheit scale sets the temperature at which water freezes at 32 degrees, or 32° F. It also measures the temperature at which water boils as 212 degrees, or 212° F. On the Celsius scale, the measurement of freezing water is set at 0 degrees, or 0° C. The boiling temperature of water is 100 degrees, or 100° C.

As a health care worker, you may need to convert between these two temperature scales. Examine the two thermometers in Figure 3-3. On the Fahrenheit scale, the difference between the boiling and freezing points of water is 180° F. On the Celsius scale, the difference between these two points is 100° C. Therefore, 180° F = 100° C and, in turn, 1.8° F = 1° C.

Figure 3-3

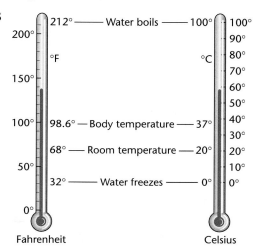

Rule 3-12

Use the following formula to convert a temperature from Fahrenheit to Celsius,

$$\frac{°F - 32}{1.8} = °C$$

EXAMPLE 1 Convert 98.6° F to °C.

Substituting 98.6 for °F in the conversion formula,

$$\frac{98.6 - 32}{1.8} = \frac{66.6}{1.8} = 37$$

98.6° F = 37° C; both measures represent normal body temperature.

Rule 3-13

Use the following formula to convert a temperature from Celsius to Fahrenheit,

$$(1.8 \times °C) + 32 = °F$$

EXAMPLE 1 Convert 37° C to °F.

Substituting 37 for °C in the conversion formula,

$$(1.8 \times 37) + 32 = 66.6 + 32 = 98.6$$

Thus 37° C = 98.6° F

You may have first learned these formulas using $\frac{9}{5}$ and $\frac{5}{9}$. Because $\frac{9}{5} = 1.8$, multiplying a quantity by $\frac{9}{5}$ is the same as multiplying it by 1.8. Multiplying a quantity by $\frac{5}{9}$ is the same as dividing it by 1.8. If you are using a calculator, you may find your work easier if you use 1.8 for your conversions.

REVIEW and PRACTICE

TEMPERATURE

In Exercises 1–8, convert the temperatures.

1. 34° C = _____ °F

2. 41° C = _____ °F

3. 95° F = _____ °C

4. 102° F = _____ °C

5. 45.3° F = _____ °C

6. 212° F = _____ °C

7. 25° C = _____ °F

8. 100° C = _____ °F

To check your answers, see page 339.

Time

Many health care facilities use the 24-hour clock, known as military or international time. A traditional 12-hour clock is a source of errors in administering medication. Using the 12-hour clock, each time occurs twice a day. For instance, the hour 10:00 is recorded as both 10:00 A.M. and 10:00 P.M. The abbreviation A.M. means "ante meridian" or "before noon"; P.M. means "post meridian" or "after noon." If these abbreviations are not clearly marked, the patient could receive medication at the wrong time.

The 24-hour clock (international time) bypasses this opportunity for error. Each time occurs only once per day. In international time, 10:00 A.M. is written as 1000, whereas 10:00 P.M. is written as 2200. (See Figure 3-4.)

Figure 3-4

International time is based on a twenty-four hour clock.

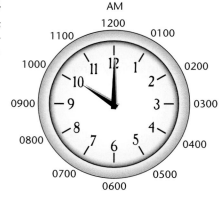

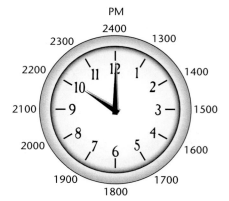

When you write the time using a 12-hour clock, you separate the hour from the minutes by a colon. You write a single digit for the hours 1 through 9. You then add A.M. or P.M. to indicate before or after noon. When you write the time using a 24-hour clock, you use a four-digit number with no colon. The first two digits represent the hour, the last two digits, the minutes.

Rule 3-14

When using a 24-hour clock for international time,

1. Write 00 as the first two digits to represent the first hour after midnight.

2. Write 01, 02, 03, . . . 09 as the first two digits to represent the hours 1:00 A.M. through 9:00 A.M.

3. Add 12 to the first two digits to represent the hours 12:00 P.M. through 11:00 P.M., so that 12, 13, 14, . . . 23 represent these hours.

4. Write midnight as either 2400 (international) or 0000 (military time).

EXAMPLE 1 Convert 9:00 A.M. to international time.

Remove the colon and the abbreviation A.M. Write the hour 9 with two digits, starting with zero.

9:00 A.M. = 0900

EXAMPLE 2 Convert 12:19 A.M. to international time.

Remove the colon and the abbreviation A.M. Because this time occurs in the first hour after midnight, use 00 for the hour.

12:19 A.M. = 0019

EXAMPLE 3 Convert 4:28 P.M. to international time.

Remove the colon and the abbreviation P.M. Because this time is after noon, add 12 to the hour.

4:28 P.M. = 1628

EXAMPLE 4 Convert 1139 to traditional time.

Insert a colon to separate the hour from the minutes. Because this time occurs before noon, add A.M. following the time.

1139 = 11:39 A.M.

EXAMPLE 5 Convert 1515 to traditional time.

Insert a colon to separate the hour from the minutes. Subtract 12 from the hour and add the abbreviation P.M.

1515 = 3:15 P.M.

Rule 3-15

To state the time using international time,

1. Say "zero" if the first digit is a zero.

2. Say "zero zero" if the first two digits are both zero.

3. If the minutes are represented by 00, then say "hundred" after you say the hour.

EXAMPLE 1 State the time 0900.

Say "zero nine" for the hours and "hundred" for the minutes. Thus, 0900 is stated as "zero nine hundred."

EXAMPLE 2 ▷ State the time 1139.

Say "eleven" for the hours and "thirty-nine" for the minutes. Thus, 1139 is stated as "eleven thirty-nine."

EXAMPLE 3 ▷ State the time 0023.

Say "zero zero" for the hours and "twenty-three" for the minutes. Thus, 0023 is stated "zero zero twenty-three."

REVIEW and PRACTICE

TIME

In Exercises 1–8, convert the times to international time.

1. 2:35 A.M.

2. 7:57 A.M.

3. 12:08 A.M.

4. 12:55 A.M.

5. 1:49 P.M.

6. 3:14 P.M.

7. 11:54 P.M.

8. 10:19 P.M.

In Exercises 9–16, convert the times to traditional time.

9. 0011

10. 0036

11. 0325

12. 0849

13. 1313

14. 1527

15. 2145

16. 2359

To check your answers, see page 339.

CHAPTER 3 REVIEW

CHECK UP

In Exercises 1–8, write the indicated amounts using numerals and abbreviations.

1. twenty-five and one-half kilograms

2. forty-five hundredths of a centimeter

3. forty micrograms

4. three-quarters of a liter

5. nine-tenths of a milligram

6. one and one-half grains

7. three hundred seventy-five thousandths of a gram

8. twelve milliliters

In Exercises 9–30, calculate the conversions.

9. 0.06 g = _____ mg

10. 125 mcg = _____ mg

11. 0.004 km = _____ m

12. 0.75 cm = _____ mm

13. 965 mL = _____ L

14. 0.008 L = _____ mL

15. 0.32 kg = _____ g

16. 0.05 mg = _____ mcg

17. 988 m = _____ km

18. 1725 cm = _____ km

19. 368 mg = _____ g

20. 247 g = _____ kg

21. 8 g = gr_____

22. gr iiss = _____ mg

23. 90 mL = _____ tbs

24. 5 tsp = _____ mL

25. 8 dr = _____ mL

26. 1200 mL = _____ oz

27. 540 mg = gr_____

28. gr $\frac{3}{4}$ = _____ mg

29. 178.2 lb = _____ kg

30. 47 kg = _____ lb

31. An order is placed for gr v of medication. If the medication is supplied in mg, how many mg should be given? (For this example, assume gr i = 65 mg.)

32. If a patient weighs 44 lb, how many kg does he weigh?

33. A physician orders $\frac{1}{2}$ oz of medication for a patient. How many mL of medication should the patient be given?

34. The maximum dose of a medication is 3 tbs. What is the maximum number of mL that the patient should be given?

35. A physician tells a patient to drink 2400 mL of fluid per day. How many quarts of liquid should this patient drink?

36. Several months ago, a patient weighed 95 kg. When he comes in for his next appointment, he tells you he has lost 11 pounds. If he is correct, how many kg should he weigh?

Convert the following temperatures to Celsius.

37. 97.6° F   **38.** 72° F   **39.** 57.4° F   **40.** 82.8° F

Convert the following temperatures to Fahrenheit.

41. 24° C   **42.** 43.8° C   **43.** 15.6° C   **44.** 8.8° C

Convert the following times to international time.

45. 3:21 A.M.   **46.** 4:42 P.M.   **47.** 10:47 P.M.   **48.** 11:20 A.M.

Convert the following times to traditional time.

49. 0029   **50.** 1417   **51.** 2053   **52.** 0912

CRITICAL THINKING

A patient suffering from a cold is given a prescription for 15 mL of cough suppressant every 8 hours for 10 days. The patient will be using a household measuring device to measure the dose of medication.

1. Which household device should the patient use?

2. How much medication should the patient take, given the device you recommend?

3. If the medication is supplied in half-pint bottles, how many bottles will the patient need during the 10 days?

CASE STUDY

The state health department requires that certain medications be stored between 36° F and 41° F. The refrigerator in the medication room has a Celsius thermometer. What temperature range is appropriate using the Celsius thermometer?

To check your answers, see page 340.

INTERNET ACTIVITY

Note: The Internet is a research tool from which to get basic information. Validate the accuracy of all Internet information.

Various sites on the Internet offer information about converting units to and from the metric system. Suppose you need to make some conversions involving units of measurement. While your conversion card is not readily available, you do have access to a computer. Locate on the Internet sites that can help you make these conversions. Suggested key words: *metric + system, metric + conversion.*

EQUIPMENT for DOSAGE MEASUREMENT

4

Objectives

When you have completed Chapter 4, you will be able to:

- Identify equipment used to administer medication.
- Indicate the appropriate equipment for delivering various types of medicine.
- Measure medications using the calibrations on the equipment.
- Describe the method of administration appropriate for each piece of measuring equipment.

Oral Administration

Many medications are available in liquid form and can be administered orally. Several types of equipment are used to measure and administer oral liquid medications. These include medicine cups, droppers, calibrated spoons, and oral syringes.

Each measuring device has a series of calibrations, or marks numbered at varying intervals. Calibrations enable you to measure the amount of liquid in the device. When choosing a measuring device, compare its calibrations with the desired dose of medication. They may represent different units of measurement. If your equipment does not match the order, then you will have to convert the order to the unit of measurement you will use to administer the medication.

Medicine Cups

Medicine cups are used to measure oral liquid medications and administer them to patients. Cups provide a measured dose that is easy for most patients to swallow. Usually, medicine cups are plastic and measure up to one fluid ounce, or its equivalent. To make dose calculation easier, most cups are typically marked with metric, household, and apothecary systems of measurement. Thus, cups include units such as tablespoons (tbs), teaspoons (tsp), milliliters (mL), drams (dr), and ounces (oz).

Use the two views of a cup shown in Figure 4-1 to compare the different calibrations. Here, milliliters are displayed in units of 5. Teaspoons and tablespoons are marked in units of 1 or $\frac{1}{2}$. Ounces are displayed in units of $\frac{1}{4}$, and drams are marked in units of 1 or 2. You can see that 5 mL is equivalent to 1 tsp. The slight curve in the surface of a liquid is the *meniscus*. Measure the quantity of liquid by the bottom of the meniscus, not by the higher levels at the edges (see Figure 4-2).

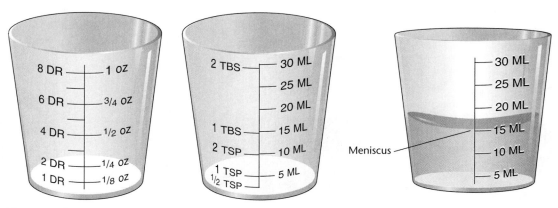

Figure 4-1 *Two views of a medicine cup.*

Figure 4-2 *Meniscus.*

Rule 4-1

Do not use medicine cups for doses less than 5 mL, even if the cup has calibrations smaller than 5 mL. Instead, use a dropper, calibrated spoon, or oral syringe to ensure accuracy.

Droppers

Droppers help you measure and administer small amounts of oral liquid medication (see Figure 4-3). You may also use them to deliver certain liquid medications to the eyes, ears, and nose. Droppers are especially helpful with oral pediatric doses. A product that requires a dropper is often packaged with one calibrated for the specified dose. The indicated units of measurement are usually milliliters, cubic centimeters (cc), or drops. Recall that 1 mL = 1 cc.

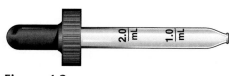

Figure 4-3

Rule 4-2

Only use the specific dropper that accompanies a particular product. Do not interchange droppers between medications.

Droppers have different-sized openings. The diameter of the opening affects the size of the individual drops. For example, three drops from a dropper with a large opening provide more medication than three drops from one with a smaller opening.

Calibrated Spoons

In some cases, you can deliver small amounts of medication by using calibrated spoons (see Figure 4-4). Spoons are often used with pediatric or elderly patients. They come in many sizes, calibrated to a variety of doses.

You can use the spoons to administer medication directly into the mouth. You can also use them to measure medication into food or a beverage for a child or elderly patient. Children who are used to being fed from a household spoon may accept medication if it comes from a calibrated spoon rather than from a dropper or a medicine cup. You can also use spoons for thick liquids that cannot be easily delivered through the small openings of a dropper.

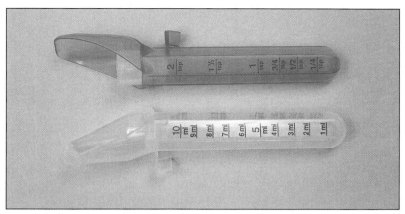

Figure 4-4 *Calibrated spoons.*

Oral Syringes

For small quantities of liquid, especially less than 5 mL, oral syringes provide accurate readings. Generic oral syringes are often calibrated for milliliters (or cc) and teaspoons, with additional calibrations between these numbers (see Figure 4-5). Oral syringes are designed with safety features to keep them from being confused with hypodermic syringes. Oral syringes often have "eccentric," or off-center, tips that have a different shape and size than the tips of hypodermic syringes. Oral syringes may be tinted, whereas hypodermic syringes are clear.

The main danger in confusing oral syringes with hypodermic syringes stems from a basic fact: oral syringes are not sterile. To administer sterile medications, you must use hypodermic syringes, not oral syringes.

Figure 4-5
Oral syringes.

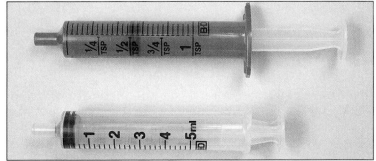

1. Never attach a hypodermic needle to an oral syringe.

2. Never inject an oral dose.

3. In emergencies, you may use a hypodermic syringe without a needle to measure and administer liquid oral doses, but never while its needle is attached.

Other Equipment for Oral Medications

Sometimes oral medications, intended for absorption in the stomach or intestines, cannot be delivered orally. The patient may have difficulty swallowing or some condition or trauma that prevents taking the medication orally. In many cases, medication is administered using a nasogastric tube that carries medication through the nose to the stomach for absorption (see Figure 4-6).

Liquid medications are preferred for nasogastric tubes. Sometimes, you can crush a solid medication, adding water to transport it through the tube. Consult your facility for the appropriate procedure. Many solid oral medications, such as gelcaps and extended-release medications, may **not** be crushed. See Chapter 9 for further discussion about these medications.

Other tubes are used to deliver medications directly to the stomach or intestines. A PEG tube delivers medication and nutrients directly to the stomach. A jejunostomy tube delivers medication and nutrients directly to the small intestine.

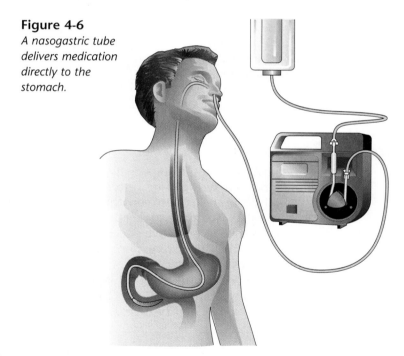

Figure 4-6
A nasogastric tube delivers medication directly to the stomach.

ERROR ALERT!
The utensil you use must provide the calibration you need to accurately measure the dose.

Suppose the volume of the dose is less than 0.5 mL. The calibrations on the utensil must measure increments of less than 0.5 mL. Otherwise, you cannot accurately measure the medication. Using a utensil that is marked in 1-mL increments and estimating the halfway point is not accurate.

Use the Correct Dropper

A baby with a fever is prescribed acetaminophen for home administration. The nurse tells the baby's father that he will be given a bottle of liquid acetaminophen and a medicine dropper for measuring the prescribed number of drops. The father is told to give the baby eight drops of medicine at regular intervals.

At home, the father accidentally drops and breaks the dropper. He remembers, though, that he has a dropper from another medication. He uses it instead to measure the acetaminophen. The second dropper is much smaller than the one that came with the acetaminophen. The baby receives a smaller dose than prescribed, even though the father administers the prescribed eight drops.

Two nights later, the baby's symptoms are not relieved. The father calls the physician, who asks if he has been delivering the number of prescribed drops. The physician prescribes a stronger medication. The baby has suffered needlessly and now is exposed to a stronger medication for no reason.

Think Before You Act

This error could easily be avoided. During the initial visit, the father should have been instructed to use *only* the dropper that accompanies the medication. When he calls two days later, he should be asked if the *correct equipment* was used.

REVIEW and PRACTICE

ORAL ADMINISTRATION

In Exercises 1–10, determine if the statement is true or false. If false, explain why it is incorrect.

1. You may use a hypodermic syringe with a needle to measure liquid for oral administration.

2. You may use a medicine cup to measure liquid doses of less than 1 mL for oral administration.

3. Oral and hypodermic syringes are identical in appearance.

4. When measuring liquid in any type of utensil for oral administration, the dose volume must be level with the corresponding calibration line on the device.

5. If the dropper supplied by a drug manufacturer for a specific medication is not available, you may substitute a dropper supplied for another medication, as long as the replacement dropper has never been used.

6. If a patient does not have a calibrated spoon, then any household spoon may be substituted.

7. Measuring utensils are often calibrated with more than one system of measurement.

8. A prescribed dose of liquid oral medication cannot be dispensed reliably without calibrated cups, spoons, oral syringes, or droppers.

9. When calculating volume and dosage, it is helpful to remember that 1 mL is equal to 1.5 cc.

10. If a prescribed dose and the calibrated device used for administering that dose use different systems of measurement, then the device cannot be used.

In Exercises 11–14, convert the dosage ordered to the same units as those marked on calibrated utensils. You may wish to refer to the conversion factors in Chapter 3. There may be more than one correct answer for each conversion.

11. The prescribed dose is 2 tbs. Which of the following is NOT equivalent, as marked on the medicine cup?
    A. 30 mL   B. 1 oz   C. 8 dr   D. 15 cc

12. An oral medication comes in a bottle labeled 10 units per cc. The dose to be administered is 50 units. Which of the following is a correct dose?
    A. 50 mL   B. 50 cc   C. 5 mL   D. 0.5 mL

13. Which of the following statements about calibrated droppers is true?
    A. 0.25 cc equals 25 drops.
    B. 0.25 cc equals five drops.
    C. 1 cc equals 10 drops.
    D. The number of drops in each cc varies per dropper.

14. The dose to be given is 5 mL. The medicine cup is labeled in tbs, tsp, oz, and dr. Which of the following is a correct dose?

    A. 5 dr   B. $\frac{1}{3}$ tbs   C. $\frac{1}{3}$ tsp   D. $\frac{1}{3}$ oz

To check your answers, see page 341.

Hypodermic Syringes

Many medications must be administered parenterally, bypassing the digestive tract. (*Parenterally* means "outside the intestines.") While parenteral dosage forms include topical and transdermal medications, inhalers, and sublingual tablets, the term most often refers to injections. The most common injection routes are intravenous (IV), intramuscular (IM), intradermal (ID), and subcutaneous (SC). See Chapters 10 and 11 for more information about these methods of injection. Different hypodermic syringes are used to administer injections. These syringes are calibrated with different measurements. The type of syringe you use depends on the type and amount of medication you must administer.

Standard Syringes

The 3-cc syringe is one of the most common standard syringes used for parenteral administration. Standard syringes have scales calibrated in cubic centimeters. Syringes with smaller capacities may have divisions of tenths, two-tenths, or even hundredths of a cubic centimeter, allowing for measurement of small doses. The 3-cc syringe in Figure 4-7 is calibrated in tenths; it has 10 calibrations for each cc. Calibrations for half and whole cubic centimeters are numbered. Standard syringes may also use the minim scale from the apothecary system. In most cases, use the metric system.

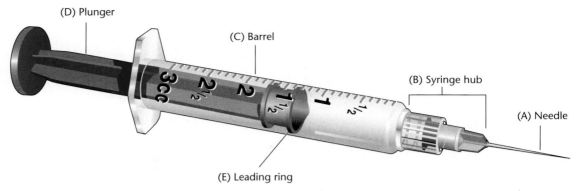

Figure 4-7 *The parts of a standard syringe include (A) the needle, (B) the syringe hub, (C) the barrel that contains the liquid, (D) the plunger, and (E) the plunger tip, also called the leading ring.*

Any health care worker who uses a syringe must be familiar with its calibrations so that the correct dose is administered. On all syringes, the zero calibration is the edge of the barrel closest to the needle. The barrel is filled with liquid up to the point of the wide ring, known as the leading ring, on the tip of the plunger closest to the needle. Liquid in the barrel does not go past this ring. While the leading ring might have a raised middle, measure from the ring itself. Do *not* measure from the trailing ring, the ring farther from the needle.

Prefilled Syringes

Prefilled syringes are shipped from the manufacturer filled with a single, standard dose of medication. They have the same parts as standard syringes: a needle, a syringe hub, a barrel, and a plunger (see Figure 4-8). Calibrations on a prefilled syringe are read similarly to those on a standard syringe. The leading ring indicates how much liquid is in the barrel. Designed to be used once and discarded, prefilled syringes are usually marked in tenths of a cc and may hold up to 2.5 cc. *Before* injecting a patient with medication from a prefilled syringe, you must discard any amount that exceeds the prescribed dose. In many cases, manufacturers routinely include 0.1 cc to 0.2 cc of excess medication to allow for air expulsion before the injection.

Figure 4-8

Prefilled syringe.

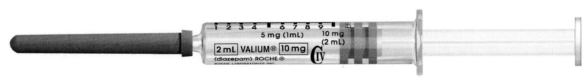

Insulin Syringes

Insulin syringes are used only to measure and administer insulin. Whether for adults or children, insulin doses are smaller than many other doses. In turn, insulin syringes are calibrated in smaller increments. Insulin is measured in Units (U). The most common form of insulin is U-100; it contains 100 Units of insulin per 1 cc.

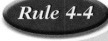 **Rule 4-4**

Never use any type of syringe other than an insulin syringe to measure and administer insulin.

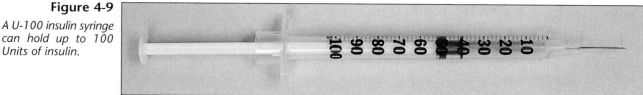

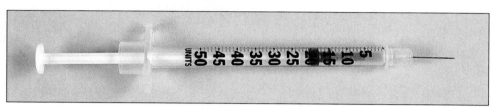

Figure 4-9 shows a standard U-100 insulin syringe. It contains up to 100 Units (1 cc) of insulin. The larger numbers mark increments of 10 Units. The smaller calibrations indicate every 2 Units. They allow you to measure smaller doses of insulin. Not all insulin syringes are marked with these increments. Figure 4-10 shows a syringe that holds up to 50 Units of insulin. The larger numbers show increments of 5 Units, and the smaller calibrations show increments of 1 Unit. This syringe is often used to measure and administer pediatric doses of insulin or adult doses less than 50 Units.

Tuberculin Syringes

Tuberculin syringes are used to administer the subcutaneous PPD skin test that determines if a person has been exposed to tuberculosis. More than that, they are simply small syringes used when small doses of medication—less than 1 mL—are administered. Vaccines, heparin, pediatric medicines, and allergen extracts are typically administered with a tuberculin syringe.

Tuberculin syringes usually hold a total volume of 1 mL and are calibrated in hundredths of a cc or mL (see Figure 4-11). The numbering is slightly different from that of the other syringes. In Figure 4-11, the marked numbers represent tenths of a cubic centimeter. The first number, located on the tenth calibration, is 0.1 cc. Each smaller calibration represents one hundredth (0.01) of a cc. Some syringes are even smaller. The tuberculin syringe in Figure 4-12 holds a total volume of 0.5 mL.

Measuring the correct dose with a tuberculin syringe requires extreme care. The calibrations are close together and marked with a number only at every one-tenth or two-tenths calibration. Be sure the leading ring is aligned with the proper calibration. Many tuberculin syringes are also calibrated with the apothecary scale in minims. You can usually disregard the apothecary scale because it is not often used today.

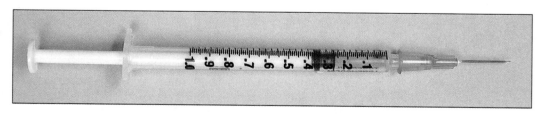

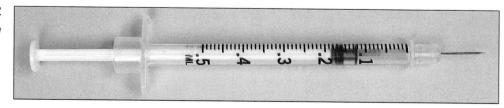

Safety Syringes

The syringes previously discussed are available as safety syringes (see Figures 4-13, 4-14, and 4-15). They have the same components as their standard counterparts: a needle, a hub, a barrel, and a plunger. However, their needles are protected by plastic shields. These shields help prevent needlestick injury. Although safety syringes do not guarantee that health care workers will not receive accidental needlesticks, they reduce the chances of such accidents. Safety syringes are calibrated in cc's or Units. Smaller-capacity safety syringes are divided into tenths, two-tenths, and hundredths of a cc.

Figure 4-13

This 100-Unit insulin safety syringe has a shield that covers the needle, minimizing needlestick injuries.

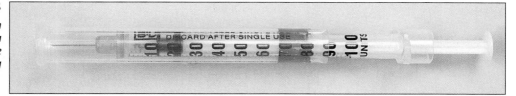

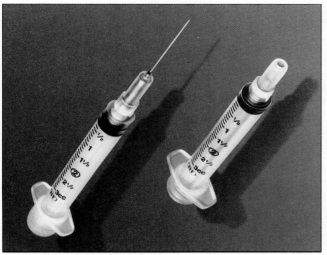

Figure 4-14

Like the safety syringe in Figure 4-15, this standard 3-cc safety syringe automatically retracts the needle into the barrel after use.

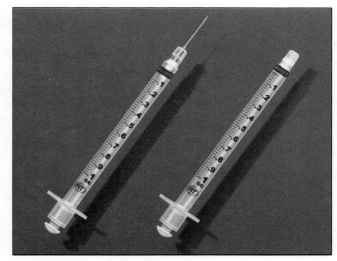

Figure 4-15

A 1-cc tuberculin safety syringe.

Syringes to Established Intravenous Lines

Some syringes are used to administer medication through already-established intravenous lines that deliver medication and fluids directly into a patient's veins. Figure 4-16 shows an example of such a syringe.

Adding medication through existing lines has several advantages. Using the injection ports, IV medications can be administered quickly without the patient being punctured repeatedly. Because the syringes do not have needles, accidental needlesticks to patients and health care workers are avoided. An intravenous system with needleless syringes allows more than one drug to be administered at a time, provided that the drugs are compatible. Needleless syringes also enable you to deliver drugs on a periodic basis and to dilute the medication.

Figure 4-16

A needleless syringe is used to inject medication into existing IV tubing.

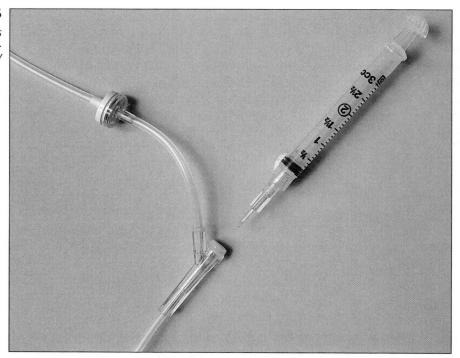

Large-Capacity Syringes

Not all medications can be delivered in doses of 3 cc or less. Therefore, syringes with 5-cc, 6-cc, 10-cc, 12-cc, or even more are available (see Figure 4-17.) As with other syringes, volume is measured in cc's and the number of calibrations between numbered cc's vary. Large-capacity syringes often have five calibrations between numbers with each mark measuring 0.2 cc.

Figure 4-17

A large-capacity syringe.

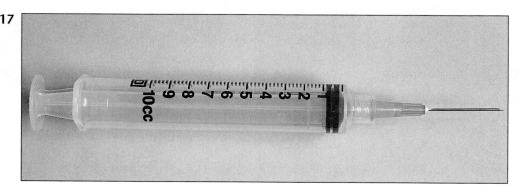

ERROR ALERT!

Pay close attention to the calibration of any syringe you use.

Perhaps the most important aspect of a syringe is its calibration. If medication is not accurately measured, serious problems can result for the patient. Do not assume the calibration of any syringe you use. Check it carefully. After determining the value of the calibration, align the plunger at the appropriate level. **Remember:** No matter what type of syringe you use, *the leading ring, closest to the needle, is the part that must be aligned with the calibration.*

Ampules, Vials, and Cartridges

Parenteral medications may be packaged in ampules, vials, or cartridges (see Figure 4-18). *Ampules* are sealed containers and usually hold one dose of liquid medication. You snap

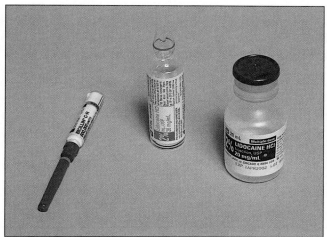

Figure 4-18

A cartridge (left), an ampule (center), and a vial (right).

them open and use any standard syringe to withdraw the medication. *Vials* are containers covered with a rubber stopper, or diaphragm. They may hold more than a single dose of medication, in either liquid or powder form. If powder, then diluent is injected in the vial to reconstitute the medication. *Cartridges* are prefilled containers shaped like syringe barrels. They generally hold one dose of medication and fit a reusable syringe. Tubex and Carpujet are examples of cartridges.

Preparing the Syringe

If you fill a syringe, you must administer it yourself or properly label the contents for the person who will use it.

Rule 4-5

In most circumstances, the person who prepares a syringe for injection should deliver the injection. Exceptions include:

1. pharmacy technicians who prefill syringes for nurses, medical assistants, or patients.

2. nurses or medical assistants preparing a syringe for a physician.

3. health care workers teaching a patient to administer his or her own medication.

This last exception occurs, for instance, when you teach a patient with diabetes how to administer insulin.

Needle Gauge and Length

When you administer an injection, you must choose a needle with an appropriate gauge. A needle's gauge is its interior diameter. Smaller gauges correspond to larger diameters; an 18-gauge needle is wider than a 22-gauge needle. The gauge you use depends on the viscosity (thickness) of the medication, as well as the injection site. More viscous drugs and deeper injections require needles with smaller gauges, as seen in Table 4-1.

The injection site also determines the length of the needle. You should select a needle that is long enough to reach the area of tissue specified. However, the needle should not be so long that it penetrates beyond that area.

Table 4-1 Needle Gauge and Length		
Type of Injection	**Gauge**	**Length (inches)**
Intradermal	25–26	$\frac{3}{8} - \frac{5}{8}$
Subcutaneous	23–27	$\frac{1}{2} - \frac{7}{8}$
Intramuscular	18–23	1–2

Finishing What You Start

A medical assistant prepares to deliver a single dose of Valium by injection. He has a prefilled syringe containing 2.5 cc, but the prescribed dose is 1.5 cc. Before he can administer the injection, his pager goes off and he rushes to another patient's room. As he does, he asks another medical assistant to administer the Valium.

She administers the Valium, assuming that the prefilled syringe contains the appropriate dose. As a result of receiving more Valium than was prescribed, the patient's blood pressure drops. The first medical assistant does not ask if the correct dose has been administered, and the patient undergoes tests to find the cause of the drop in blood pressure.

Think Before You Act

This overdose could be avoided. The first medical assistant should check the prescribed dose and immediately discard the extra medication from the syringe. He should also either personally deliver the dose or identify its contents properly before handing it over to another assistant. The second medical assistant also should take extra precautions. She should confirm directly with the first medical assistant the amount to deliver. She also should check the patient's chart before administering medication.

REVIEW and PRACTICE

HYPODERMIC SYRINGES

In Exercises 1–4, provide a brief answer.

1. What is the standard calibration of a 3-cc syringe?

2. What is the standard calibration of a 50-Unit insulin syringe?

3. What is the standard calibration of a tuberculin syringe?

4. What is the standard calibration of a large-capacity syringe?

In Exercises 5–12, determine if the statement is true or false. If false, explain why it is incorrect.

5. Any extra medication in a syringe should be discarded before the injection is given.

6. The first calibration on any syringe is always zero (0).

7. When measuring a dose in a syringe, read the calibration that aligns with the trailing ring on the plunger.

8. Some prefilled syringes are overfilled with 0.1 to 0.2 cc of medication to allow for air expulsion from the needle.

9. Prefilled syringes and standard syringes do not have the same calibrations.

10. You can use an insulin syringe to measure 6 cc of medication.

11. A patient is punctured each time a syringe is used with an established intravenous line.

12. Safety syringes are a guaranteed way to avoid accidental needlestick injuries.

In Exercises 13–22, identify the type of syringe and the volume of the dosage it contains. Identify the correct units of measurement.

Example: Refer to the sample syringe below:

Sample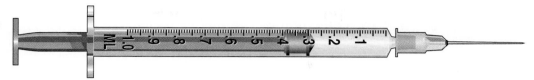

Type: <u>tuberculin</u> Volume: <u>0.3 cc</u>

13. Refer to syringe A:

Type: _____ Volume:_____

A.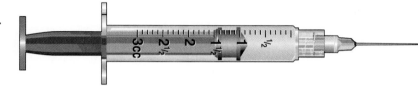

14. Refer to syringe B:

Type: _____ Volume:_____

B.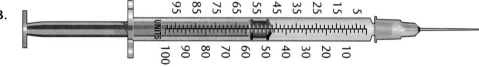

15. Refer to syringe C:

Type: _____ Volume:_____

C.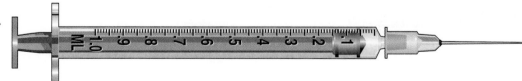

16. Refer to syringe D:

Type: _____ Volume:_____

D.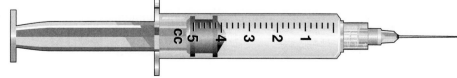

17. Refer to syringe E:

Type: _____ Volume: _____

E.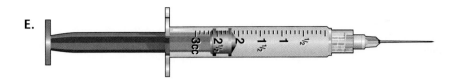

18. Refer to syringe F:

Type: _____ Volume: _____

F.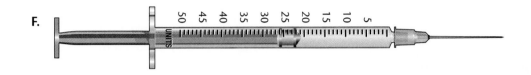

19. Refer to syringe G:

Type: _____ Volume: _____

G.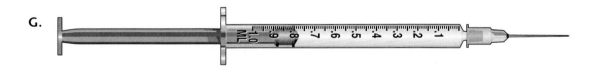

20. Refer to syringe H:

Type: _____ Volume: _____

H.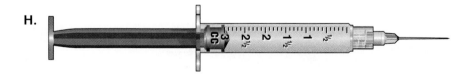

21. Refer to syringe I:

Type: _____ Volume: _____

I.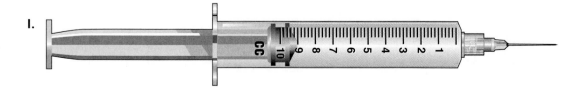

22. Refer to syringe J:

Type: _____ Volume: _____

J.

To check your answers, see page 341.

Other Administration Forms

You can administer medications in other ways. You need to become familiar with them in order to correctly measure and administer each dose of medication.

Topical Medications

Topical medications, such as gels, creams, ointments, and pastes, are applied directly to or through the skin. You administer the drug with a glove, tongue blade, or cotton-tipped applicator. Topical medications are usually given for their therapeutic effect in or on the skin. Follow the instructions that accompany the product to determine how to remove the medication from its container and administer it. Avoid letting any of the medication contact your own skin.

Transdermal Medications

A transdermal medication is a form of topical medication in which the medication is absorbed through the skin. Often you administer a transdermal medication by using a self-adhesive patch (see Figure 4-19). You place the medication-filled patch on clean, dry, hairless skin that has no rash or irritation, and with good circulation. The medication is then released continuously through the skin to the entire body for a specified period. The package is marked with the dose rate.

Because patches allow for continuous regular absorption, they maintain consistent levels of the medication in the blood. Patches are beneficial for people who have trouble

Figure 4-19

A transdermal patch.

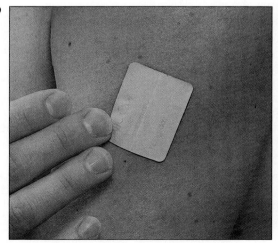

swallowing oral drugs. Patches bypass the gastrointestinal (GI) system, where the medication could cause digestive and other problems. Because they do not involve injection, you can easily administer patches on an outpatient basis.

When you administer a patch, you must document its placement so that other health care providers can readily find it. Mark each new patch with your initials, the date, and the time of administration. Rotate placement sites. Remove older patches and dispose of them safely. Medications commonly administered through the transdermal method include cardiovascular drugs, hormones, and allergy and pain medications.

Drops, Sprays, and Mists

Different types of equipment are used to deliver medication to the nose, ears, eyes, and throat in the form of drops, sprays, and mists. Drops, also called instillations, deliver medication to the nose, eyes, and ears. Sprays deliver medication to the nose and throat. Drops and sprays are measured according to the dose prescribed and the manufacturer's instructions. Therefore, be sure to use the equipment that accompanies the drug when you administer these medications.

Droppers, similar to those for oral medications, are used to administer drops. Plastic squeeze bottles are used for drops and sprays. Atomizers deliver sprays by using a rubber bulb to propel the spray from a medicine container into the nose.

Another way to administer medication is to use a mist which the patient inhales. Vaporizers, or steam inhalers, use boiling water to create a mist from liquid medication. Nebulizers, often used by patients with asthma, and metered dose inhalers (MDI) also help deliver medication to the patient.

Vaginal and Rectal Medications

You administer some medications vaginally or rectally. Suppositories are available for vaginal and rectal administration, and tablets are available for vaginal administration. These medications are usually solid dosage forms administered into the patient's vagina or rectum, depending on the product. Each suppository or vaginal tablet contains a pre-determined dose. Some of the vaginal medications are available in oral form, but the vaginal form is preferred for patients who have difficulty with oral medications, or need the medication directly on the site.

Whereas suppositories deliver medication in solid forms, liquid forms of medication can also be administered. Douches deliver liquid vaginal medication through a special nozzle. Enemas deliver liquid rectal medication through a tube inserted into the patient's rectum. Other medications are administered through creams and foams.

CRITICAL THINKING ON THE JOB

Document the Use of Patches

An elderly nursing home patient with cancer has chronic pain. She is receiving oral codeine and morphine, but still has debilitating pain between doses. She complains about the problem to the nurse, who suggests to the physician that the patient may benefit from a more continuous administration of medication.

The doctor prescribes a transdermal Fentanyl patch. The patch contains enough medication for three days. The nurse applies the patch to the right side of the patient's back. Later that night, another nurse checks to see whether the patient's patch has been applied. It is difficult to roll the patient on her side to examine her back. Because the patch is not readily visible, the second nurse assumes the patch has not been placed and puts another patch on the patient's chest.

The next morning, the first nurse notes that the patient is barely breathing and can't be awakened. She quickly finds the patch on her chest. She remembers placing a patch on the back, not the chest. She confirms that two patches are in place, strips off both, and calls the physician. Narcan is administered to reverse the drug's effects; the patient quickly becomes more coherent.

Think Before You Act

This problem could be avoided if the second nurse is more careful assessing the patient before placing a second patch. The second nurse should not assume that the patch is not in place. At the same time, the first nurse should indicate clearly on the patient's chart when the patch was placed and its exact location. Because patches are so potent, they make it easy for health care workers to give an overdose of the drug. You must carefully document the placement of patches and ensure that no patch is already in place when you administer a new one.

CHAPTER 4 REVIEW

CHECK UP

In Exercises 1–10, answer the multiple choice questions. More than one answer may be correct.

1. Which of the following equals 1 oz?
   - A. 2 tbs
   - B. 20 mL
   - C. 8 dr
   - D. 2 tsp

2. A patient is supposed to receive 15 mL of Mylanta. A measuring cup cannot be found. What is an equivalent dose?
   - A. 1 tsp
   - B. 2 tsp
   - C. 3 tsp
   - D. 5 tsp

3. The dose of a liquid medication for oral administration is $\frac{3}{4}$ oz. Which is the correct equivalent dose?
   - A. 20 mL
   - B. 25 mL
   - C. 7.5 dr
   - D. 1.5 tbs

4. The ordered dosage of a liquid medication for oral administration is 2.5 mL. What is the appropriate method of oral administration?
   - A. $\frac{1}{8}$ oz as measured in a medicine cup
   - B. 1 dr as measured in a medicine cup
   - C. $\frac{1}{2}$ tsp as measured in a calibrated spoon
   - D. 2.5 mL as measured in a calibrated dropper

5. The prescribed dosage of a medication is 5 drops. Which of the following is an appropriate method of administering the dose?
   - A. 0.5 mL using only the calibrated dropper that accompanies the medicine bottle
   - B. 5.0 mL using the calibrated dropper that accompanies the medicine bottle
   - C. 5 drops using any calibrated dropper
   - D. 5 drops using only the calibrated dropper that accompanies the medicine bottle

6. The ordered oral dosage of a medication is 5 mL. Which of the following is an appropriate method of administering the dose?
   - A. 1 tsp using a calibrated spoon
   - B. 5 mL using a syringe for parenteral administration with the needle removed
   - C. 25 drops using a calibrated dropper
   - D. 5 tsp using a calibrated spoon

7. The ordered dosage of a medication is 10 mg. The medication is mixed at a strength of 5 mg per mL. Using a 2.5 cc prefilled syringe, how much medication should be discarded before administration?
   - A. 0.2 cc
   - B. 1 cc
   - C. 0.5 cc
   - D. 2 cc

8. A tuberculin syringe is being used to administer 0.25 cc of a given medication. Which of the following is the equivalent dose?
   - A. 2.5 hundredths of a cc
   - B. 25 hundredths of a cc
   - C. 250 hundredths of a cc
   - D. 2.5 drops using a calibrated dropper

9. Which of the following can be used to administer a 7 cc dose via the parenteral route?
   - A. A large-capacity syringe
   - B. A standard syringe
   - C. A tuberculin syringe
   - D. An insulin syringe

10. Which of the following has the most precise and accurate calibrations?
    A. A 5-cc syringe to an established intravenous line
    B. A 3-cc syringe to an established intravenous line
    C. A 3-cc safety syringe
    D. A 1-cc tuberculin syringe

In Exercises 11–20, determine if the statement is true or false. If false, explain why it is incorrect.

11. It is apparent from the calibrations on the medicine cups that 30 mL is equivalent to 1 oz.

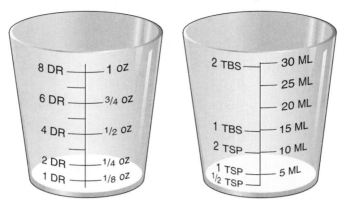

12. If an ordered dose calls for 3 mL, a medicine cup may be used to measure it.

13. A calibrated dropper dispenses a standard drop of 3 mL.

14. The standard syringe can hold more than 1 cc.

15. The standard syringe is calibrated in tenths of a cc.

16. Prefilled, single-dose syringes can be used more than once.

17. The standard U-100 insulin syringe can hold up to 100 Units or 1 cc.

18. The tuberculin syringe is used to measure doses of drugs larger than 3 mL.

19. The syringes used to deliver medication through already established intravenous systems are hypodermic syringes.

20. You may administer an oral medication by injecting it parenterally.

In Exercises 21–36, use the accompanying illustrations of equipment. For each question, mark with a line or with shading where you would measure the required dose:

21. 30 mL (Refer to medicine cup A.)

22. $\frac{1}{2}$ ounce (Refer to medicine cup B.)

23. 1 mL (Refer to calibrated dropper C.)

24. 0.6 mL (Refer to calibrated dropper D.)

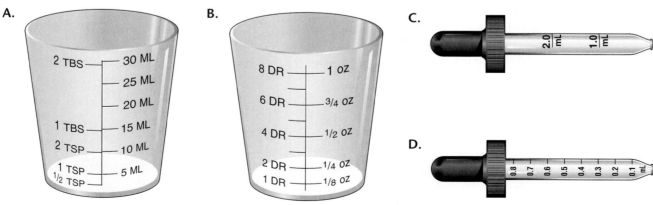

25. 2 mL (Refer to syringe E.)

26. $1\frac{1}{2}$ tsp (Refer to syringe F.)

E.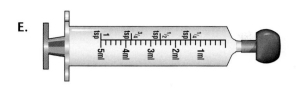

F.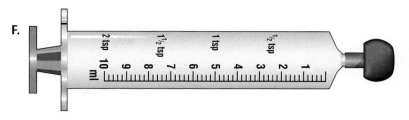

27. 1.5 cc (Refer to syringe G.)

G.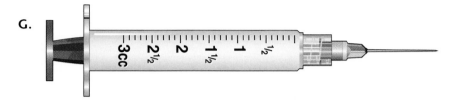

28. 2.3 cc (Refer to syringe H.)

H.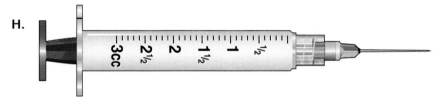

29. 80 Units (Refer to syringe I.)

I.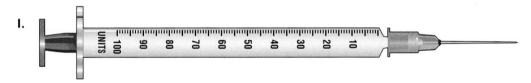

30. 45 Units (Refer to syringe J.)

J.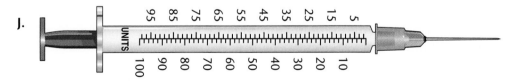

31. 35 Units (Refer to syringe K.)

K.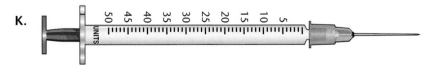

32. 27 Units (Refer to syringe L.)

L.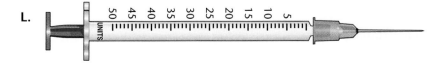

33. 0.5 cc (Refer to syringe M.)

M.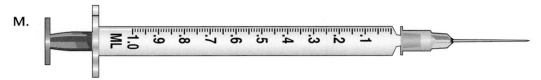

34. 0.25 cc (Refer to syringe N.)

N.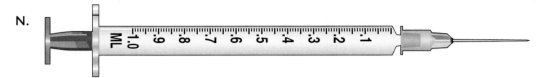

35. 5 cc (Refer to syringe O.)

O.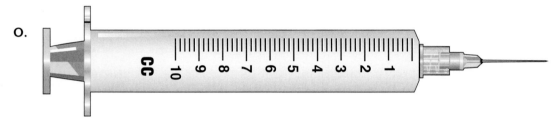

36. 7.2 cc (Refer to syringe P.)

P.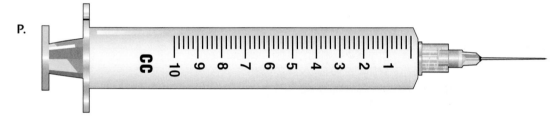

CRITICAL THINKING

What are the best utensils for measuring and administering the doses in each of the following situations? Choose from any of the equipment discussed in this chapter.

A. 1.5 cc, to be delivered parenterally

B. 29 Units of insulin, to be delivered parenterally

C. 0.3 mL, to be delivered parenterally

D. oral liquid dose of 29 mL

E. oral liquid dose of 1 tbs

F. parenteral dose of 1.25 mL

G. oral liquid dose of 2 tbs

H. 8 mL, to be administered parenterally

I. 0.3 milligrams (mg), to be administered transdermally

J. 0.4 mL, to be administered orally

CASE STUDY

An emergency medical technician (EMT) must administer 10 drops of an oral medication. In attempting to administer the dose, the EMT breaks the calibrated dropper. Instructions on the bottle say that 20 drops is equal to 1.5 tsp. What is the dose to be administered, and what is the best utensil for measuring it, now that the dropper is broken?

To check your answers, see page 341.

INTERNET ACTIVITY

Note: The Internet is a research tool from which to get basic information. Validate the accuracy of all Internet information.

In the medical practice where you work, one of your coworkers has developed a real fear of accidentally getting stuck by a syringe needle. Although your practice does not have safety syringes, you know they are available and might help to ease your coworker's fears.

You approach the office manager about ordering safety syringes. The manager tells you that she does not know enough about them to purchase them. She asks you to gather information about them so that she can make a wise purchase choice.

Assignment: Search the Internet for information about safety syringes. Include information about price, brand names, and safety statistics.

Suggested key words: safety syringe, needlestick injuries, parenteral administration.

DRUG ORDERS

5

Objectives

When you have completed Chapter 5, you will be able to:

- Summarize the Seven Rights of Medication Administration.
- Interpret a written drug order.
- Identify on physicians' orders and prescriptions the information needed to dispense medication.
- Locate on Medication Administration Records or medication cards the information needed to administer medication.
- Recognize drug orders that do not contain all of the necessary information to carry out the orders safely.
- Select appropriate action for confusing, incomplete, or illegible drug orders.

The Seven Rights of Medication Administration

When you carry out a medication order, you can be held responsible if an error occurs, regardless of its source. You must be able to interpret and confirm physicians' orders. To assist you, the medical field has created seven guidelines, called the Seven Rights (see Table 5-1).

Right Patient. Before giving medication to a patient, check that the name on the original order is *exactly the same* as the name on the Medication Administration Record (MAR), medication card, or prescription. Verify the full name. Two patients with the same last name may have the same first initials, or even the same first name. Ask the patient for his or her name. (Ask "What is your name?") For inpatient settings, also check the bed number and the patient's identification bracelet number.

Table 5-1 The Seven Rights of Medication Administration

1. Right Patient	5. Right Time
2. Right Drug	6. Right Technique
3. Right Dose	7. Right Documentation
4. Right Route	

Right Drug. To be certain that a patient receives the *right drug,* administer only drugs you have prepared yourself or that are clearly and completely labeled. Check that the drug order has not expired and that the medication is still in date. (See Chapter 6 for more on drug labels.)

If a patient questions a medication, recheck the original order. Be sure you have the correct drug. Patients are often familiar with their medications. Listening to them may prevent an error. A patient **always** has the right to refuse medication. If this happens, do not return the medication to its container. Instead, follow your facility's guidelines for disposing of it. Record the patient's refusal and notify the physician.

Right Dose. The patient is entitled to the *right dose* of medication. In later chapters, you will learn to convert from the *dosage ordered* by the physician to the *desired dose*—the amount of drug that a patient should receive at any one time. You will also learn to calculate the *amount to administer* to a patient, factoring in the strength of the medication and the equipment you are using.

Use extreme caution when you calculate the desired dose and the amount to administer. Pay special attention to decimal points. They can easily be placed in the wrong location or missed altogether when an order is copied. If you misread a decimal point, then the patient could receive a dose significantly different than the one ordered.

Right Route. You must give patients drugs by the *right route.* A drug intended for one route is often not safe if administered via another route. For example, only drugs labeled "for ophthalmic use" should be instilled (applied with a dropper) into the eye.

Some medications are produced in different versions for different routes. The drug label (see Chapter 6) will indicate the intended route. For example, Compazine is available as a suppository, a tablet, and an injection. Always check that the route listed on the drug label matches the route ordered by the physician.

Right Time. Give medications at the *right time.* In most cases, to be "on time," you must administer medications within 30 minutes of schedule. The right time may refer to an absolute time, such as 6:00 P.M., or to a relative time, such as "before breakfast."

Some medications, such as insulin, antibiotics, and antidysrhythmic drugs, must be given at specific times because of how they interact with food or the patient's body. Other medications may be spaced over waking hours without changing their effectiveness. The MAR or medication card must identify special timing considerations to be followed. If a medication is ordered PRN (whenever necessary), a time interval or condition must usually be specified (e.g., for temperature > 101 or BP > 120). Before administering such a PRN drug, check that enough time has passed since the previous dose was given. Otherwise, the patient could receive the medication too soon, leading to severe consequences.

Right Technique. Be familiar with the *right technique* to administer a medication. For example, both buccal and sublingual medications are applied to the mucous membranes of the mouth. A buccal medication, such as Cepacol lozenges, is placed between the cheek and the gum, whereas a sublingual medication, such as nitroglycerin, is placed under the tongue. If you are not familiar with the correct technique to use, check resources such as the *Physicians' Desk Reference* (PDR) or a nursing drug reference for more information.

Right Documentation. Be sure that the *right documentation* is completed. For example, if you administer a medication, you must sign the MAR (or similar form) *immediately after* the patient takes the medication. Until a procedure is documented, it is not complete. Document that you have administered a medication *only after* and *immediately after* you have actually administered it. If the patient declines the medication, consumes only part of the dose, or vomits shortly after taking the medication, document that information as well.

PATIENT EDUCATION

Even though patient education is not listed specifically as one of the rights of medication administration, you should provide patients with basic information regarding their drugs.

1. Explain the purpose of a medication and its side effects.

2. Review the dose, route, frequency, and time that the physician has prescribed.

3. When appropriate, be certain that the patient understands how to self-administer the medication.

4. If the patient is taking liquid oral medications at home, emphasize the importance of using calibrated spoons and measuring cups.

Physicians' Orders and Prescriptions

Physicians use abbreviations when writing orders. Memorize the commonly used ones and have available a complete list of those accepted at your facility. (See Table 5-2.) Approved abbreviations vary among facilities. You may encounter either upper case or lower case letters and orders with or without punctuation marks. You may also notice slight differences in the way that the abbreviations are spelled.

Table 5-2 Abbreviations Commonly Used in Drug Orders

General Abbreviations

Abbreviation	Meaning		
aq	water	NKDA	no known drug allergies
aq dist	distilled water	NPO, n.p.o.	nothing by mouth
a, $\bar{a}$	before, ante	$\bar{p}$, p	after
aa, $\overline{aa}$	of each	q, q., $\bar{q}$	every
BP	blood pressure	qs	quantity sufficient
c, $\bar{c}$	with	R	take
d.c., D/C	discontinue	$\bar{s}$	without
disp	dispense	sig. s	write on label
et	and	ss, $\overline{ss}$	one-half
iss, $\overline{iss}$	one and one-half	sys	systolic
NKA	no known allergies	tbs, T	tablespoon
		tsp, t	teaspoon
		ut dict, ud	as directed

Table 5-2 (Continued)

Form of Medication

Abbreviation	Meaning
cap, caps	capsule
comp	compound
dil, dil.	dilute
EC	enteric coated
elix, elix.	elixir
ext, ext.	extract
fld., fl	fluid
gtt, gtts	drop, drops
H	hypodermic
LA	long acting
liq	liquid
MDI	metered dose inhaler
sol, soln.	solution
SR	slow release
supp, supp.	suppository
susp, susp.	suspension
syr, syp.	syrup
syr	syringe
tab	tablet
tr, tinct, tinc.	tincture
ung, oint	ointment

Route (Where to Administer)

Abbreviation	Meaning
ad, A.D., AD	right ear
as, A.S., AS	left ear
au, A.U., AU	both ears
GT	gastrostomy tube
ID	intradermal
IM, I.M.	intramuscular
IV, I.V.	intravenous
IVP	intravenous push
IVPB	intravenous piggyback
IVSS	intravenous soluset
KVO, TKO	keep vein open
NG, NGT, ng	nasogastric tube
NJ	nasojejunal tube
od, O.D., OD	right eye
os, O.S., OS	left eye

ou, O.U., OU	both eyes
per	per, by, through
po, p.o., PO, P.O.	by mouth; orally
R, P.R., p.r.	rectally
sc, SC, s.c., sq, SQ, sub-q	subcutaneous, beneath the skin
SL, sl	sublingually, under the tongue
top, TOP	topical, applied to skin surface

Frequency

Abbreviation	Meaning
a.c., ac, AC, $\overline{ac}$	before meals
ad. lib., ad lib	as desired, freely
b.i.d., bid, BID	twice a day
b.i.w.	twice a week
h, hr	hour
h.s., hs, HS	hour of sleep, at bedtime
LOS	length of stay
min	minute
non rep	do not repeat
n, noc, noct	night
od	every day
p.c., pc, PC, $\overline{pc}$	after meals
p.r.n., prn, PRN	when necessary, when required
qam, q.a.m.	every morning
qpm, o.n., q.n.	every night
q.d., qd	once every day
q.h., qh	every hour
q.___hrs, q___h	every _____ hours
qhs, q.h.s.	every night, at bedtime
q.i.d., qid, QID	4 times a day
q.o.d., qod	every other day
rep	repeat
SOS, s.o.s.	once if necessary, as necessary
stat	immediately
t.i.d., tid, TID	3 times a day
t.i.w.	3 times a week

Some physicians use lowercase Roman numerals, such as ii, to indicate numbers. You may see these numerals with a line over them, such as ī͞i. Physicians often use this format for apothecary measurements such as grains. They may also put a line over general and frequency abbreviations, such as *a, ac, c, p,* and *s,* when the abbreviations are lowercase.

Always verify that a drug order contains all information needed to carry it out safely and accurately. It should include the full name of the patient, the full name of the drug, the dose, the route, the time and frequency, the signature of the prescribing physician, and the date of the order. A prn order must include the reason for administering the medication. If an order is unclear, talk with the physician before carrying it out.

Outpatient Settings

For outpatient settings, physicians' orders are given as prescriptions that are filled at a pharmacy or through the mail. Prescriptions include all the elements of a physician's order, as well as the physician's name and prescriber number, the quantity to be dispensed, the number of refills permitted, and instructions for the label of the container. These instructions are preceded by the word *sig* (see Figure 5-1).

Figure 5-1
Prescription form.

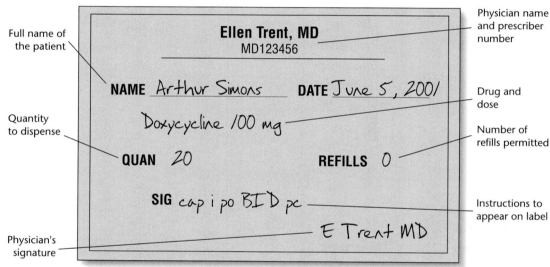

The patient is Arthur Simons. The drug is Doxycycline. The dose is 100 mg. From the *sig* line, the instructions on the label should read "Take one capsule twice a day after meals" or one capsule (cap i), twice a day (BID), by mouth (po), after meals (pc). Form, number, route, frequency, and timing are all shown. The quantity (quan) of capsules is 20. The prescription cannot be refilled. The physician's name, prescriber number, and signature are present. This order contains all of the required elements.

Inpatient Settings

For inpatient settings, drug orders are usually written on physicians' order forms, with space for multiple orders. Orders may also be entered into a computer. The patient's name and the physician's signature appear once on the form. Under *Medication Orders,* the physician writes the components of each medication requested in the following sequence: name of drug, dose, route, frequency, and additional instructions.

The form in Figure 5-2 shows several medication orders; some are correct and others have errors. Order #1 contains all necessary components. The drug is Lasix, the dose is 20 mg, the route is oral (po), and the frequency is once a day (qd).

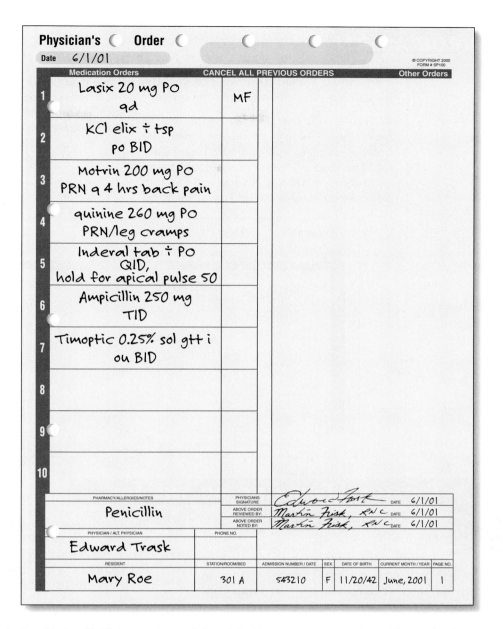

Figure 5-2

Physician's order form.

Physician's Order

Date 6/1/01

© COPYRIGHT 2000
FORM # SP100

Medication Orders	CANCEL ALL PREVIOUS ORDERS	Other Orders

1. Lasix 20 mg PO qd — MF
2. KCl elix ÷ tsp po BID
3. Motrin 200 mg PO PRN q 4 hrs back pain
4. quinine 260 mg PO PRN/leg cramps
5. Inderal tab ÷ PO QID, hold for apical pulse 50
6. Ampicillin 250 mg TID
7. Timoptic 0.25% sol gtt i ou BID
8.
9.
10.

PHARMACY/ALLERGIES/NOTES
Penicillin

PHYSICIANS SIGNATURE: *Edward Trask* DATE 6/1/01
ABOVE ORDER REVIEWED BY: *Martin Frisk, RNC* DATE 6/1/01
ABOVE ORDER NOTED BY: *Martin Frisk, RNC* DATE 6/1/01

PHYSICIAN / ALT. PHYSICIAN — Edward Trask — PHONE NO.

RESIDENT	STATION/ROOM/BED	ADMISSION NUMBER / DATE	SEX	DATE OF BIRTH	CURRENT MONTH / YEAR	PAGE NO.
Mary Roe	301 A	543210	F	11/20/42	June, 2001	1

Order #2, for K Cl (potassium chloride) elixir, is not complete. The order lists one teaspoon as the amount, but K Cl elixir is available in strengths of 10, 20, 30, or 40 mEq per 15 mL. Each strength provides a different dose per teaspoon.

Order #3 is correct. The drug is Motrin, the dose is 200 mg, the route is oral (po), and the frequency is whenever necessary (PRN) every 4 hours (q 4 hrs). For PRN drugs, the physician must specify how often it may be given. Here, Motrin may not be administered more often than every 4 hours.

Order #4 is not complete because it does not include an adequate frequency. The quinine is ordered PRN, when necessary for leg cramps. Yet no minimum time interval is specified.

In Order #5, the physician has included instructions for "holding" (not administering) the medication. You need to check if the patient's apical pulse is below 50 before administering Inderal. The order is not complete because the physician has ordered one tablet, not the actual dose. Inderal is available in 10-, 20-, 40-, 60-, and 90-mg tablets.

Order #6 does not specify the route for 250 mg Ampicillin, available in oral, intramuscular, and intravenous forms. Consult the physician to find the intended route.

Unlike Order #6, Order #7 is complete. The physician specified the number of drops, as well as the strength of Timoptic desired.

Never guess what the prescriber meant.

If an order is not legible, always contact the prescribing physician to clarify the order.

In Figure 5-3, the physician intended to order *Zyrtec 10 mg po qd.* However, the order is illegible, and you could read Zantac. The loop on the *m* in *mg* could be an extra zero, or 100 mg. A small extra loop in *qd* makes it hard to tell if the order is qd (once every day) or qod (every other day). Because you bear the responsibility of administering the correct dose at the correct frequency, you must contact the physician to clarify the order. Also contact the physician if any part of the order is missing.

Figure 5-3

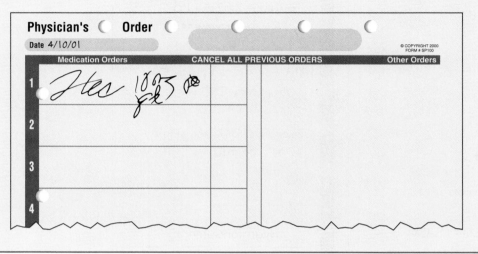

CRITICAL THINKING ON THE JOB

The Importance of the Right Dose

A physician's order reads: *Compazine supp i pr q4h PRN/nausea.* The pharmacy technician interprets this order as "administer 1 Compazine suppository rectally every four hours as necessary for nausea."

The pharmacy technician assumes that the patient is an adult and dispenses 25-mg suppositories, the normal adult dose. In turn the nurse, who does not notice that the dose is not specified in the order, administers the 25-mg suppository to the patient, a 6-year-old boy.

The usual dose of Compazine for children is a 2.5-mg suppository. The pediatrician who wrote the order did not include the dose, assuming the staff would know this information. The child receives ten times the normal dose of Compazine. He has a seizure and develops fever, respiratory distress, severe hypotension, and tachycardia because of drug toxicity. He is admitted to the intensive care unit for treatment.

Think Before You Act

The pediatrician made the initial error by not specifying the dose. This error does not relieve either the pharmacist, pharmacy technician, or the nurse of their responsibilities. All of them should have recognized that one of the seven rights—the right dose—was missed in this order. They should have called the physician to clarify the desired dose.

Verbal Orders

Usually, orders must be written or personally signed by a physician. However, if a physician is not able to write an order that must be carried out quickly, verbal orders may be permitted. State laws govern which personnel may accept such orders and how soon the physician must countersign them.

If you are legally permitted to accept a telephone order, write it carefully and legibly *as* you receive it, *not after* the call. In some cases, you may write the order on the physician's order form, identifying it as a verbal order. Always read the order back to the physician. Verify that you have transcribed it correctly. If you are not certain of the spelling of the drug name, ask the physician to spell it. Many drugs have names that are pronounced or spelled similarly (Table 5-3).

If you must prepare a medication from a verbal order, take special precautions. Double check that you have prepared the medication accurately. If a physician is present, show the label before administering the medication or before handing it to the physician to administer. State the medication and the dose so that the physician can verify that what you have prepared is what was ordered.

Table 5-3 Look-Alike and Sound-Alike Drug Names

This list provides some examples. It is not meant to be a complete list of drugs with similar names.

Acular - Ocular	digitoxin - digoxin	Persantine - Persistin
Adderall - Inderal	dobutamine - dopamine	Phenaphen - Phenergan - Theragran
Aldara - Alora	Equagesic - EquiGesic	
Allegra - Viagra	Eurax - Urex	phentermine - phentolamine
alprazolam - lorazepam	Flomax - Fosamax	Pitocin - Pitressin
Alupent - Atrovent	glipizide - glyburide	prednisolone - prednisone
Amcill - Amoxil	glutethimide - guanethidine	Proscar - Prozac
Anaspaz - Antispas	Humalog - Humulin	Psorex - Serax - Xerac
Aralen - Arlidin	Hycodan - Vicodin	Pyridium - pyridoxine
Asacol - Os-Cal	Hygroton - Regroton	quinidine - quinine
Bacitracin - Bactrim	Hyperstat - Nitrostat	Remeron - Zemuron
Banthine - Brethine	iodine - Lodine	rifabutin - rifampin
Benadryl - Bentyl	Isordil - Isuprel	Rifadin - rifampin - Ritalin
Benylin - Ventolin	lamivudine - lamotrigine	Serentil - sertraline - Sinequan
Betagan - Betagen	Lasix - Luvox	selegiline - sertraline
Cafergot - Carafate	Mebaral - Mellaril - Moderil	Serax - Psorex - Xerac
calcitonin - calcitriol	Mephyton - methyldopa	Tagamet - Tegretol
Cardene - codeine	mesantoin - Mestinon	Tegretol - Toradol
Cardiem - Cardizem	Myleran - Mylicon	Theolair - Thyrolar - Theodur
Celebrex - Celexa - Cerebyx	Narcan - Norcuron	thiamine - Tenormin
centoxin - Cytoxan	Nasarel - Nizoral	Tobradex - Tobrex
chlorpromazine - chlorpropamide	Nembutal - Myambutol	Tuinal - Tylenol
cimetidine - simethicone	Neurontin - Noroxin	Ultane - Ultram
Clinoril - Clozaril	Nicobid - Nitro-Bid	Uracel - uracil
clonidine - Klonopin	Nilstat - Nitrostat	Uracid - Urised
Coumadin - Kemadrin	Ornade - Orinase	Vepesid - Versed
Cytosar - Cytoxan	oxycodone - OxyContin	Vibramycin - Viomycin
Danazol - Dantrium	Parlodel - pindolol	vinblastine - vincristine
Darvon - Diovan	Pathocil - Pitocin - Pitressin	Xanax - Zantac
Diamox - Dobutrex	Pavabid - Pavased	Zofran - Zosyn
diazepam - diazoxide	Paxil - Taxol	Zyprexa - Zyrtec

The Importance of the Right Drug

A patient is brought to the hospital with a severe thumb laceration. The attending physician verbally orders lidocaine 1% solution 2 mL as a local anesthetic. The medical assistant picks up a vial labeled lidocaine 1% with epinephrine and draws up 2 cc (equal to 2 mL). He then says, "This is lidocaine 1% solution 2 mL," but neither mentions the epinephrine nor shows the physician the label.

A while later, the patient expresses concern about continuing numbness in his thumb. After locating the vial, the staff member realized that the patient received epinephrine, a vasoconstricting drug, in addition to the lidocaine. The patient is reassured that feeling will return to his thumb, though not quite as quickly as was first anticipated.

Think Before You Act

The medical assistant should have read the label three times to be certain that he had the correct drug. If he had also shown the label to the physician, the error could have been avoided.

REVIEW and PRACTICE

PHYSICIANS' ORDERS AND PRESCRIPTIONS

In Exercises 1–5, refer to Prescription A. In Exercises 6–10, refer to Prescription B.

1. What components, if any, are missing from Prescription A?

2. How many Lopressor tablets should the pharmacy technician dispense?

3. How often should the patient take Lopressor?

4. What strength tablets should be dispensed?

5. If the patient gets all of the refills permitted, how long will the medication covered by this prescription last?

6. What components, if any, are missing from Prescription B?

Alan Capsella, MD
MD398475

DATE _July 9, 2001_

NAME _Ann Pechin_

Lopressor   50 mg

SIG _tab i po tid_

QUAN _90_   REFILLS _5_

Alan Capsella MD

Prescription A

Alan Capsella, MD
MD398475

DATE _April 10, 2001_

NAME _Mark Ward_

Amoxil   oral susp

SIG _i tsp po q8h_

QUAN _100 mL_   REFILLS _0_

Alan Capsella MD

Prescription B

7. How much Amoxil should the pharmacy technician dispense?

8. How much Amoxil should the patient take at one time?

9. How many times can this prescription be refilled?

10. How often should the patient take Amoxil?

In Exercises 11–20, refer to Physician's Order Form 1.

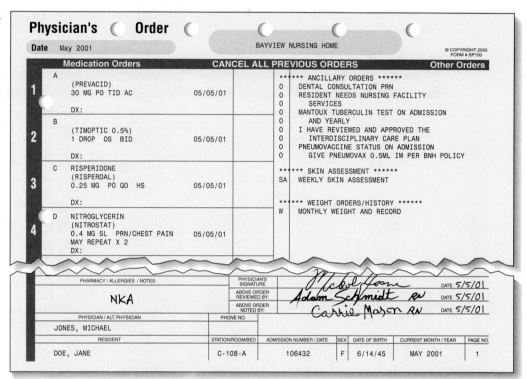

Physician's Order Form 1

11. When should Prevacid be administered?

12. By what route should Timoptic be given?

13. How often should Risperdal be administered?

14. How much Nitrostat should be given in a single dose?

15. By what route should Prevacid be given?

16. How often should Timoptic be administered?

17. How much Risperdal should be given in a single dose?

18. When should Risperdal be given?

19. By what route should Nitrostat be given?

20. If medications are delivered once a week to this facility, how many doses of Risperdal should be dispensed?

To check your answers, see page 344.

Medication Administration Systems

Most facilities have a standard schedule for administering medication (see Table 5-4). To minimize errors, many of them use the 24-hour clock (see Chapter 3). The person who verifies the transcription ensures that the times listed are appropriate for the medications. For example, some medications need to be given with food or after a meal, others on an empty stomach. Times may need to be adjusted to accommodate a patient's meals. A patient may take two or more medications with conflicting schedules. Again, the timing may need to be adjusted.

Table 5-4 Sample Times for Medication Administration

Frequency Ordered	Times to Administer
qd	0800
bid	0800 - 2000
tid	0800 - 1400 - 2000
qid	0800 - 1200 - 1600 - 2000
q 12 hrs	0800 - 2000
q 8 hrs	2400 - 0800 - 1600
q 6 hrs	2400 - 0600 - 1200 - 1800
qhs	2000

Medication Administration Records

Medication Administration Records (MAR) are legal documents that may be handwritten forms or computerized printouts. An MAR contains the same information as a physicians' order form. It specifies the actual times to administer the medication. It also provides a place to document that each medication has been given. Remember: by law, when you administer medication, you must *immediately* document this step.

Rule 5-2

An MAR must include the following information:

1. The full name of the medication, the dose, the route, and the frequency.
2. Times that accurately reflect the frequency specified.
3. The full name and identification number of the patient.
4. The date the order was written. If no start date is listed, then the assumption is that the date of order is the start date. Orders for narcotics and antibiotics should include end dates, according to your facility's policies.
5. Any special instructions or information as required by your facility. This includes, but is not limited to, the patient's diagnosis and weight.

EXAMPLE 1 Determine whether the MAR in Figure 5-4 is complete.

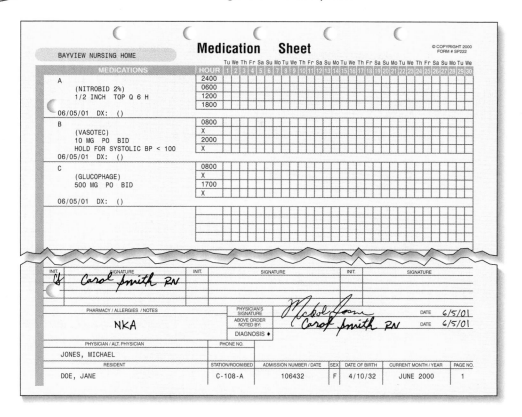

Figure 5-4 *Medication Administration Record (MAR)*

In Figure 5-4 all three orders are written correctly. In Order A, the drug is Nitrobid 2% cream, the dose is $\frac{1}{2}$ inch, the route is topical, and the frequency is every 6 hrs. The scheduled times are 2400 (midnight), 0600 (6:00 A.M.), 1200 (12:00 P.M.), and 1800 (6:00 P.M.).

In Order B, the drug is Vasotec, the dose is 10 mg, the route is oral, and the frequency is twice a day. This order includes a special instruction to hold the medication if the systolic blood pressure is below 100.

In Order C, the drug is Glucophage, the dose is 500 mg, the frequency is twice a day, and the route is oral. Glucophage must be administered with meals. Therefore, the times have been adjusted to fit the facility's meal schedule.

EXAMPLE 2 Determine whether MAR in Figure 5-5 is complete.

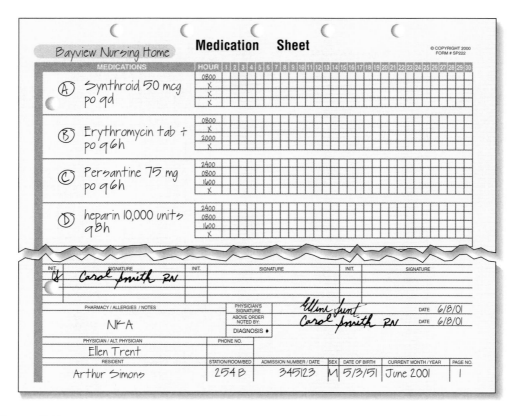

Figure 5-5

In Figure 5-5 Order A is correct. The drug is Synthroid, the dose is 50 mcg, the route is oral, and the frequency is daily. Order B may seem to have all required information, but the dose, 1 tablet, is not adequate. Erythromycin is available in several strengths. The order does not specify which dosage strength is intended. Order C contains an error in the times listed. Persantine 75 mg is to be given q6h, or every 6 hours. The times (2400 - 0800 - 1600) are for every 8 hours. If the error is not recognized, then the patient may not receive a therapeutic level of the drug. Order D does not include a route. Heparin can be administered either subcutaneously or intravenously. This order cannot be carried out as written.

Medication Cards

Some facilities use medication cards. Each drug order is listed on its own card. The cards for all patients are stored on a special rack according to the time of the next medication administration. At these specified hours, a health care worker gathers the cards and prepares the medications. After the medications have been administered, the cards are refiled based on the next set of administration times. Most medication cards have a grid representing all of the hours of the day. The times that medication is to be given are marked on the grid.

A medication card must contain the patient's name and room number, the full name of the drug, the dose, the route, the frequency, any special instructions, the administration times, and the date ordered.

Medication card systems have several disadvantages. Because of their small size, the cards are easily misplaced. Each medication is listed separately, increasing the potential for omitting a medication. Also, medication cards generally do not list allergies or diagnoses. By contrast, MARs list all drugs together where health care workers can see the big picture, including orders for medications that should not interact with each other.

EXAMPLE 1 Determine if medication card A below is complete.

Card A lists the patient's complete name, the room number, the physician who wrote the order, the date of the order, and the initials of the person who transcribed the order. According to the card, the drug is Zithromax, the dose is 250 mg, the route is oral, and the frequency is daily. The medication time of 8:00 A.M. is checked and is consistent with the frequency of the drug. The card is complete.

EXAMPLE 2 Determine if medication card B below is complete.

Card B lists the patient's complete name, the room number, the name of the physician who wrote the order, the date of the order, and the initials of the person who transcribed the order. The drug is Pathocil, the dose is 125 mg, the route is oral, and the frequency is three times a day after meals. Yet only two medication times are listed: 10:00 A.M. and 8:00 P.M. Moreover, neither time corresponds to the instruction to provide the medication after meals (p.c.). The card will need to be corrected before medication can be administered.

NAME	Melton, Lee
ROOM 118D	DR. Pringle

MEDICATION

Zithromax 250 mg
po qd

DATE ORDERED	INITIALS
4/17/01	GRT

A								X			
M	12	1	2	3	4	5	6	7	8	9	10	11
P											
M	12	1	2	3	4	5	6	7	8	9	10	11

Medication Card A

NAME	Jones, Sally
ROOM 322E	DR. Summer

MEDICATION

pathocil 125 mg
po tid pc

DATE ORDERED	INITIALS
8/22/01	MLC

A										X	
M	12	1	2	3	4	5	6	7	8	9	10	11
P								X			
M	12	1	2	3	4	5	6	7	8	9	10	11

Medication Card B

Computerized Medical Records

In order to provide the most effective care, health care providers should be aware of a patient's complete medical history, including information about earlier reactions to medications and any previously diagnosed medical conditions. In the past, this information was recorded on paper.

Now patient information is often entered directly into a computer either via a hand module or console at the patient's bedside or at a centralized console. Information can be easily updated and is accessible from these same locations. All information can be stored on disk. Hard copies can be printed at will and used for backup copies.

A computerized medical record (see Figure 5-6) includes all orders for a medication, administration times, and the patient's reaction to that medication. Lab results and observations, information about allergies, and other records can be obtained immediately. A computerized record can even be used to schedule anticipated procedures or to plan for the patient's eventual discharge. It is not, however, an MAR. A computerized record is not used as the ongoing working document that records signatures and initials whenever medications are administered.

```
6K   -0626                    CENTRAL CITY HOSPITAL                 PAGE 001
09/14/01  07:05
========================================
SMITH, JOHN                         M      39
SSN: 123456789   ACCT#: 501330269251
SERV: MULT     6K      067999
MD: JONES, MARY                                      PATIENT CARE WORKSHEET
DX: STAB WOUND IN ABD                                      TEMPORARY
SHORT STAY:
========================================
WORKSHEET: 09/14 07:15   TO 15:15
    DATA RETRIEVED ACROSS ALL ADMISSIONS:
        09/08/01     DRUG ALLERGY: NO KNOWN ALLERGY
    PATIENT IMFORMATION:
        09/08         ADMIT DX:STAB WOUND IN ABD
        09/08         PRINCIPAL DX:S/P EX LAP, DUODENAL REPAIR, MESENTERIC VESSEL REPAIR
        09/08         WT: ADM WT: 77.1 KG
    ALL CURRENT MEDICAL ORDERS:
      DOCTOR TO NURSE ORDERS:
        09/09  85.00 ACTIVITY, OUT OF BED, AMBULATE IN HALL TID, <09/09/01>
        09/08         --ALL ORDERS ON MULTIPLE TRAUMA PATIENTS TO BE WRITTEN OR COUNTERSIGNED
                      BY TRAUMA SERVICE EXCEPT FOR ICP MANAGEMENT ORDERS
        09/08         --NURSING CARE PER BURN/TRAUMA STANDARD OF CARE
        09/08         NOTIFY MD --FOR TEMP GREATER THAN 101.5
        09/08         --PNEUMATIC STOCKINGS THIGH -- FOR DVT PROPHYLAXIS
        09/08         --NG TO LCS.
        09/08         INCENTIVE SPIROMETER Q1H W/AWAKE
        09/08         JEJUNOSTOMY TUBE --FLUSH W/20CC NS Q6HRS.
        09/09         INCENTIVE SPIROMETER Q1H --COUGH/DEEP BREATH
        09/10         --INCREASE TF BY 20CC Q4HR UNTIL REACH GOAL OF 110/HR DONT CHECK
                      RESIDUALS --DECREASE IVF PROPORTIONAL TO TF
        09/12         --GLYCERIN SWABS TO BEDSIDE
        09/14         --HEP.LOCK IV
    DIET:
        09/08         DIET: NPO, <09/08/01>
    SCHEDULED MEDICATIONS:
    *   09/08         (ZANTAC) RANITIDINE IVPB 50 MG, IN 50ML 1/2 N/S, Q8H,
                      (09/08/01 13:00-..) 13
    F   09/13         (ATIVAN) *LORAZEPAM INJ (2MG/1ML) 0.5 MG, IV, NOW, --FOR AGITATION,
                      (09/13/01 05:24)
    *   09/13         THIAMINE TAB 100MG,, #1, (GIVE 1 TAB) JT, DAILY, (09/13/01 09:00-..) 09
    *   09/13         (FOLATE) FOLIC ACID TAB 1MG,, #1 (GIVE 1 TAB) JT, DAILY
                      (09/13/01 09:00-..) 09
    *   09/13         MULTIVIT THERAPEUTIC LIQ 5ML, JT, DAILY, (09/13/01 09:00-..) 09
    F*  09/13         (ATIVAN) *LORAZEPAM INJ (2MG/1ML) 0.5 MG, IV, Q6H, STARTING AT 14:00,
                      START TODAY, (09/13/01 14:00-..) 09 14
    *   09/14         (DEMEROL +**MEPERIDINE INJ (50MG/1ML) 50MG, IM, NOW, (09/14/01 05:10)
    PRN MEDICATIONS:
        09/14         (DEMEROL) +** MEPERIDINE 50MG, IM, (GIVE: 50MG TO 75MG), Q3H, PRN,
                      PAIN, <09/14/01 05:10-..>
        09/14         +**MEPERIDINE 75MG, IM, (GIVE: 50MG TO 75MG), Q3H, PRN, PAIN, <09/14/01
                      05:10-..>

        R=TIME TO RENEW    U=UNVERIFIED    F=REFRIGERATE    *=SCHEDULED MED
        APOSTROPHE=BILL ON ORDER    +=MED TEACHING SHEET AVAILABLE
        ++=PROVIDE PT W/DRUG LEAFLET OBTAINED FROM PHARMACY
    IV-S: (WITH OR WITHOUT ADDITIVES):
    U   09/13         IV SALINE LOCK CONVERT TO
    U   09/12         DRUG --KCL20MEQ/MVI5ML/THIAMINE10 OMG/MGSO4 2GM, $25.00. 00999 D5-
                      1/2NS, 1000ML, 100ML/H, DAILY, CONT TIL DC'D (MISC MED), <09/12/01
                      09:14-..>
    U   09/12         KCL 20MEQ, PREMIXED/D5-1/2NS 1000ML, IV 40ML/H, CONT TIL DC'D
                      (MISC MED), <09/12/01 12:56-..>
================================================================================
SMITH, JOHN                                              PATIENT CARE WORKSHEET
```

Figure 5-6 *A computerized medical record contains all information connected with a patient's hospital stay, including all ordered medications.*

When in Doubt, Check

A nurse is preparing medications. An entry in the MAR calls for 600 mg of Lasix IV, higher than what she usually administers. She checks the *Physicians' Desk Reference*. It indicates that doses this high may be used for congestive heart failure, the patient's diagnosis. Still, the nurse is not comfortable with this level. She checks the original order on the Physician's Order Form and discovers a potential error (see Figure 5-7).

Think Before You Act

By using her critical thinking skills, the nurse has prevented a serious error. The Lasix order appears to be 600 mg. However, the nurse realizes that the second zero of 600 is actually the loop of the *q* from the Digoxin order. The intended dose of Lasix is 60 mg. If the nurse had not checked the physician's orders, she might have given ten times more than the physician intended. When in doubt, always verify the order written on the chart.

Figure 5-7

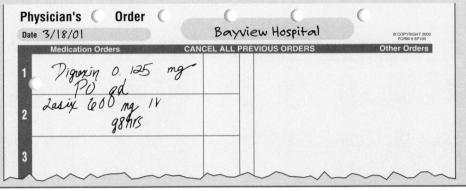

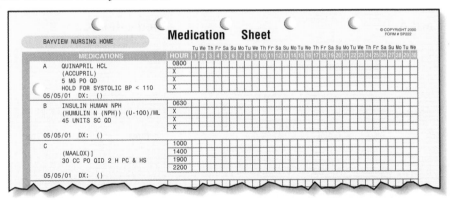

REVIEW and PRACTICE

MEDICATION ADMINISTRATION SYSTEMS

Exercises 1–6 refer to MAR 1 for Jane Doe.

1. What action must you take before administering Accupril?

2. What dose of Accupril should this patient receive?

3. At what time is the insulin to be given?

4. By what route is the insulin given?

5. This unit's schedule for QID medications is 0800 - 1200 - 1700 - 2000. Why is Maalox scheduled for different times?

6. How much Maalox will this patient receive at 1400?

Exercises 7–20 refer to Medication Cards A through J.

7. When should Gina Pilotti be given Furosemide?

8. What is the route of administration for Cecile Parsons's Viroptic?

9. Why are no times marked on medication card C?

10. What is the route of administration for Ann Briggs's Ancef?

11. Which cards list medications that should be given at 0800?

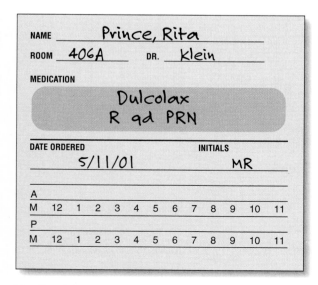

Medication Card A

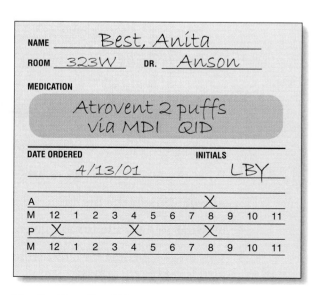

Medication Card B

Medication Card C

Medication Card D

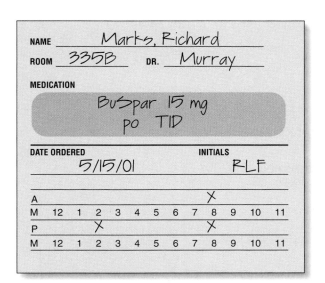

Medication Card E

NAME Marks, Richard
ROOM 335B   DR. Murray
MEDICATION
BuSpar 15 mg
po TID

| DATE ORDERED | INITIALS |
| 5/15/01 | RLF |

A								X			
M	12	1	2	3	4	5	6	7	8	9	10	11
P		X						X			
M	12	1	2	3	4	5	6	7	8	9	10	11

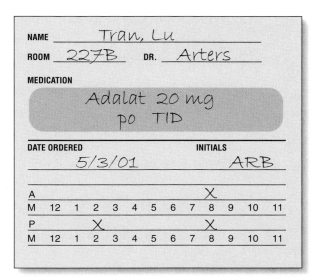

Medication Card F

NAME Tran, Lu
ROOM 227B   DR. Arters
MEDICATION
Adalat 20 mg
po TID

| DATE ORDERED | INITIALS |
| 5/3/01 | ARB |

A								X			
M	12	1	2	3	4	5	6	7	8	9	10	11
P		X						X			
M	12	1	2	3	4	5	6	7	8	9	10	11

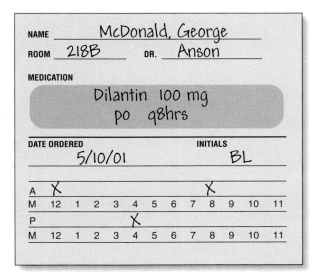

Medication Card G

NAME McDonald, George
ROOM 218B   DR. Anson
MEDICATION
Dilantin 100 mg
po   q8hrs

| DATE ORDERED | INITIALS |
| 5/10/01 | BL |

A	X							X			
M	12	1	2	3	4	5	6	7	8	9	10	11
P				X							
M	12	1	2	3	4	5	6	7	8	9	10	11

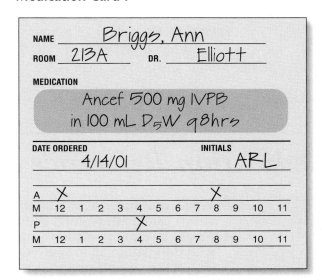

Medication Card H

NAME Briggs, Ann
ROOM 213A   DR. Elliott
MEDICATION
Ancef 500 mg IVPB
in 100 mL D₅W q8hrs

| DATE ORDERED | INITIALS |
| 4/14/01 | ARL |

A	X							X			
M	12	1	2	3	4	5	6	7	8	9	10	11
P				X							
M	12	1	2	3	4	5	6	7	8	9	10	11

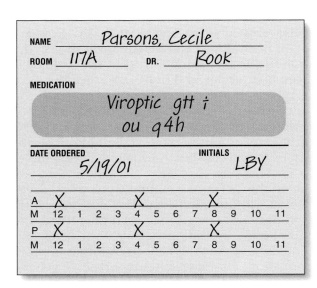

Medication Card I

NAME Parsons, Cecile
ROOM 117A   DR. Rook
MEDICATION
Viroptic gtt ī
ou q4h

| DATE ORDERED | INITIALS |
| 5/19/01 | LBY |

A	X			X				X			
M	12	1	2	3	4	5	6	7	8	9	10	11
P	X			X				X			
M	12	1	2	3	4	5	6	7	8	9	10	11

Medication Card J

NAME Pillotti, Gina
ROOM 220B   DR. Gee
MEDICATION
Furosemide 80 mg
IV stat

| DATE ORDERED | INITIALS |
| 4/18/01 | NLS |

A											
M	12	1	2	3	4	5	6	7	8	9	10	11
P											
M	12	1	2	3	4	5	6	7	8	9	10	11

12. Which cards do *not* include all of the required elements for a drug order?

13. What is the frequency for Lu Tran's Adalat?

14. What is the route for Richard Marks's BuSpar?

15. What medication should George McDonald receive at 1600?

16. What dose of Humulin N should Tom Beiler receive at 0700?

17. What is the route for Anita Best's Atrovent?

18. What dose of Ancef should Ann Briggs receive at 0800?

19. How often does Anna Ott receive Normodyne?

20. If medications are delivered daily, how many doses of Dilantin should be supplied for George McDonald for 24 hours?

To check your answers, see page 345.

Medication Reference Materials

When you dispense or administer medications, you are responsible for knowing their effects. Hundreds of drugs exist. New ones are produced all the time. You cannot memorize all of the information you might need to know. Therefore, you need to be familiar with drug information sources.

Package inserts provided by the manufacturers with each medication are important reference tools. They describe intended effects, possible side effects, typical doses, dosage forms available, conditions under which the drug should not be used, and special precautions to be taken while using the drug. See Chapter 6 to learn more.

Information from package inserts is also printed in the *Physicians' Desk Reference* (PDR). Other versions feature nonprescription medications and herbal medications. The PDR has information about most currently available prescription drugs. A new volume is produced each year. Many physicians' offices, pharmacies, and health care facilities have the PDR available for employee use.

Many other guides for health care professionals are available, including the United States Pharmacopeia/National Formulary. Most are updated every year or two. Although many of these books have titles suggesting they are for nurses, they are useful to all health care workers. Their information is similar to the PDR's, but they often have simpler language.

Internet users can access information about the 200 most commonly prescribed drugs at www.rxlist.com/top200.htm. This site provides information about the most frequently prescribed drugs based on a list published in *American Druggist*. For each drug listed, the site lists appropriate doses of the drug for specific indications, available dosages and dosage forms, descriptions of the pills or liquids, and the drug's effects. Another Internet site, www.druginfonet.com, lists drug information, allows searches by brand or generic names, and provides many other useful features.

CHAPTER 5 REVIEW

CHECK UP

1. What action should you take when you receive this drug order: *Dilaudid tab 2 mg po PRN for pain q4h*

2. What action should you take when you receive this drug order: *Codeine tab 30 mg po qid*

In Exercises 3–6, refer to Prescription 1.

3. What instructions should be printed for the patient?

4. How many times can this prescription be refilled?

5. By what route should this medication be administered?

6. What information should be on the drug label to verify that this medication is appropriate for the ordered route?

In Exercises 7–12, refer to Physician's Order Form 2.

7. How often should Theodur be given?

8. By what route is Serevent administered?

9. If Jane Doe receives Percocet for pain at 4:00 A.M., when will she be permitted to have another dose?

10. If medications are delivered to this unit once daily, how many Percocet tablets should be dispensed at one time?

11. What dose of Theodur should Jane Doe be given?

12. How often should Serevent be given?

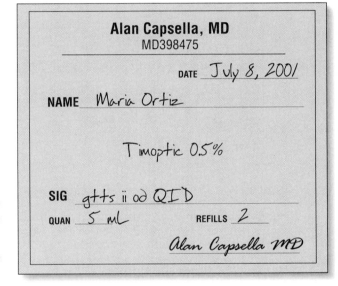

Prescription 1

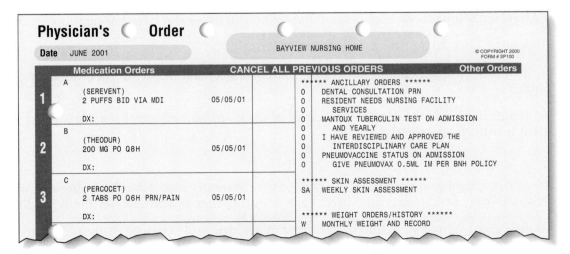

Physician's Order Form 2

In Exercises 13–18, refer to MAR 3 for Arthur Simons.

13. By what route is the tobramycin to be given?

14. What dose of Propulsid does Mr. Simons receive?

15. What medications does Mr. Simons receive at 8:00 P.M.?

16. How frequently does Mr. Simons receive Trental?

17. Should Mr. Simons be served breakfast at 7:00 A.M., 7:30 A.M., or 8:00 A.M.?

18. Which orders do *not* have all of the essential elements for an MAR order? State what is missing from each of them.

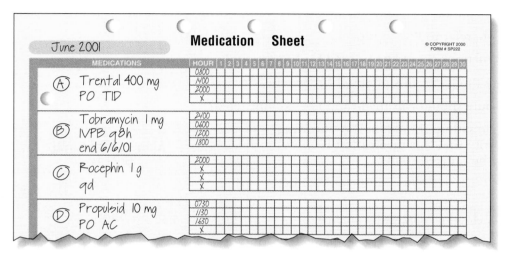

MAR 3

In Exercises 19–26, refer to Medication Cards A through F.

19. By what route is Adam Trask's Bleph-10 given?

20. What dose of Premarin does Marla O'Brien receive?

21. At what times should Roger Ellis be given Sinemet?

22. Which cards list orders to be administered at 1600?

23. If Margaret Bell had a dose of Benadryl at 0200, when can she have her next dose?

24. How often does Angel Corazon receive heparin?

25. How would Mark Eshelman's medication card be different if the drug order called for q6h instead of qid?

26. Which medication cards do *not* include all of the essential elements for a drug order? Which element is missing from each?

27. At 1:30 P.M., you are preparing medications for patients who have just returned from lunch. Describe some precautions you might take to ensure that you administer the right dose.

28. You have just started your shift on a unit with geriatric and pediatric patients. You are scheduled to administer drugs to several elderly patients with Alzheimer's as well as to several children. What steps should you take to ensure that you administer the right drugs to the right patients?

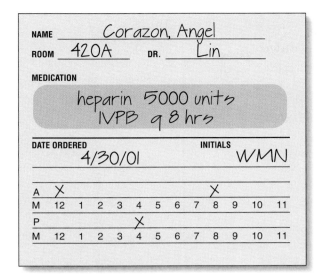

Medication Card A

NAME	Corazon, Angel											
ROOM	420A	DR.	Lin									

MEDICATION

heparin 5000 units
IVPB q 8 hrs

DATE ORDERED						INITIALS						
4/30/01						WMN						

A	X					X						
M	12	1	2	3	4	5	6	7	8	9	10	11
P					X							
M	12	1	2	3	4	5	6	7	8	9	10	11

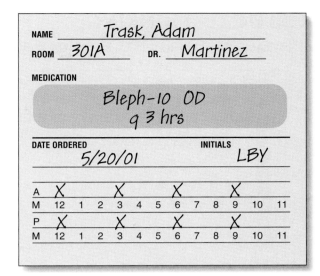

Medication Card B

NAME	Trask, Adam											
ROOM	301A	DR.	Martinez									

MEDICATION

Bleph-10 OD
q 3 hrs

DATE ORDERED						INITIALS						
5/20/01						LBY						

A	X			X			X			X		
M	12	1	2	3	4	5	6	7	8	9	10	11
P	X			X			X			X		
M	12	1	2	3	4	5	6	7	8	9	10	11

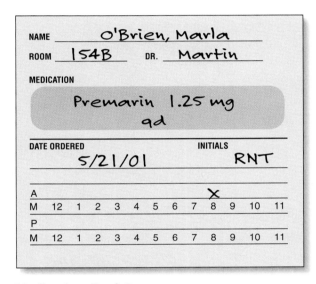

Medication Card C

NAME	O'Brien, Marla											
ROOM	154B	DR.	Martin									

MEDICATION

Premarin 1.25 mg
qd

DATE ORDERED						INITIALS						
5/21/01						RNT						

A							X					
M	12	1	2	3	4	5	6	7	8	9	10	11
P												
M	12	1	2	3	4	5	6	7	8	9	10	11

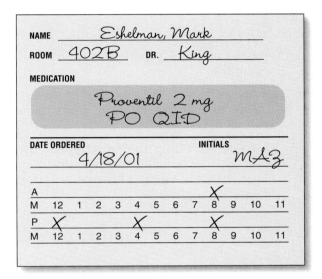

Medication Card D

NAME	Eshelman, Mark											
ROOM	402B	DR.	King									

MEDICATION

Proventil 2 mg
PO QID

DATE ORDERED						INITIALS						
4/18/01						MAZ						

A								X				
M	12	1	2	3	4	5	6	7	8	9	10	11
P	X				X				X			
M	12	1	2	3	4	5	6	7	8	9	10	11

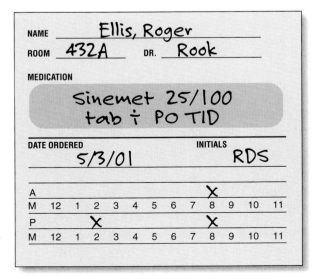

Medication Card E

NAME	Ellis, Roger											
ROOM	432A	DR.	Rook									

MEDICATION

Sinemet 25/100
tab ī PO TID

DATE ORDERED						INITIALS						
5/3/01						RDS						

A								X				
M	12	1	2	3	4	5	6	7	8	9	10	11
P			X					X				
M	12	1	2	3	4	5	6	7	8	9	10	11

Medication Card F

NAME	Bell, Margaret											
ROOM	221D	DR.	Roe									

MEDICATION

Benadryl 25 mg
PO q4h PRN/itch

DATE ORDERED						INITIALS						
4/29/01						WC						

A												
M	12	1	2	3	4	5	6	7	8	9	10	11
P												
M	12	1	2	3	4	5	6	7	8	9	10	11

CRITICAL THINKING

What action should you take with the following drug order?

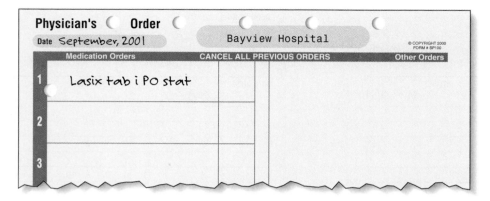

Physician's Order — Bayview Hospital
© COPYRIGHT 2000 FORM # SP100

Date September, 2001

Medication Orders | CANCEL ALL PREVIOUS ORDERS | Other Orders

1. Lasix tab i PO stat
2.
3.

CASE STUDY

A physician gives a patient the following prescription:

1. One of your jobs is to instruct patients how to take prescription drugs. What should you tell Martin Burke?

2. If you are filling the prescription, how many tablets will you dispense to the patient? Will you refill the prescription?

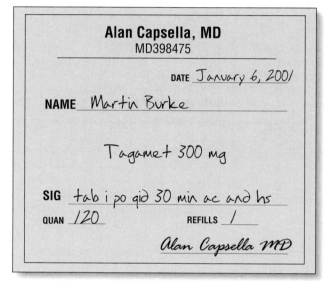

Alan Capsella, MD
MD398475

DATE January 6, 2001

NAME Martin Burke

Tagamet 300 mg

SIG tab i po qid 30 min ac and hs

QUAN 120   REFILLS 1

Alan Capsella MD

To check your answers, see page 345.

INTERNET ACTIVITY

Note: The Internet is a research tool from which to get basic information. Validate the accuracy of all Internet information.

You receive a physician's order for cephalexin 500 mg q6h. In the past, you have given only 250 mg doses. You want to verify that 500 mg is safe. Use the Top 200 Prescribed Drugs list from the Internet to check the safety of this dose.

Assignment: Type *www.rxlist.com/top200.htm* in the address bar of your Internet search program. Find cephalexin, then read about "Dosage and Administration." Determine whether the ordered dose is safe.

DRUG LABELS and PACKAGE INSERTS

Objectives

When you have completed Chapter 6, you will be able to:

- Identify on a drug label the drug name, form, dosage strength, route, warnings, and manufacturing and storage information.
- Locate directions on drug labels and package inserts for reconstituting and diluting medications.
- Recognize different types of tablets and capsules.
- Distinguish administration routes for medications.
- Locate additional information in a package insert.

Locating Information on Drug Labels and Package Inserts

In order to prepare and administer drugs, you must understand information that appears on drug labels, including the drug name, form, dosage strength, total amount in the container, route of administration, warnings, storage requirements, and manufacturing information.

Below are four drug labels. Several items are marked to guide you through the following discussion.

Drug Name

Every drug has an official name—its generic name. By law, this name must appear on the drug's label. It is also recorded with a national listing of drugs: the United States Pharmacopeia (USP) and the National Formulary (NF). In Figures 6-1, 6-2, 6-3, and 6-4, letter A points to each drug's generic name. Letter B points to USP, which indicates that this drug's name is recorded with the United States Pharmacopeia.

Some drug labels list only a generic name (see Figure 6-4). Many include the trade, or brand name used to market the drug. Letter C in Figures 6-1, 6-2, and 6-3 points to the trade name, which is listed before the generic name. A trade name is the property of a specific drug company. The registered mark ® indicates the name has been legally registered with the U.S. Patent and Trademark Office. Several companies may manufacture a drug but market it under different trade names.

Figure 6-1

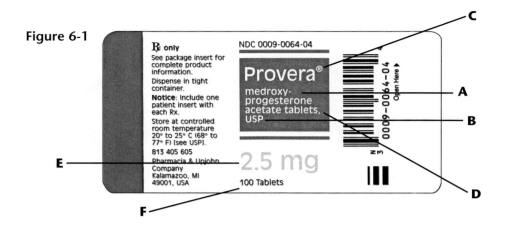

C

NDC 0009-0064-04

℞ only
See package insert for complete product information.

Dispense in tight container.

Notice: Include one patient insert with each Rx.

Store at controlled room temperature 20° to 25° C (68° to 77° F) [see USP].

813 405 605

Pharmacia & Upjohn Company
Kalamazoo, MI
49001, USA

Provera®
medroxy-
progesterone
acetate tablets,
USP — A

— B

2.5 mg

100 Tablets

E

D

F

Figure 6-2

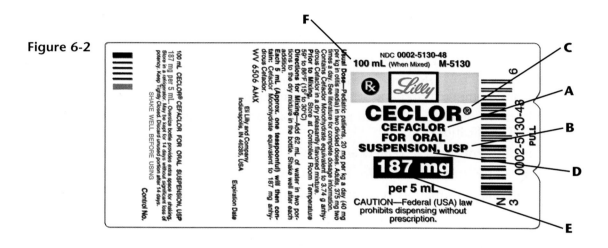

F

NDC 0002-5130-48
100 mL (When Mixed) M-5130

℞ *Lilly*

CECLOR® — A
CEFACLOR
FOR ORAL
SUSPENSION, USP — B

187 mg — D

per 5 mL — E

CAUTION—Federal (USA) law prohibits dispensing without prescription.

C

100 mL CECLOR® CEFACLOR FOR ORAL SUSPENSION, USP 187 mg per 5 mL. Oversize bottle provides extra space for shaking. Store in a refrigerator. May be kept for 14 days without significant loss of potency. Keep Tightly Closed. Discard unused portion after 14 days.

SHAKE WELL BEFORE USING

Control No.

WV 6506 AMX

Eli Lilly and Company
Indianapolis, IN 46285, USA

Expiration Date

Usual Dose—Pediatric patients, 20 mg per kg a day (40 mg per kg in otitis media) in two divided doses. Adults, 375 mg two times a day. See literature for complete dosage information.

Contains Cefaclor in a dry pleasantly flavored mixture.

Prior to Mixing, Store at Controlled Room Temperature 59° to 86°F (15° to 30°C).

Directions for Mixing—Add 62 mL of water in two portions to the dry mixture in the bottle. Shake well after each addition.

Each 5 mL (Approx. one teaspoonful) will then contain: Cefaclor Monohydrate equivalent to 187 mg anhydrous Cefaclor.

Figure 6-3

ucb Pharma — F

PHARMACIST: Dispense in a tight, light-resistant container with a child-resistant closure.

Store at controlled room temperature, 15°-30°C (59°-86°F).

NDC 50474-902-50   500 TABLETS

LORTAB® 5/500 — C

HYDROCODONE BITARTRATE — A
AND ACETAMINOPHEN
TABLETS, USP — B
5 mg/500 mg

USUAL DOSAGE: See package insert for complete dosage recommendations.

COPY   1/2"

Lot No.:
Exp. Date:

Manufactured for
UCB Pharma, Inc.
Smyrna, GA 30080
by Mallinckrodt Inc.
Hobart, NY 13788

Each scored, white with blue specks tablet contains:

Hydrocodone Bitartrate . . . . 5 mg
Acetaminophen . . . . 500 mg

℞ only

3 50474-902-50 9

Rev. 2/99
P/N 1002570

D

E

Physicians can write drug orders using either generic or trade names. Some companies produce drugs under their generic names and market them at a lower cost than the trade-name equivalents. For example, ibuprofen is sold under its generic name as well as trade names such as Advil and Motrin.

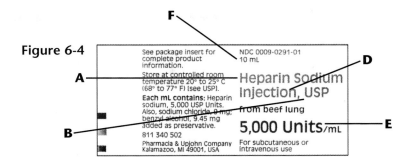

Figure 6-4

Rule 6-1

You must know both the generic and trade names of drugs.

EXAMPLE 1 Suppose a patient is allergic to Vicodin, a narcotic painkiller. The generic drugs in Vicodin, hydrocodone bitartrate and acetaminophen, are also found in the trade-name drugs Anexsia, Lortab, and Zydone. If you administer one of these drugs as an alternative to Vicodin, the patient may have a similar allergic reaction. When you record a patient's drug allergy, include both the trade and generic names. Resources such as the PDR (*Physicians' Desk Reference*) provide information about a drug's ingredients.

Form of the Drug

Manufacturers may offer the same drug in different forms. For example, penicillin is available as a tablet, a capsule, a liquid for oral administration, and an injection. Every label indicates the drug's form. Solid oral medications come in the form of tablets, capsules, gelcaps, and caplets. Liquid forms include oral, injections, inhalants, drops, sprays, and mists. Other forms of medication include ointments, creams, lotions, patches, suppositories, and shampoos. See letter D in Figures 6-1, 6-2, 6-3, and 6-4.

Dosage Strength

Drug labels include information about the amount of the drug present. This amount, combined with information about the form of the drug, identifies the drug's *dosage strength*. On the label, the dosage strength is stated as the amount of drug per dosage unit. In most cases, the amount of the drug is listed in grams (g), milligrams (mg), micrograms (mcg or μg), or grains (gr). In certain cases, such as insulin, the amount is listed in Units. Certain liquid drugs, such as hydrogen peroxide and glycerin, may list the amount in milliliters (mL).

For solid medications, the dosage strength is the amount of drug present per tablet, capsule, or other form. In Figure 6-1, letter E notes the amount of Provera (2.5 mg) present in a tablet, the form of medication. The dosage strength is 2.5 mg/tablet. *Note: For most solid medications, if the unit is not listed, assume it is one tablet, one capsule, one gelcap, and so forth.*

For liquid medications, the dosage strength is the amount of the drug present in a certain quantity of solution. Recall from Chapter 2 that a solute (the drug) is mixed with a solvent or diluent (such as saline) to create a solution. You need to know both the amount of the drug and the amount of the total solution in which it is contained.

The amount of solution that is considered a dosage unit varies. For example, in Figure 6-2 (letter E), when Ceclor is prepared properly, 187 mg of drug are present in every 5 mL of solution. In this case, 5 mL is the dosage unit. The dosage strength is 187 mg/5 mL. In Figure 6-4 (letter E), however, 5000 Units of Heparin Sodium are present in every 1 mL of solution. Here, 1 mL is the dosage unit. The dosage strength for this medication is 5000 Units/mL.

Pharmaceutical companies manufacture medications with dosage strengths corresponding to commonly prescribed doses. This practice reduces the risk of medical error by reducing the number of dosage calculations.

Combination Drugs

The generic names and dosage strengths of all components of a combination drug must appear on the label. The label in Figure 6-3 lists the components of Lortab 5/500: hydrocodone bitartrate and acetaminophen. It also provides information about the individual drugs' dosage strengths. The line 5 mg/500 mg indicates that Lortab 5/500 contains 5 mg of hydrocodone bitratrate *and* 500 mg of acetaminophen per tablet. All combination drugs have a trade name, usually used in drug orders. For example, a drug order might read *Lortab 5/500 1 tab q 4-6h PRN for pain*. The order would *not* read *hydrocodone bitartrate 5 mg, acetaminophen 500 mg, q 4-6h PRN for pain*.

Total Number or Volume in Container

Many oral medications are packaged separately in *unit doses*. These packages may contain a single dosage unit, for example, a single tablet or a vial with 2 mL of solution for injection. If the container holds more than one dosage unit, the total number or volume must be listed on the label. See letter F in Figures 6-1, 6-2, 6-3, and 6-4. Nonprescription medications are often packaged in multiple-dose containers. Figure 6-5 indicates that nonprescription Motrin IB is available in containers of 50 gelcaps (see letter F), each gelcap with 200 mg of drug.

Figure 6-5

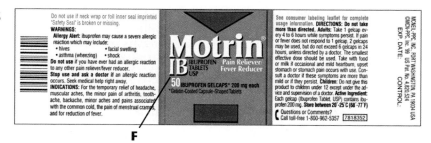

F

Figure 6-6 shows the label for Theo-24, a prescription medication. The container has 100 capsules, each one packaged as a unit dose (see letter F). In Figure 6-7, the container of Synthroid provides a unit-dose of 200 mcg. The term *unit dose* is not on the label. However, the label's directions indicate that you reconstitute the drug, administer it intravenously, and discard any unused portion. The container is used once.

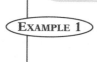

Rule 6-2

Do not confuse the total amount of drug in the container with the dosage strength.

EXAMPLE 1 According to Figure 6-1, the Provera container holds 100 tablets, with a dosage strength of 2.5 mg per tablet. The entire container holds 100 × 2.5 mg, or 250 mg of drug, whereas an individual tablet holds 2.5 mg of drug.

According to Figure 6-2, each 5 mL of Ceclor solution contains 187 mg of drug when mixed. The entire amount of solution, when mixed, is 100 mL, not 5 mL. The entire container, therefore, holds 100 mL ÷ 5 mL, or 20 unit doses. Even though you mix the entire contents of the container, you will only administer a small portion of it at a time.

Figure 6-6

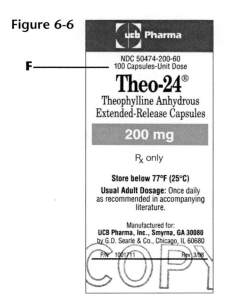

F——

Figure 6-7

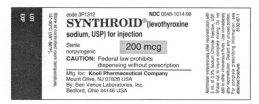

Route of Administration

Directions for the route of administration may be specified on the label. This information may not be included for oral medications. However, if a tablet or a capsule is not to be swallowed, additional information will be provided. For example, the label for Nitrostat shows it is administered sublingually, under the tongue (Figure 6-8, letter G). Chewable tablets will be labeled as such (Figure 6-9, letter G).

Liquid medications may be given orally or injected. Labels will indicate whether an injection is given intradermally (ID), intravenously (IV), intramuscularly (IM), or subcutaneously (SC) (see Figures 6-10 and 6-11, letter G). Labels will indicate other routes as well. For example, Vanceril is an aerosol that is inhaled (see Figure 6-12, letter G).

Figure 6-8

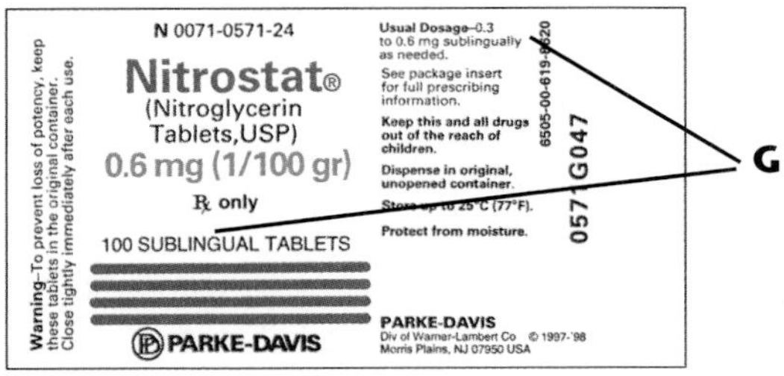

Figure 6-9

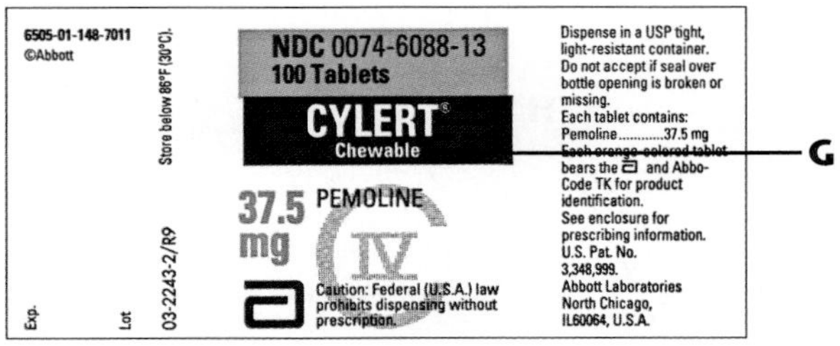

Figure 6-10

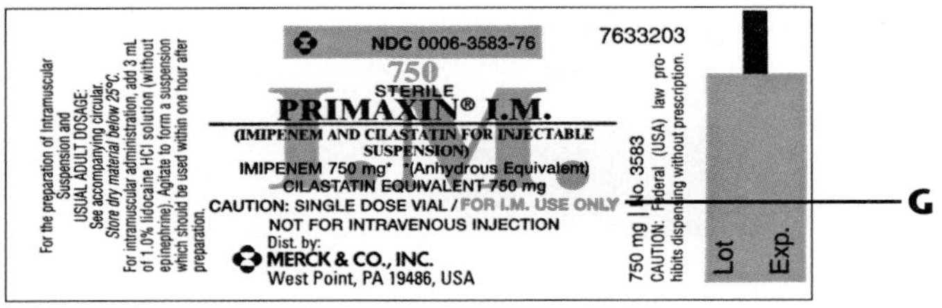

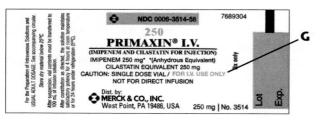

Figure 6-11

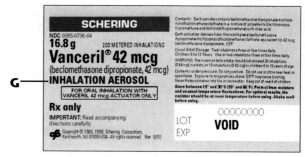

Figure 6-12

ERROR ALERT!

Give the right medication by the right route.

Cortisporin is an anti-inflammatory medication that is available in a variety of forms, including an antibacterial suspension for otic (ear) use and an antimicrobial suspension for ophthalmic (eye) use. The usual dosage of the otic suspension is 4 drops instilled three to four times a day into the affected ear. The usual dosage of the ophthalmic suspension is one or two drops instilled every 3 or 4 hours. If you were to carry out an order for the otic suspension by administering it to the patient's eye, you would not only fail to provide appropriate care for the ear, you would also cause considerable irritation to the eye. *The bottom line: do not administer drugs by any route other than intended, as described in the drug label and on the order.*

Warnings

Warnings on labels help health care workers administer drugs safely. They include statements such as, "This is a high potency product. Keep patient under close observation of a physician." (See Figure 6-13, letter H.) Controlled substances such as phenobarbital warn: "May be habit forming." Other labels indicate that the contents are poisonous (Figure 6-14, letter H). Labels may carry warnings for specific groups of patients. Some labels state that the product is not safe for pregnant women or for children. Other labels describe harmful effects from combinations with other products.

Every facility follows guidelines for disposing of drugs that are not used. The guidelines for medications that carry warnings are especially strict. For example, in some cases, you destroy (e.g., flush) narcotics with a co-worker as witness, then provide appropriate documentation.

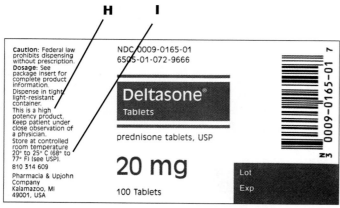

Figure 6-13

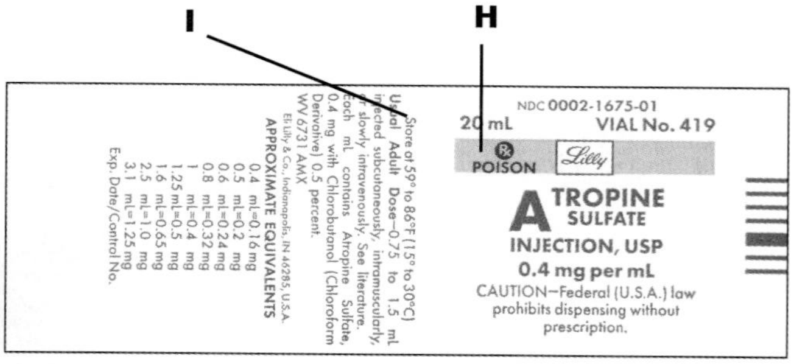

Figure 6-14

Storage Information

Some drugs must be stored under specific conditions to maintain their potency and effectiveness. Storage information will appear on the drug's label. The label may have information about storage temperature, exposure to light, or the length of time the drug will remain potent after the container has been opened. Storage at the wrong temperature or exposure to light can trigger a chemical reaction that makes the drug unusable. (See Figures 6-13 and 6-14, letter I, for storage information.)

Manufacturing Information

Pharmaceutical manufacturers are strictly regulated by the U.S. Food and Drug Administration (FDA). FDA regulations state that every drug label must include the name of the manufacturer (Figure 6-15, letter J); an expiration date, abbreviated EXP, after which the drug may no longer be used (letter K); and the lot number (letter L).

Figure 6-15

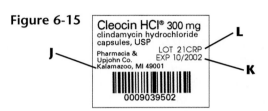

Medications are produced in batches, known as lots. The lot number is a code that indicates when and where a drug was produced. It allows the manufacturer to trace problems linked to a particular batch. If a manufacturer has to remove an entire lot from the market because of contamination, suspected tampering, or unexpected side effects, the lot number helps identify which batch to recall.

Rule 6-3

Never use a drug after the expiration date has passed.

Older drugs may become chemically unstable or altered. As a result, they may not provide the correct dosage strength. Worse, they could have an effect different from the intended one. Advise patients to check the expiration dates on all drug labels. If they have not used a product by the date listed, they should discard it. At an inpatient setting, the medication may need to be returned to the pharmacy, depending on the facility's policy.

Information About Reconstituting Drugs

Some drugs, such as antibiotics for pediatric use, are packaged in powder form. You reconstitute the drug (add liquid to the powder) shortly before administering it. Reconstituted medications remain potent for only a short amount of time. The label indicates the time period within which they can be safely administered (see Figures 6-16 and 6-17, letter M).

Figure 6-16

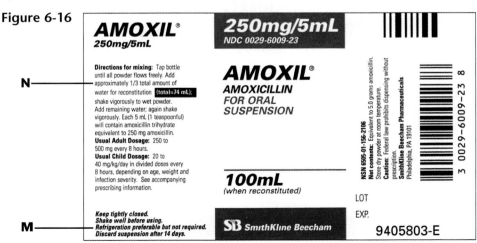

Figure 6-17

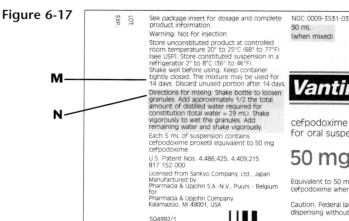

See package insert for dosage and complete product information.

Warning: Not for injection

Store unconstituted product at controlled room temperature 20° to 25°C (68° to 77°F) [see USP]. Store constituted suspension in a refrigerator 2° to 8°C (36° to 46°F). Shake well before using. Keep container tightly closed. The mixture may be used for 14 days. Discard unused portion after 14 days.

Directions for mixing: Shake bottle to loosen granules. Add approximately 1/2 the total amount of distilled water required for constitution (total water = 29 mL). Shake vigorously to wet the granules. Add remaining water and shake vigorously.

Each 5 mL of suspension contains cefpodoxime proxetil equivalent to 50 mg cefpodoxime.

U.S. Patent Nos. 4,486,425; 4,409,215 817 152 000

Licensed from Sankyo Company, Ltd., Japan Manufactured by Pharmacia & Upjohn S.A.-N.V., Puurs - Belgium for Pharmacia & Upjohn Company Kalamazoo, MI 49001, USA

5Q4992/1

NDC 0009-3531-03
50 mL
(when mixed)

Pharmacia & Upjohn

Vantin™ For Oral Suspension

cefpodoxime proxetil for oral suspension

50 mg per 5 mL

Equivalent to 50 mg per 5 mL cefpodoxime when constituted

Caution: Federal law prohibits dispensing without prescription.

M

N

Other drugs must be diluted before they are administered; they too must be used within a limited time. Directions for reconstituting or diluting a drug appear on the label (see Figures 6-16 and 6-17, letter N). Additional information can be found in the package insert, discussed below.

ERROR ALERT!

Consider the age and health needs of your patient when you administer a drug.

Suppose the drug order reads *Biaxin 250 mg po b.i.d.* Biaxin, an antibiotic, is available in 250-mg tablets and as an oral suspension with a reconstituted dosage strength of 125 mg per 5 mL. (An oral suspension is a liquid that contains solid particles of medication. You shake the medication before administering it, suspending the particles.)

It may seem logical to fill the order with one tablet. Yet the age or health of the patient may make a liquid the better choice, especially for children or patients who have difficulty swallowing. If you see a situation where another form of a drug may work better, consult the physician or pharmacist about changing the form of the drug.

Package Inserts

Package inserts provide complete and authoritative information about a medication. The information in package inserts can also be found in the PDR and other guides. Figure 6-18 shows a portion of a package insert. Table 6-1 summarizes the sections of a package insert.

Figure 6-18

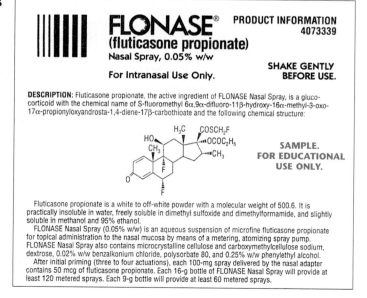

FLONASE®
(fluticasone propionate)
Nasal Spray, 0.05% w/w

PRODUCT INFORMATION
4073339

For Intranasal Use Only.

SHAKE GENTLY BEFORE USE.

DESCRIPTION: Fluticasone propionate, the active ingredient of FLONASE Nasal Spray, is a glucocorticoid with the chemical name of S-fluoromethyl 6α,9α-difluoro-11β-hydroxy-16α-methyl-3-oxo-17α-propionyloxyandrosta-1,4-diene-17β-carbothioate and the following chemical structure:

SAMPLE. FOR EDUCATIONAL USE ONLY.

Fluticasone propionate is a white to off-white powder with a molecular weight of 500.6. It is practically insoluble in water, freely soluble in dimethyl sulfoxide and dimethylformamide, and slightly soluble in methanol and 95% ethanol.

FLONASE Nasal Spray (0.05% w/w) is an aqueous suspension of microfine fluticasone propionate for topical administration to the nasal mucosa by means of a metering, atomizing spray pump.

FLONASE Nasal Spray also contains microcrystalline cellulose and carboxymethylcellulose sodium, dextrose, 0.02% w/w benzalkonium chloride, polysorbate 80, and 0.25% w/w phenylethyl alcohol.

After initial priming (three to four actuations), each 100-mg spray delivered by the nasal adapter contains 50 mcg of fluticasone propionate. Each 16-g bottle of FLONASE Nasal Spray will provide at least 120 metered sprays. Each 9-g bottle will provide at least 60 metered sprays.

Table 6-1 Sections of a Package Insert

Description	Chemical and physical description of the drug
Clinical Pharmacology	Description of the actions of the drug
Indications and Usage	Medical conditions in which the drug is safe and effective; instructions for usage
Contraindications	Conditions and situations under which the drug should not be administered
Warnings	Information about serious, possibly fatal, side effects
Precautions	Information about drug interactions and other conditions that may cause unwanted side effects
Adverse Reactions	Less serious, anticipated side effects that can be caused by the drug
Overdosage	Effects of overdoses and instructions for treatment
Dosage and Administration	Recommended dosages under various conditions and recommendations for administration routes
Preparation for Administration	Directions for reconstituting or diluting the drug, if necessary
Manufacturer Supply	Information on dosage strengths and forms of the drug available

CRITICAL THINKING ON THE JOB

Read Labels Carefully

A nurse is filling the order *Synthroid 0.025 mg p.o. q.d.* Synthroid is available in tablets of 11 different strengths; each in a different color. The nurse has access to tablets in 0.025 mg (orange), 0.050 mg (white), 0.125 mg (brown), and 0.150 mg (blue) doses.

Looking quickly at the labels, the nurse sees a Synthroid label with "25" on it. Without realizing it is for 0.125 mg, he removes a tablet. When he tries to administer it, the patient tells him that her usual pill is orange, not brown. The nurse checks the order and replaces the incorrect tablet with the correct one.

Think Before You Act

In this example, the nurse made an initial mistake. He did not carefully compare the drug order with the drug label. He did, however, listen to the patient and recheck his work. Looking at Figures 6-19 and 6-20, you may think that the nurse's error was reasonable given the similarity between the labels. Still, this error should have been avoided. The nurse should have read the label three times before trying to administer the drug. This rule is especially important when you administer a drug that is available in different dosage strengths or is designed for different route of administration.

Fortunately, the patient gave the nurse an opportunity to catch the error. When she questioned the color, the nurse listened. However, if he had not listened, or the patient had not alerted him, he may have administered five times the amount of the drug that was ordered.

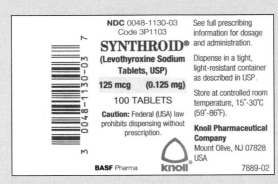

Figure 6-19

Figure 6-20

LOCATING INFORMATION ON DRUG LABELS AND PACKAGE INSERTS

In Exercises 1–6, refer to Label A.

1. What is the trade name of the drug?

2. What is the generic name of the drug?

3. Does this container hold multiple doses or a Unit dose? How do you know?

4. What is the name of the manufacturer?

5. What is the dosage strength?

6. At what temperature should the drug be stored?

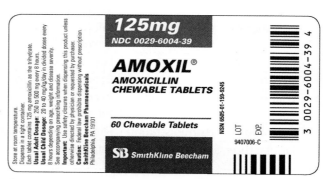

A

In Exercises 7–12, refer to label B.

7. What is the generic name of the drug?

8. What is the trade name of the drug?

9. What is the dosage strength?

10. What special information can you learn about the appearance of the drug from the label?

11. What is the lot number?

12. What are the storage requirements for this drug?

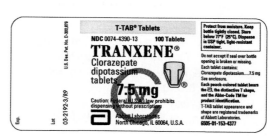

B

In Exercises 13–18, refer to label C.

13. What is the trade name of the drug?

14. How many doses are in the container?

15. What is the dosage strength?

16. How would you administer this drug?

17. How would you store this drug?

18. When would you read the package insert for this drug?

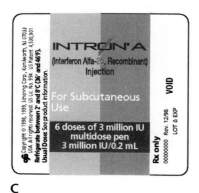

C

In Exercises 19–24, refer to label D.

19. What is the generic name of the drug?

20. By what route is this drug administered?

21. What is the usual dose?

22. What is the dosage strength?

23. If you had a drug order for 6 mg of Ventolin, how many teaspoons would you administer to the patient?

24. How long would this bottle last if you administered 3 doses of 15 mL daily?

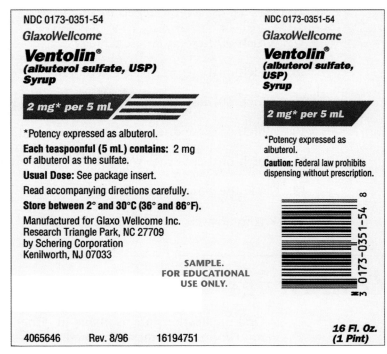

D

In Exercises 25–30, refer to label E.

25. What is the generic name of the drug?

26. What is the trade name of the drug?

27. By what route is this drug administered?

28. What special instructions are provided on the label?

29. What is the dosage strength?

30. What is the maximum number of times you should administer this drug to an individual patient daily?

E

In Exercises 31–36, refer to label F.

31. Why is Augmentin considered to be a combination drug?

32. How would you reconstitute this drug?

33. How much water should initially be added to the powder?

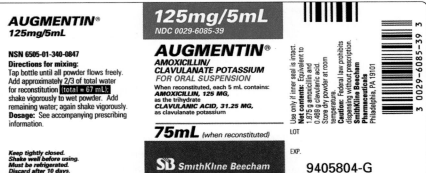

F

34. When reconstituted, what is the dosage strength?

35. What are two conditions under which you could not use the drug?

36. If the usual dose is 5 mL, how many doses are in this container?

In Exercises 37–42, refer to labels A through F.

37. Which of these drugs are tablets?

38. Which of these drugs are given orally?

39. Which of these are combination drugs?

40. Which of these drugs must be refrigerated?

41. Which of these drugs would be administered parenterally?

42. Name the generic drug that is present in two of the containers. How does its use vary?

To check your answers, see page 346.

Oral Drugs

Oral medications are available in either solid or liquid form. Tablets are the most common form. They may be scored, chewable, or enteric-coated. Scored tablets can be broken into equal portions so that you can administer a partial dosage, if necessary. Chewable tablets must be chewed to be effective. Enteric-coated tablets must be swallowed whole. Chewing them or dividing them breaks the seal provided by their coating, allowing the drug to be absorbed sooner than intended.

Capsules have a gelatin shell that contains the drug. In most cases, they should be swallowed whole. In some cases, capsules may be opened and mixed with food. Controlled-release capsules, also called sustained-release or extended-release capsules, release the drug over a long period of time. If these capsules are not swallowed whole, they may release too much of the drug too quickly for absorption. See Chapter 9 for more information about solid oral medications.

Rule 6-4

You may break tablets to give a partial dose *only* when the tablets are scored. Enteric-coated, controlled-release, extended-release, and sustained-release medications should *never* be crushed or broken.

Abbreviations such as SR, CR, and ER listed after the drug name indicate a special drug action. In Figure 6-21, letter O, *SR* following the brand name Isoptin means the drug is designed for sustained release. *CR* means that a drug is controlled release, *ER* that a drug has an extended-release mechanism.

Liquid oral medications are described as oral solutions, syrups, elixirs, oral suspensions, and simply liquids (see Figures 6-22, 6-23, and 6-24, letter P). In liquid medications, the dosage strength corresponds to a specific volume of the solution, for example, 250 mg/5 mL.

If a medication needs to be reconstituted, the instructions will be on the label.

Rule 6-5

When you reconstitute a drug, you must write your initials as well as the time and date of reconstitution on the label.

Oral liquids may be measured in droppers, calibrated spoons, medicine cups, or oral syringes. Calibrated cups and spoons are available at most pharmacies and sometimes come with the medication. Advise patients who take oral liquid medications at home to use a medicine cup or baking measuring spoon—not a household cup or spoon—if they do not have calibrated cups or spoons.

Figure 6-21

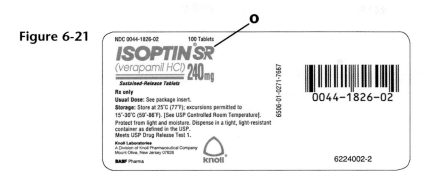

Figure 6-22

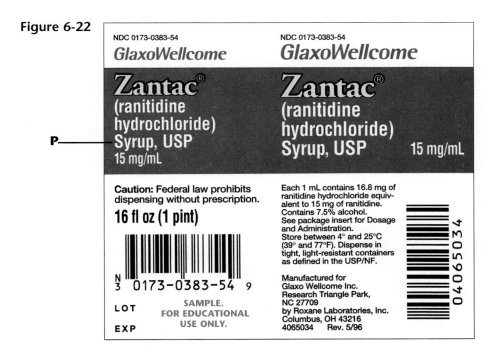

Figure 6-23

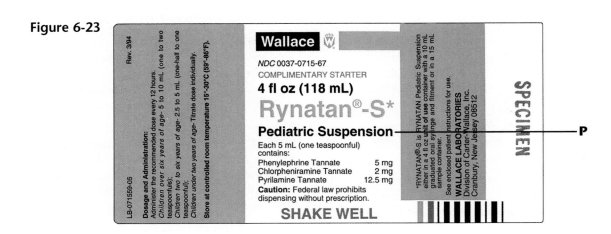

Figure 6-24

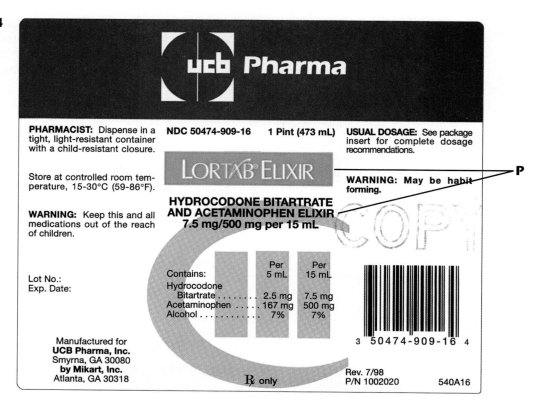

PATIENT EDUCATION

Health care workers often educate patients about the proper way to take drugs at home. In some outpatient settings, this responsibility may be the duty of the pharmacy technician, the office nurse, or the certified medical assistant, when permitted. If you are authorized to provide patient education, you should take the following steps:

1. Make sure the patient understands English. Otherwise, you may need to include an English-speaking member of the patient's household in the patient education process.

2. Be sure the patient or caretaker can read and understand the label. Some patients cannot see the fine print on labels. Others do not have the necessary literacy skills.

3. Ask the patient about drug allergies and any medications that he or she may be taking. Check the label or the package insert for drug interactions. Also check with the patient about any over-the-counter medications and herbal remedies being taken.

4. Review the dose, frequency, and length of time the drug is to be taken. Have the patient or caretaker repeat this information to you.

5. Review any special written instructions.

6. Describe any adverse effects of the drug that are serious enough to warrant prompt medical attention. Encourage the patient to seek help immediately if these side effects occur. Also discuss side effects that are considered normal.

7. Remind the patient to refer to the label when needed. Emphasize that the patient should call the pharmacy or physician with any questions that cannot be answered from the label. Many pharmacies provide additional written instructions.

ORAL DRUGS

A

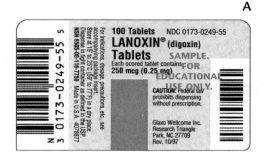

In Exercises 1–4, refer to label A.

1. Can these tablets be divided?

2. What is the dosage strength?

3. Can you store this drug on a shelf in the storeroom?

4. How might you administer a dose of Lanoxin 0.375 mg?

B

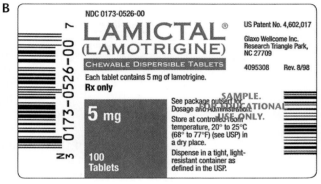

In Exercises 5–8, refer to label B.

5. What is the trade name of this drug?

6. How should these tablets be administered?

7. What is the dosage strength?

8. What is the usual dosage to administer?

In Exercises 9–12, refer to label C.

C

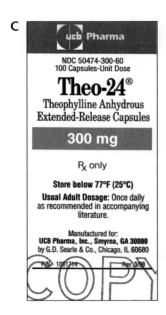

9. What is the generic name of this drug?

10. How many capsules are in this container?

11. What might the "24" in the trade name represent?

12. Can these capsules be broken or divided?

In Exercises 13–16, refer to Label D.

13. How many mL of water should be used to reconstitute this drug?

14. What is the dosage strength when the drug is reconstituted?

15. What is the total volume in the container when the drug is reconstituted?

16. How long can this drug be stored after it is reconstituted?

D

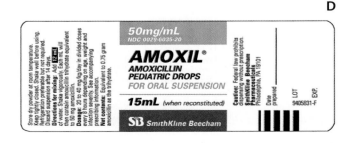

In Exercises 17–20, refer to labels A through D.

17. Which of these drugs could be divided to give a partial dose? Why?

18. According to the labels alone, which of these drugs can be safely administered to children?

19. Which of these drugs can be stored at room temperature?

20. Which tablets should not be broken or divided?

To check your answers, see page 347.

Parenteral Drugs

Figure 6-25

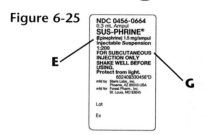

NDC 0456-0664
0.3 mL Ampul
SUS-PHRINE®
(Epinephrine) 1.5 mg/ampul
Injectable Suspension
1:200
**FOR SUBCUTANEOUS
INJECTION ONLY
SHAKE WELL BEFORE
USING.
Protect from light.**
602409330456*D
mfd by Steris Labs., Inc.
Phoenix, AZ 85043 USA
mfd for Forest Pharm., Inc.
St. Louis, MO 63045

Lot

Ex

Parenteral drugs may be packaged in single-use ampules or vials, single-use prefilled syringes, or multi-use vials. These small containers have small labels that have limited space for providing comprehensive information (Figure 6-25). You must read these labels with extra care. You will often need to review the package insert to obtain complete drug information.

Most parenteral drugs can be injected intradermally (ID), intramuscularly (IM), intravenously (IV), or subcutaneously (SC). Recall that inhalants and transdermal medications are also considered parenteral. The drug label specifies the appropriate route. Primaxin is a drug that can be administered either intramuscularly or intravenously (see Figures 6-10 and 6-11). SUS-PHRINE is administered only subcutaneously (see Figure 6-25, letter G).

The dosage strength of parenteral drugs (see letter E) can be expressed as a ratio (Figure 6-25), in mg (Figure 6-26), in Units (Figures 6-27 and 6-28), or as a percent (Figure 6-29). In some cases, the strength is expressed in both mg and mcg. Dosage strength may also be expressed in mEq.

Look at the labels for insulin in Figures 6-27 and 6-28. In addition to the standard components, these labels contain information about the origin of the medication (letter Q) and how quickly the insulin takes effect (letter R). Insulin can be made from human sources (recombinant DNA origin, or rDNA) or animal sources (beef or pork). Most animal-source insulin is being phased out in the United States. Different types of insulin take effect over different time periods. NPH insulin (Figure 6-27) is an intermediate-acting insulin. Regular insulin (Figure 6-28) is fast-acting. See Chapter 10 for more information about insulin.

Figure 6-26

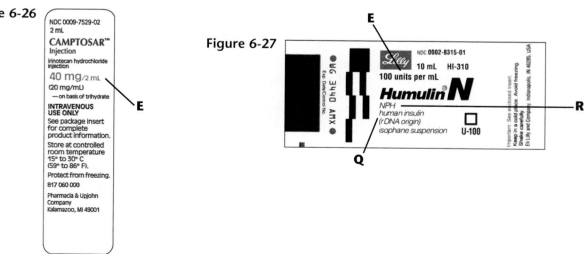

NDC 0009-7529-02
2 mL

CAMPTOSAR™
Injection

irinotecan hydrochloride
injection

40 mg/2 mL
(20 mg/mL)
—on basis of trihydrate

**INTRAVENOUS
USE ONLY**

See package insert
for complete
product information.

Store at controlled
room temperature
15° to 30° C
(59° to 86° F).

Protect from freezing.

817 060 000

Pharmacia & Upjohn
Company
Kalamazoo, MI 49001

Figure 6-27

NDC 0002-8315-01
10 mL   HI-310
100 units per mL

Humulin® N

NPH
human insulin
(rDNA origin)
isophane suspension   U-100

OMG 3440 XMA
Exp. Date/Control No.

Important: See enclosed insert
Keep in a cold place. Avoid freezing.
Shake carefully.
Eli Lilly and Company, Indianapolis, IN 46285, USA

Figure 6-28

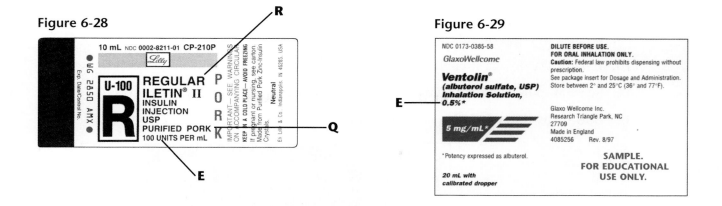

```
                                          R
10 mL NDC 0002-8211-01 CP-210P

        Lilly

U-100   REGULAR      P
        ILETIN® II   O
  R     INSULIN
        INJECTION    R
        USP
        PURIFIED PORK K
        100 UNITS PER mL
                              E

Exp. Date/Control No.   ●WG 2850 AMX ●
IMPORTANT—SEE WARNINGS
ON ACCOMPANYING CIRCULAR
KEEP IN A COLD PLACE—AVOID FREEZING
If pregnant or nursing, see carton
Made from Purified Pork Zinc-Insulin
Crystals.                    Neutral
Eli Lilli & Co. Indianapolis IN 46285. USA
                                          Q
```

Figure 6-29

```
NDC 0173-0385-58          DILUTE BEFORE USE.
                          FOR ORAL INHALATION ONLY.
GlaxoWellcome             Caution: Federal law prohibits dispensing without
                          prescription.
Ventolin®                 See package insert for Dosage and Administration.
(albuterol sulfate, USP)  Store between 2° and 25°C (36° and 77°F).
Inhalation Solution,
0.5%*                     Glaxo Wellcome Inc.
                          Research Triangle Park, NC
 5 mg/mL*                 27709
                          Made in England
                          4085256    Rev. 8/97
*Potency expressed as albuterol.
                                    SAMPLE.
                                FOR EDUCATIONAL
 20 mL with                         USE ONLY.
 calibrated dropper
E
```

REVIEW and PRACTICE

PARENTERAL DRUGS

In Exercises 1–4, refer to label A.

1. What is the dosage strength?

2. By what route of administration is this drug given?

3. What other instructions does this label provide?

4. What is the trade name of the drug?

In Exercises 5–8, refer to label B.

5. What is the dosage strength of this drug?

6. What are the storage requirements for this drug?

7. What is the generic name of this medication?

8. If you were not familiar with this drug, would you be able to administer it with only the information on the label? Why?

A

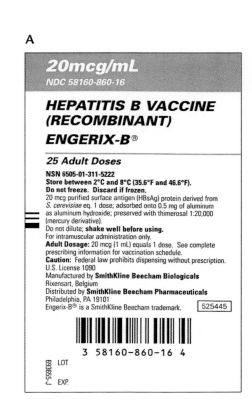

```
20mcg/mL
NDC 58160-860-16

HEPATITIS B VACCINE
(RECOMBINANT)
ENGERIX-B®

25 Adult Doses
NSN 6505-01-311-5222
Store between 2°C and 8°C (35.6°F and 46.6°F).
Do not freeze. Discard if frozen.
20 mcg purified surface antigen (HBsAg) protein derived from
S. cerevisiae eq. 1 dose; adsorbed onto 0.5 mg of aluminum
as aluminum hydroxide; preserved with thimerosal 1:20,000
(mercury derivative).
Do not dilute; shake well before using.
For intramuscular administration only.
Adult Dosage: 20 mcg (1 mL) equals 1 dose. See complete
prescribing information for vaccination schedule.
Caution: Federal law prohibits dispensing without prescription.
U.S. License 1090
Manufactured by SmithKline Beecham Biologicals
Rixensart, Belgium
Distributed by SmithKline Beecham Pharmaceuticals
Philadelphia, PA 19101
Engerix-B® is a SmithKline Beecham trademark.   525445

   3 58160-860-16 4

LOT
EXP.
```

B

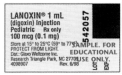

```
LANOXIN® 1 mL
(digoxin) Injection
Pediatric   Rx only
100 mcg (0.1 mg)         542057
Store at 15° to 25°C (59° to 77°F).
PROTECT FROM LIGHT.   SAMPLE. FOR
Dist.: Glaxo Wellcome Inc.  EDUCATIONAL
Research Triangle Park, NC 27709 USE ONLY.
4098907        Rev. 6/98
```

In Exercises 9–12, refer to label C.

9. What warning is on this label?

10. What is the dosage strength?

11. By what route of administration is this drug given?

12. How many doses does this container hold?

C

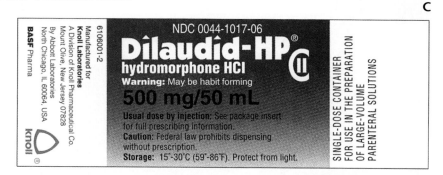

In Exercises 13–16, refer to label D.

13. What is the origin of this insulin?

D

14. What is the dosage strength of the insulin?

15. What is the generic name of this insulin?

16. If the usual dose is 10 Units, how many doses are in this container?

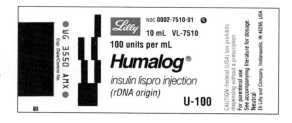

To check your answers, see page 348.

CRITICAL THINKING ON THE JOB

Avoid Unnecessary Risks

A drug order calls for the nurse to administer an IV preparation of Mefoxin on May 31. The pharmacy sends a vial with a label that reads *Mefoxin 10 g Merck*. Written by hand on the label is "5/23, 8 A.M." The nurse sends the vial back to the pharmacy with the note, "Please replace. Past expiration date."

Think Before You Act

By using her critical thinking skills, the nurse has prevented a serious error. When the nurse read the drug label, she noticed that once Mefoxin is reconstituted, it must be used within 1 week if refrigerated and 24 hours if stored at room temperature. According to the note on the label, the drug was reconstituted on May 23. Even if it had been refrigerated, it expired by May 30 and should not have been used. The nurse observed the special instructions on the drug label and, in turn, protected the patient's rights.

Drugs Administered by Other Routes

Although many drugs use oral and parenteral routes of administration, other routes exist. They include sublingually (under the tongue), buccally (between the tongue and cheek), rectally, and vaginally. Drugs may also be administered as topical ointments (used on the skin), eye or ear drops, patches applied to the skin (transdermal delivery), or nasal and throat inhalants (see Figures 6-30, 6-31, and 6-32, letter G).

Figure 6-30

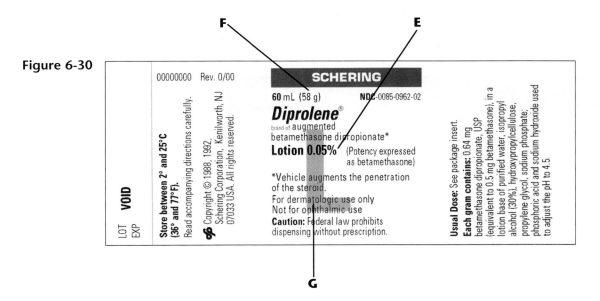

Figure 6-31

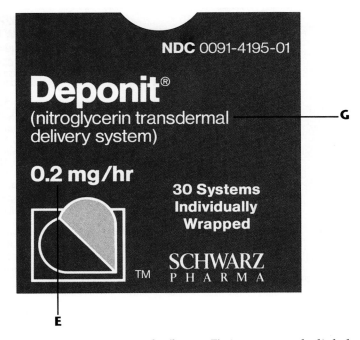

The dosage strength (letter E) is expressed slightly differently on these labels. In Figure 6-30, the dosage strength is the percentage that the active ingredient beta-methasone makes up of the entire lotion. The total amount of lotion is given in both grams and milliliters. In Figure 6-31, the dosage strength is given as 0.2 mg/hr; this drug is absorbed over time through the skin. In Figure 6-32, the dosage strength is simply 84 mcg. The delivery system contains 120 metered sprays. The dosage strength is actually 84 mcg/metered spray.

Figure 6-32

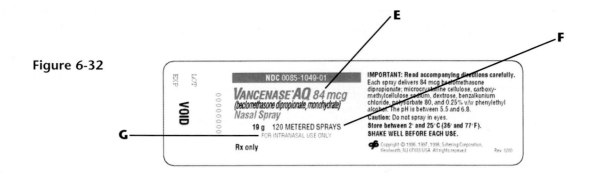

REVIEW and PRACTICE

DRUGS ADMINISTERED BY OTHER ROUTES

In Exercises 1–4, refer to label A.

1. What is the generic name?

2. What is the dosage strength?

3. What percent of the total solution is the inhalation solution?

4. What are the dilution instructions?

A

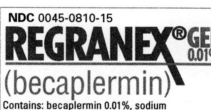

B

In Exercises 5–8, refer to label B.

5. By what route is this drug to be administered?

6. What are the drug's storage requirements?

7. What is the dosage strength?

8. On what ingredient is the dosage strength based?

NDC 0045-0810-15

REGRANEX®GEL 0.01%

(becaplermin)

Contains: becaplermin 0.01%, sodium carboxymethylcellulose, sodium chloride, sodium acetate trihydrate, glacial acetic acid, L-lysine hydrochloride, and water for injection, with preservatives: methylparaben 0.156%, propylparaben 0.017%, and m-cresol 0.086%.

P Rx only.
Dosage and Administration: See package insert.
STORE REFRIGERATED, 2° - 8°C (36° - 46°F).
DO NOT FREEZE.
Warning: Keep out of reach of children.
Important: Do not use if seal has been punctured or is not visible.
To open: Use cap to puncture seal.
To close: Recap tightly after each use.

DIN 02239405
NET WT. 15g
For Topical Use Only
Multi-dose tube
See crimp end for lot number and expiration date.

ORTHO-McNEIL

Distributed by:
ORTHO-McNEIL
PHARMACEUTICAL, INC.
Raritan, New Jersey 08869
and JANSSEN-ORTHO INC.
Toronto, Canada M3C 1L9

Manufactured by:
OMJ Pharmaceuticals, Inc.
U.S. Lic. #1196
San German,
Puerto Rico 00683
© OMP 1998
Made in U.S.A.

107-10-247-3

In Exercises 9–12, refer to label C.

9. What is the route of administration?

10. What is the dosage strength?

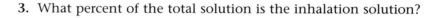

C

11. How many metered sprays are in this container?

12. Can this spray be delivered through more than one route?

In Exercises 13–16, refer to label D.

13. By what route is this drug delivered?

14. What is the dosage strength?

15. What dosage instructions are given?

16. How many doses are in this box?

To check your answers, see page 348.

D

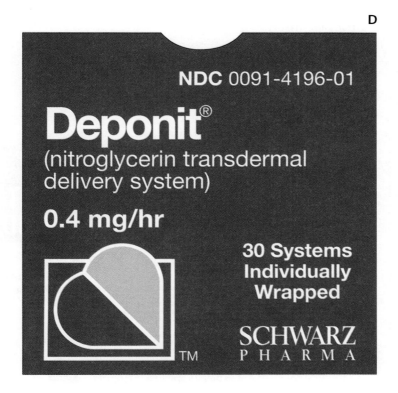

CHAPTER 6 REVIEW

CHECK UP

1. Distinguish a drug's trade name from its generic name.

2. Explain why a drug order might be written using only the trade name of a drug.

3. Explain the difference between IM and IV.

4. List the types of tablets that cannot be divided, broken, or crushed for administration, and explain why.

5. Describe when you would use a package insert.

6. Explain the importance of a lot number.

In Exercises 7–10, refer to label A.

7. What name would be used in writing a drug order for this medication?

8. What is the amount of the drug in the container?

9. What is the name of the manufacturer of this drug?

10. How is this drug administered?

A

Do not accept if ⊒-imprinted band on cap is broken or missing.

For conditions in which iron deficiency and vitamin C deficiency occur concomitantly with deficient intake or increased need for the B-complex vitamins.

Usual Dosage: Adults, including pregnant females and children 4 years of age and older — 2 teaspoonfuls (10 mL) three times daily, after meals;

Children 1-3 years of age — 1 teaspoonful (5 mL) three times daily, after meals. Otherwise as directed by the physician.

Each teaspoonful (5 mL) provides:
Elemental Iron
(as ferrous sulfate) .... 26.25 mg
Vitamin C (Ascorbic Acid) .... 37.5 mg
Niacinamide .... 7.5 mg
Dexpanthenol .... 2.5 mg
Vitamin B₁ (Thiamine
Hydrochloride) .... 1.5 mg
Vitamin B₂ (as riboflavin 5' phosphate
sodium) .... 1.5 mg
Vitamin B₆ (Pyridoxine
Hydrochloride) .... 1.25 mg
Vitamin B₁₂
(Cyanocobalamin) .... 6.25 mcg

Inactive Ingredients:
Alcohol 1%, methylparaben, propylparaben, sorbitol, water, natural and artificial flavors.

Warning: Close tightly and keep out of reach of children. Contains iron, which can be harmful or fatal to children in large doses. In case of accidental overdose, seek professional assistance or contact a Poison Control Center immediately.
Protect from temperatures above 77°F (25°C). Dispense in amber bottle only.
©Abbott
02-7610-4/R23
Abbott Laboratories
North Chicago, IL 60064, U.S.A.

NDC 0074-7173-01
Oral Solution

IBERET®-LIQUID

Hematinic
Supplying
Iron, Vitamin C
and Vitamin
B-Complex

**8 fl oz
(236 mL)**

N 3 0074-7173-01 3

Exp.
Lot   SPECIMEN

In Exercises 11–14, refer to label B.

11. What is the generic name of this drug?

12. How is this drug administered?

13. What is the dosage strength?

14. How many doses are in the container?

B

NDC 0456-0670-98
3.5 g 50 metered inhalations
AEROBID®-M
(flunisolide)
Inhaler System
FOR ORAL INHALATION ONLY
CAUTION: Federal law prohibits dispensing without prescription.
mfd for
FOREST PHARMACEUTICALS, INC.
Subsidiary of Forest Laboratories, Inc
St. Louis, MO 63045

Shake Well Before Using.
Contains flunisolide as the hemihydrate suspended in propellants (trichloromonofluoromethane, dichlorodifluoromethane and dichlorotetrafluoroethane) with sorbitan trioleate as a dispersing agent, and menthol as a flavoring agent. Each activation delivers approximately 250 mcg flunisolide to the patient.

Usual Dose: Two inhalations twice daily, morning and evening. SEE ACCOMPANYING PACKAGE INSERT FOR FULL PRESCRIBING INFORMATION.

CONTENTS UNDER PRESSURE. Do not puncture. Do not use or store near heat or open flame. Exposure above 120° F (49° C) may cause container to burst. Never throw container into fire or incinerator.
Keep out of reach of children.
mfd by 3M Pharmaceuticals St. Paul, MN   L 7820 594

Lot No.
Exp. Date

In Exercises 15–18, refer to label C.

15. Can this medication be divided to give a partial dose?

16. What is the dosage strength?

17. What special precautions should be taken in storing the drug?

18. How many capsules are in the container?

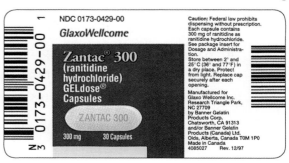

In Exercises 19–23, refer to label D.

19. What is the origin of this insulin?

20. What word on the label describes the time frame in which this insulin acts?

21. How is this drug administered?

22. What is the dosage strength?

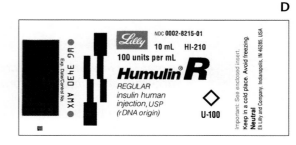

CRITICAL THINKING

You are working in a clinic that serves many adult homeless people. Two forms of Ceclor are available (see labels below). If the patient needs *Ceclor 250 mg t.i.d.,* which form do you think is preferable and why?

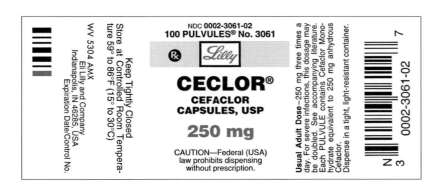

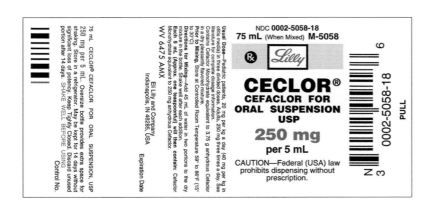

CASE STUDY

A drug order reads, *Dilaudid-HP 8 mg IM stat.* You have available a drug with the following label:

   a. What would you do to prepare for administering this drug?

   b. How would you administer the drug?

   c. What would you do with the vial after administering a dose of the drug?

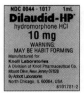

To check your answers, see page 348.

INTERNET ACTIVITY

Note: The Internet is a research tool from which to get basic information. Validate the accuracy of all Internet information.

  Mr. Liu is about to be discharged from the hospital with instructions to take *Coumadin 1 mg bid.* Mr. Liu is an elderly, easily confused man who will be cared for by his daughter. Although you have reviewed his medication instructions with him several times, you are not completely confident he understands that he should not drink alcohol or take any self-prescribed over-the-counter medications or herbal cures while he is taking Coumadin.

Assignment: Conduct an Internet search to find information in plain language regarding the importance of not taking any over-the-counter medications while taking Coumadin.

METHODS of DOSAGE CALCULATIONS

7

Objectives

When you have completed Chapter 7, you will be able to:

- Describe how the information on a physician's order, medication administration record (MAR), or prescription, along with the drug label and package insert, are used to calculate the *desired dose.*

- Convert the *dosage ordered* to the *desired dose,* using both fraction and ratio proportions.

- Calculate the *amount to administer* of a drug, using both proportion and formula methods.

- Recognize common errors that occur during dose calculations.

In this chapter and the next, you will calculate the correct amount of medication to administer to a patient. You will bring together information from both the physician's order (Chapter 5) and the drug label (Chapter 6). Earlier, you reviewed how to find a missing value in a proportion (Chapter 2) and to convert quantities from one unit of measurement to another (Chapter 3). As you master various calculations in this chapter, refer back to these earlier chapters as needed.

Dosages and Doses

Before you can calculate in practical terms how many dosage units of a medication to administer to a patient, you must first find the *desired dose*: the amount of the actual drug that the patient is to be given at one time. To determine the *desired dose,* you must know the following information: the *dosage ordered* and the *dose on hand.*

The *dosage ordered* is the amount of drug the physician has ordered along with the frequency with which it is given. You will find this information on the physician's order or prescription, the medication administration record (MAR), or the medication card. You may also receive this information verbally from a physician, especially in emergency situations. (Remember to check a verbal order by repeating it as you are writing it down.) *Always check the physician's original order the first time you administer a medication to a patient or if you have any questions about the information on the MAR or medication card.*

Recall from Chapter 6 that dosage strength measures the amount of drug per dosage unit. Many medications are available in different dosage strengths. For example, a medication may be produced in two versions, 75 mg per tablet and 100 mg per tablet. In both of these versions, the dosage unit is a tablet.

The *dose on hand* is the specific amount of drug that is present in a dosage unit. In this example, the *dose on hand* for the first tablet is 75 mg. The *dose on hand* for the second tablet is 100 mg. For any medication you have available, you can read the drug label to determine the *dose on hand*. Dosage strength, then, is the *dose on hand* per *dosage unit*.

Rule 7-1

1. The *dosage ordered* is found on the physician's order or prescription, the medication administration record (MAR), the medication card, or the physician's verbal order.

2. The *dose on hand* is found on the drug label.

EXAMPLE 1 ▷ Determine the *dosage ordered* and the *dose on hand* from the following information:

MAR reads: *Paxil 40 mg p.o. q.d.*

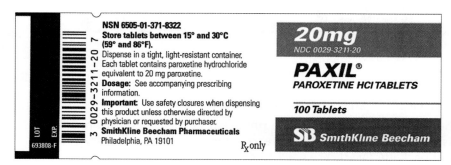

The *dosage ordered* is 40 mg (from the MAR).

The *dose on hand* is 20 mg (from the drug label). It is provided in tablet form.

Table 7-1 The Language of Dosage Calculations

Dosage Ordered	The total amount of drug the physician has ordered, along with the frequency. Its unit of measurement may not be the same as that of the dosage unit.
Desired Dose	The amount of drug to be administered at a single time. Its unit of measurement must be the same as the dosage unit.
Dosage Unit	The volume of medication that contains a quantity of drug, such as a tablet, a capsule, 1 mL, or 5 mL. This volume is listed on the drug label. If a medication has 250 mg of drug per tablet, the dosage unit is one tablet.
Dose on Hand	The amount of drug contained within a dosage unit of medication. If a medication has 250 mg of drug per tablet, the dose on hand is 250 mg.
Dosage Strength	The dose on hand per dosage unit. If the dose on hand is 250 mg and the dosage unit is one tablet, the dosage strength is 250 mg/tablet.
Amount to Administer	The volume of medication that contains the desired dose. In practical terms, the number of tablets or mL of solution that you administer at one time to provide an amount of drug.

Rule 7-2

The *desired dose* must be in the same unit of measurement as the *dose on hand*.

Sometimes the *dosage ordered* and the *dose on hand* have the same unit of measurement. In these cases, the *desired dose* is the same as the *dosage ordered* and no conversion is necessary. Frequently, however, the *dosage ordered* and the *dose on hand* are expressed in different units of measurement. In these cases, you must convert the *dosage ordered* so that it has the same unit of measurement as the *dose on hand*. This conversion leads you to the *desired dose*.

EXAMPLE 1 Suppose the *dosage ordered* is nitroglycerin gr $\frac{1}{200}$. The *dose on hand* is 0.3 mg, available in nitroglycerin tablets. To find the *desired dose,* you would need to convert *gr* (the *dosage ordered*) to *mg* (the *dose on hand*).

Conversion Factors

Recall from Chapter 3 that conversion factors are expressions that allow you to switch from one unit of measurement to another. The numerator and denominator of a conversion factor are equivalent; the factor itself equals 1.

In some cases, you convert between units in the same system of measurement; you will use conversion factors such as $\frac{1 \text{ mg}}{1000 \text{ mcg}}$ and $\frac{1000 \text{ mcg}}{1 \text{ mg}}$. In other cases, you convert between systems, using conversion factors such as $\frac{1 \text{ tsp}}{5 \text{ mL}}$ and $\frac{5 \text{ mL}}{1 \text{ tsp}}$.

Calculating the Desired Dose

This section presents two methods for calculating the *desired dose*. The first, the conversion factor method, uses fraction proportions. The second is the ratio proportion method. Both lead to the same result. Which method you use is a matter of personal preference.

The amount of medication that a physician orders for a patient equals the amount that you give to a patient. Thus,

dosage ordered = desired dose and $\frac{dosage\ ordered}{desired\ dose} = 1$

In these equations, *dosage ordered* is the amount of medication given at one time (a dose), not its frequency.

The Conversion Factor Method

Recall from Rule 3-5 in Chapter 3 that you can use fraction proportions to convert a quantity from one unit of measure to another. Knowing that a conversion factor equals 1, and that $\frac{dosage\ ordered}{desired\ dose} = 1$, leads to the following conversion factor method for finding the *desired dose*.

Rule 7-3

Solve for the *desired dose* in the proportion
$$\frac{dosage\ ordered}{desired\ dose} = \text{conversion factor, where}$$

1. the numerator of the conversion factor must have the same unit of measurement as the *dosage ordered,* and

2. the denominator of the conversion factor must have the same unit of measurement as the *desired dose.*

Here, the *dosage ordered* is the quantity you know. The *desired dose* is the quantity you want (the missing value).

EXAMPLE 1 The *dosage ordered* is 0.2 mg. The *dose on hand* is in mcg. Find the *desired dose.*

The *desired dose* must be in the same unit of measurement as the d*ose on hand.* Because, the *dose on hand* is in mcg, the *desired dose* can be expressed as ? mcg.

$$\frac{dosage\ ordered}{desired\ dose} = \frac{0.2 \text{ mg}}{? \text{ mcg}}$$

Therefore, according to Rule 7-3,

$$\frac{0.2 \text{ mg}}{? \text{ mcg}} = \text{conversion factor}$$

The conversion factor should relate mg to mcg. Its numerator should be mg, its denominator mcg. Use $\frac{1 \text{ mg}}{1000 \text{ mcg}}$.

$$\frac{0.2 \text{ mg}}{? \text{ mcg}} = \frac{1 \text{ mg}}{1000 \text{ mcg}}$$

Now, cross multiply to solve.

$$\frac{0.2 \text{ mg}}{? \text{ mcg}} \diagdown\!\!\!\!\diagup \frac{1 \text{ mg}}{1000 \text{ mcg}}$$

$$0.2 \times 1000 = ? \times 1$$

$$200 = ?$$

The *dosage ordered,* 0.2 mg, equals the *desired dose,* 200 mcg, which is in the same unit of measure as the *dose on hand.*

EXAMPLE 2 The order reads: *ASA gr v po qd.* The drug label indicates 325 mg tablets. Find the *desired dose.*

The *dosage ordered,* gr v, is in grains. The *dose on hand* is in mg; thus the *desired dose* must be in mg, and is expressed as ? mg. The conversion factor $\frac{\text{gr i}}{65 \text{ mg}}$ relates gr and mg.

$$\frac{\text{gr v}}{? \text{ mg}} = \frac{\text{gr i}}{65 \text{ mg}}$$

Cross multiply: $5 \times 65 = ? \times 1$ so that $325 = ?$

The *desired dose* is 325 mg.

The reciprocal of $\frac{\text{gr i}}{65 \text{ mg}}$, or $\frac{65 \text{ mg}}{\text{gr i}}$, also relates gr and mg. For this example, though, you want grains in the numerator of the conversion factor and mg in the denominator, matching the units of the other fraction $\frac{\text{gr v}}{? \text{ mg}}$.

Recall from Chapter 3 that the relation between *gr* and *mg* is approximate, not exact. Different medications use different conversion factors (see Table 7-2).

Table 7-2 Selected Conversion Factors For Grains	
aspirin, iron	$\frac{\text{gr i}}{65 \text{ mg}}$
nitroglycerine, codeine, morphine	$\frac{\text{gr i}}{60 \text{ mg}}$

EXAMPLE 3 Find the *desired dose.*

Ordered: *codeine gr ss PO PRN pain*

On Hand:

The *dosage ordered* is gr ss, or $\frac{1}{2}$ grain. From the label, the *dose on hand* is 30 mg. In turn, the *desired dose* must be in mg. The conversion factor $\frac{\text{gr i}}{60 \text{ mg}}$ relates gr and mg.

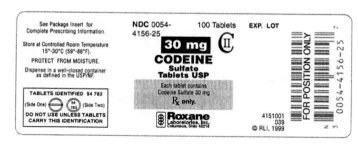

$$\frac{dosage\ ordered}{desired\ dose} = \frac{gr\ ss}{?\ mg} = \frac{gr\ i}{60\ mg}$$

$$\frac{1}{2} \times 60 = ? \times 1$$

$$30 = ?$$

The *dosage ordered,* gr ss, equals the *desired dose,* 30 mg, which is in the same unit of measurement as the *dose on hand.* Had you used the conversion factor $\frac{gr\ i}{65\ mg}$, your calculation would have led to a *desired dose* of 32.5 mg, within 10% of 30 mg.

EXAMPLE 4 ▷ Find the *desired dose.*

Ordered: *Vicodin Tuss Expectorant 1 tsp q4h ac & hs*

On hand:

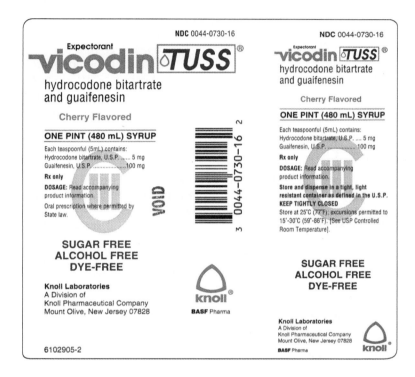

In the previous two examples, the medication was supplied in tablet form. Here, however, the medication is liquid. The *dosage ordered* is 1 tsp. The *dose on hand* is in mL. Therefore, the *desired dose* must be in mL. Earlier, you learned that one of the basic conversions you should memorize is 1 tsp = 5 mL. Remembering this conversion, you should be able to establish quickly that the *desired dose* is 5 mL.

EXAMPLE 5 ▷ The order reads *Codimal DM Syrup 10 cc t.i.d. p.c.* The patient will be using a calibrated teaspoon at home to measure the medication. Express the *desired dose* in teaspoons.

The *dosage ordered* is 10 cc. The *desired dose* is ? tsp. Recall that 1 cc = 1 mL and that 1 tsp = 5 mL = 5 cc. Thus,

$$\frac{dosage\ ordered}{desired\ dose} = \frac{10\ cc}{?\ tsp} = \frac{5\ cc}{1\ tsp}$$

$$10 \times 1 = ? \times 5$$

$$2 = ?$$

The *desired dose* is 2 tsp.

In Examples 4 and 5, you are not calculating the actual amount (weight) of the drug itself. You are calculating the amount of solution (volume) that contains the drug. In both cases, the *dosage ordered* is based on volume, not weight.

ERROR ALERT!

In a fraction proportion, the units of the numerators match each other. The units of the denominators match each other.

If you set up a proportion with mismatched units, you will calculate the *desired dose* incorrectly. In an earlier example, the *dosage ordered* was 10 cc and the *desired dose* was ? tsp. Suppose you used the conversion factor $\frac{1 \text{ tsp}}{5 \text{ cc}}$ instead of $\frac{5 \text{ cc}}{1 \text{ tsp}}$. Then your proportion would be

$$\frac{10 \text{ cc}}{? \text{ tsp}} = \frac{1 \text{ tsp}}{5 \text{ cc}}$$

Here, the units are mismatched. If you solve for ? (ignoring the units for the moment), you would calculate

$$10 \times 5 = ? \times 1$$
$$50 = ?$$

You would reach the conclusion that the patient should be given 50 tsp of medication, an inappropriate amount. Always check that the units of measurement in a proportion match correctly.

The Ratio-Proportion Method

Recall from Chapters 2 and 3, that you can write a proportion using ratios rather than fractions. Instead of cross-multiplying, you use the means and extremes to solve for the missing value (again, the *desired dose*). Rule 7-4 describes the ratio-proportion method, also known as the colon method.

Rule 7-4

Solve for the *desired dose* in the proportion A:B::C:D, where

1. A is the *dosage ordered,* the quantity you know

2. B is the *desired dose,* the quantity you want

3. C is the numerator of the conversion factor

4. D is the denominator of the conversion factor

EXAMPLE 1 The *dosage ordered* is 0.2 mg. The *dose on hand* is in mcg. Find the *desired dose.*

The *desired dose* must be in the same unit of measurement as the *dose on hand,* mcg. The ratio A:B can be expressed

A:B = dosage ordered:desired dose = 0.2 mg:? mcg

The second ratio is the conversion factor. Its units must match the units of the first ratio. The ratio C:D can be expressed

C:D = 1 mg:1000 mcg

In turn, write the proportion as

A:B::C:D = 0.2 mg:? mcg::1 mg:1000 mcg

Use the means and extremes to solve for the missing value.

$$? \times 1 = 0.2 \times 1000$$
$$? = 200$$

Therefore, the *desired dose* is 200 mcg.

EXAMPLE 2 The order reads: *ASA gr v po qd.* The drug label indicates 325 mg tablets. Find the *desired dose.*

The *dosage ordered,* gr v, is in grains. Because the *dose on hand* is in mg, the *desired dose* will also be in mg. The first ratio can be written

A:B = *dosage ordered:desired dose* = gr v:? mg

The second ratio, the conversion factor, relates gr to mg. Its units must match the units of the first ratio.

C:D = gr i:65 mg

The proportion, therefore, is

A:B::C:D = gr v:? mg::gr i:65 mg

Using means and extremes to find the missing value,

$? \times 1 = 5 \times 65$

$? = 325$

The *desired dose* is 325 mg. Examples 1 and 2 are the same as Examples 1 and 2 in the previous section. The calculations lead to the same results, simply using different methods. You can choose the method which is most comfortable for you.

EXAMPLE 3 The *dosage ordered* is Hivid 375 mcg. The *dose on hand* is 0.375 mg tablets. Find the *desired dose.*

The *dosage ordered* is in mcg. Because the *dose on hand* is in mg, the *desired dose* will also be in mg.

A:B = *dosage ordered:desired dose* = 375 mcg:? mg

The conversion factor relates mcg to mg.

C:D = 1000 mcg:1 mg

The proportion is

A:B::C:D = 375 mcg:? mg::1000 mcg:1 mg

Using means and extremes to find the missing value,

$? \times 1000 = 375 \times 1$

$? = \dfrac{375}{1000} = 0.375$

The *desired dose* is 0.375 mg.

REVIEW and PRACTICE

CALCULATING THE DESIRED DOSE

In Exercises 1–10, convert the *dosage ordered* to the same unit as that of the *dose on hand* or measuring device. Use conversion tables from Chapter 3 as needed.

1. Ordered: *amoxicillin 0.25 g*   Desired Dose:_____
   On hand: amoxicillin 125 mg capsules

2. Ordered: *erythromycin 0.5 g*   Desired Dose:_____
   On hand: erythromycin 500 mg tablets

3. Ordered: *phenobarbital gr ss*   Desired Dose:_____
   On hand: phenobarbital 15 mg tablets

4. Ordered: *Levoxyl 0.15 mg* Desired Dose:_____
   On hand: Levoxyl 300 mcg tablets

5. Ordered: *Duratuss HD 5 cc* Desired Dose:_____
   Available measuring device is marked in teaspoons.

6. Ordered: *Robitussin DM 2 tsp* Desired Dose:_____
   Available measuring device is marked in cc.

7. Ordered: *Seconal gr v* Desired Dose:_____
   On hand: Refer to label A.

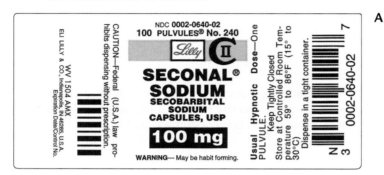

A

8. Ordered: *morphine gr $\frac{1}{4}$* Desired Dose:_____
   On hand: Refer to label B.

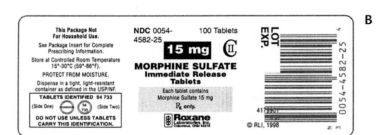

B

9. Ordered: *Synthroid 0.05 mg* Desired Dose:_____
   On hand: Refer to label C.

10. Ordered: *Synthroid 0.09 mg* Desired Dose:_____
    On hand: Refer to label D.

To check your answers, see page 350.

C

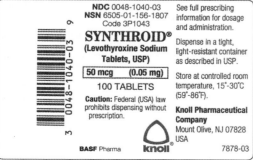

D

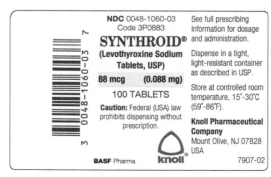

Calculating the Amount to Administer

Once you have determined the *desired dose,* you still have one more step. You must calculate the *amount to administer* to the patient. For example, do you give a patient 1 or 2 tablets, or some other amount? How many mL of solution do you draw into a syringe or mix in an intravenous bag?

In this section, you will learn different methods for calculating the *amount to administer:* fraction proportions, ratio proportions, and a formula. All lead to the same result.

Knowing the *dosage strength* from a drug label gives you two important pieces of information: the *dose on hand* and the *dosage unit.* A third piece of information is the *desired dose,* which you have already learned to calculate. You can use this information to calculate a fourth: *the amount to administer.*

The Proportion Method

The dosage strength of a drug does not change based on the amount that you administer. Whether you administer 50 mg of a drug in 1 tablet or 100 mg in 2 tablets, the dosage strength remains 50 mg per 1 tablet. Thus, you can set up the proportion:

$$\frac{50 \text{ mg}}{1 \text{ tablet}} = \frac{100 \text{ mg}}{2 \text{ tablets}}$$

You can also write this proportion in its general form as:

$$\frac{dose\ on\ hand}{dosage\ unit} = \frac{desired\ dose}{amount\ to\ administer}$$

Suppose in this example that you wanted to give a patient 100 mg of medication, but did not know how many tablets to administer. Using a fraction proportion, you would write

$$\frac{50 \text{ mg}}{1 \text{ tablet}} = \frac{100 \text{ mg}}{? \text{ tablets}}$$

Cross-multiply to find the number of tablets to administer.

$$50 \times ? = 1 \times 100$$
$$? = 2$$

Rule 7-5

To calculate the amount of medication to administer using a fraction proportion,

1. Convert the *dosage ordered* to the *desired dose,* using the same unit of measurement as the *dose on hand.*

2. Set up a fraction proportion in the form

$$\frac{dose\ on\ hand}{dosage\ unit} = \frac{desired\ dose}{amount\ to\ administer}$$

3. Cross-multiply to solve for the amount to administer.

4. Use critical thinking skills to evaluate your answer before administering the drug.

> **EXAMPLE 1** Find the amount of medication to administer.
>
> Ordered: *Famvir 500 mg PO q8h*
>
> On hand:

40069US1
40069US1
40069US1

0007-4116-13

250mg
NDC 0007-4116-13

FAMVIR®
FAMCICLOVIR
TABLETS

30 Tablets

SB SmithKline Beecham

LOT
EXP.

Store between 15° and 30°C (59° and 86°F).
Each tablet contains famciclovir, 250 mg.
Dosage: See accompanying prescribing information.
Important: Use safety closures when dispensing this product unless otherwise directed by physician or requested by purchaser.
Caution: Federal law prohibits dispensing without prescription.
Manufactured by **SmithKline Beecham Pharmaceuticals,** Crawley, UK, for **SmithKline Beecham Pharmaceuticals** Philadelphia, PA 19101
670705-A

1. The *dosage ordered* (500 mg) and the *dose on hand* (250 mg) are already in the same unit of measurement, mg. Therefore, no additional conversion is needed. The *desired dose* is 500 mg.

2. The dosage strength is 250 mg per 1 tablet. The *dosage unit* is 1 tablet. Now set up the proportion

$$\frac{dose\ on\ hand}{dosage\ unit} = \frac{desired\ dose}{amount\ to\ administer} \text{ so that}$$

$$\frac{250\ mg}{1\ tablet} = \frac{500\ mg}{?\ tablet}$$

3. Solve by cross-multiplying.

$$250 \times ? = 1 \times 500$$

$$? = 2$$

Administer 2 Famvir 250 mg tablets orally every 8 hours.

4. Evaluate the answer. 500 mg is twice 250 mg. Therefore, the number of tablets for 500 mg should be twice the number needed for 250 mg. Because 1 tablet is needed to deliver 250 mg, it is sensible that 2 tablets are needed to deliver 500 mg.

EXAMPLE 2 ▷ Find the amount of medication to administer.

Ordered: *Prozac Liquid 40 mg PO qd*

On hand:

1. The *dosage ordered* is 40 mg. The *dose on hand* is 20 mg. They are already in the same unit of measurement. Therefore, the *desired dose* is 40 mg.

2. The dosage strength is 20 mg per 5 mL. Therefore, the *dosage unit* is 5 mL.

$$\frac{20\ mg}{5\ mL} = \frac{40\ mg}{?\ mL}$$

3. $20 \times ? = 5 \times 40$

$$? = 10$$

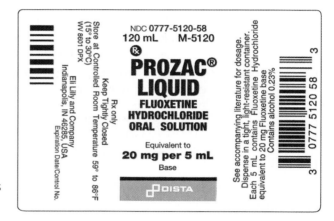

Administer 10 mL of Prozac Liquid orally once every day.

4. The *dosage ordered* is twice the amount of the *dose on hand*. The *amount to administer* should be twice the *dosage unit*.

You can also use ratio proportions to find the amount of medication to administer.

Rule 7-6

To calculate the amount of medication to administer using a ratio proportion,

1. Convert the *dosage ordered* to the *desired dose,* using the same unit of measurement as the *dose on hand.*

2. Set up a ratio proportion in the form

   dose on hand:dosage unit::desired dose:amount to administer

3. Use means and extremes to solve for the *amount to administer.*

4. Use critical thinking skills to evaluate your answer before administering the drug.

EXAMPLE 1 Find the amount of medication to administer. The tablets are scored.

Ordered: *Brethine 2.5 mg tid PO*

On hand:

1. The *dosage ordered* is 2.5 mg. The *dose on hand* is 5 mg. They are already in the same unit of measurement. Therefore, the *desired dose* is 2.5 mg.

2. The dosage strength is 5 mg per tablet. The *dosage unit* is 1 tablet. The proportion is:

    5 mg:1 tablet::2.5 mg:? tablet

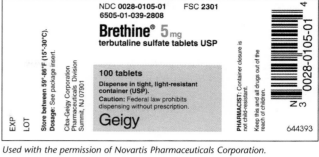

Used with the permission of Novartis Pharmaceuticals Corporation.

3. Use means and extremes to solve.

    $1 \times 2.5 = 5 \times ?$

    $\frac{1}{2} = ?$

You should administer $\frac{1}{2}$ tablet of Brethine 5 mg scored tablets orally three times a day. Note that the tablets are scored. You may break them in order to administer $\frac{1}{2}$ tablet.

4. The *dosage ordered,* 2.5 mg, is half the *dose on hand,* 5 mg. The *amount to administer,* therefore, should be half the *dosage unit.*

EXAMPLE 2 Find the amount of medication to administer.

Ordered: *phenobarbital gr $\frac{3}{4}$ PO stat*

On hand:

1. The *dosage ordered* is gr $\frac{3}{4}$. The *dose on hand* is 15

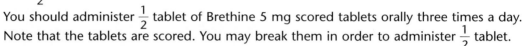

mg. You must convert the *dosage ordered* to the *desired dose* with the same unit as the *dose on hand.*

   gr $\frac{3}{4}$:? mg::gr i:60 mg

Using means and extremes,

   $? \times 1 = \frac{3}{4} \times 60$

   $? = 45$

The *desired dose* is 45 mg.

2. The dosage strength is 15 mg per tablet. The *dosage unit* is 1 tablet. The proportion is

    15 mg:1 tablet::45 mg:? tablet

3. Use means and extremes to solve.

    $1 \times 45 = 15 \times ?$

    $3 = ?$

Administer 3 phenobarbital 15 mg tablets by mouth immediately.

4. From Chapter 3, you can confirm that gr $\frac{1}{4}$ = 15 mg. Because gr $\frac{3}{4}$ is three times as much, 45 mg is a correct answer. At first, 3 tablets may seem like a lot. However, you can confirm that phenobarbital is available in 30 mg and 60 mg tablets. Thus, a total amount of 45 mg seems reasonable.

THE PROPORTION METHOD

In Exercises 1–10, use either fraction proportions or ratio proportions to find the amount of medication to administer.

1. Ordered: *Thorazine 20 mg PO t.i.d.* On hand: Thorazine 10 mg tablets

2. Ordered: *ranitidine hydrochloride 150 mg PO b.i.d.* On hand: Zantac syrup 15 mg ranitidine hydrochloride per mL

3. Ordered: *Ceclor 0.375 g PO b.i.d.* On hand: Ceclor Oral Suspension 187 mg per 5 mL

4. Ordered: *nitroglycerin gr $\frac{1}{100}$ SL stat* On hand: nitroglycerin 0.3 mg tablets

5. Ordered: *amoxicillin 250 mg po t.i.d.*
   On hand: Refer to label A.

6. Ordered: *Ceclor 500 mg p.o. b.i.d.*
   On hand: Refer to label B.

7. Ordered: *Procardia 20 mg PO t.i.d.*
   On hand: Refer to label C.

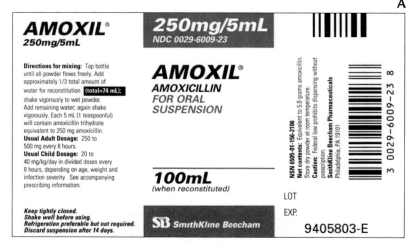

A

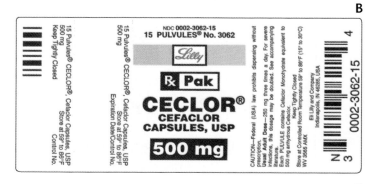

B

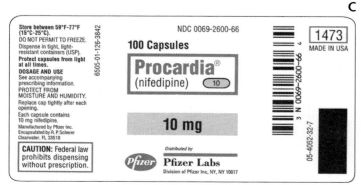

C

8. Ordered: *moexipril hydro-chloride 15 mg p.o. q.d. a.c.*
   On hand: Refer to label D.

9. Ordered: *Synthroid 0.3 mg PO q.d.*
   On hand: Refer to label E.

10. Ordered: *Wellbutrin 0.15 g po b.i.d.*
    On hand: Refer to label F.

To check your answers, see page 350.

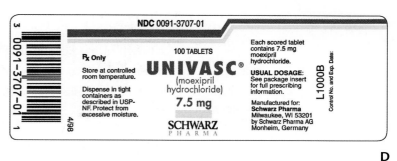

D

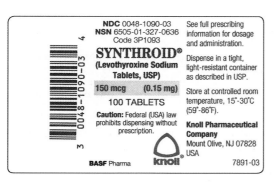

E

F

The Formula Method

Another way to find the amount of medication to administer is to use the formula

$$D \times \frac{Q}{H} = A$$

In this formula, D is the *desired dose,* H is the *dose on hand,* Q is the *dosage unit* (also called quantity on hand), and A is the *amount to administer.* You may also see this formula in two other versions:

$$\frac{D}{H} \times Q = A \quad \text{or} \quad \frac{DQ}{H} = A$$

You can find this formula by starting with the fraction proportion from the previous section.

$$\frac{dose\ on\ hand}{dosage\ unit} = \frac{desired\ dose}{amount\ to\ administer}$$

First, substitute H for the *dose on hand,* Q for the *dosage unit,* D for the *desired dose,* and A for the *amount to administer,*

$$\frac{H}{Q} = \frac{D}{A}$$

Now, cross-multiply.

$$HA = DQ$$

This becomes

$$A = \frac{DQ}{H} = \frac{D}{1} \times \frac{Q}{H} = D \times \frac{Q}{H}$$

Thus,

$$\frac{dose\ on\ hand}{dosage\ unit} = \frac{desired\ dose}{amount\ to\ administer} \rightarrow D \times \frac{Q}{H} = A$$

To calculate the amount of medication to administer using the formula method,

1. Convert the *dosage ordered* to the *desired dose*.

2. Substitute D for the *desired dose,* H for the *dose on hand,* and Q for the *dosage unit* in the formula

$$D \times \frac{Q}{H} = A$$

3. Solve for A, the *amount to administer*.

4. Use critical thinking skills to evaluate your answer before administering the drug.

EXAMPLE 1 Find the *amount to administer*.

Ordered: *Levsin 0.5 mg IM stat*

On hand:

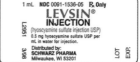

1. The *dosage ordered* (0.5 mg) and the *dose on hand* (0.5 mg) are already in the same unit of measurement. No additional conversion is needed. The *desired dose* is 0.5 mg.

2. The *desired dose* (D) is 0.5 mg, the *dose on hand* (H) is 0.5 mg, and the dosage unit (Q) is 1 mL. Substitute these values into the formula

$$D \times \frac{Q}{H} = A \rightarrow 0.5 \text{ mg} \times \frac{1 \text{ mL}}{0.5 \text{ mg}} = A$$

3. Solve for A.

$$^{1}\cancel{0.5 \text{ mg}} \times \frac{1 \text{ mL}}{\cancel{0.5 \text{ mg}}_{1}}$$

$$1 \times 1 \text{ mL} = A$$

$$A = 1 \text{ mL}$$

The *amount to administer* is 1 mL. According to the label, the entire package contains 1 mL. Therefore, you would administer the entire contents of the package.

You can see from this example that the units of measurement for D and H are the same; these units cancel themselves out. In turn, the unit of measurement for Q becomes the unit of measurement for A, the amount to administer.

4. The drug label indicates that the dosage strength is 0.5 mg per mL and that the package contains 1 mL. Therefore, the package contains 0.5 mg. This amount, 0.5 mg, matches the *desired dose.* The calculations should confirm that the amount to administer is one package.

EXAMPLE 2 Find the amount of medication to administer.

Ordered: *Monoket 15 mg po BID*

On hand:

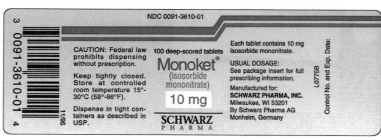

1. The *dosage ordered* (15 mg) and the *dose on hand* (10 mg) are already in the same unit of measurement. No additional conversion is needed.

2. The *desired dose* (D) is 15 mg, the *dose on hand* (H) is 10 mg, and the *dosage unit* (Q) is 1 tablet. Substitute these values into the formula

$$D \times \frac{Q}{H} = A \rightarrow 15 \text{ mg} \times \frac{1 \text{ tablet}}{10 \text{ mg}} = A$$

3. $^3\cancel{15}\text{ mg} \times \dfrac{1 \text{ tablet}}{\cancel{10}\text{ mg}_2} = A$

$\dfrac{3}{2} \times 1 \text{ tablet} = A$

$A = 1\dfrac{1}{2}$ tablets

You would administer $1\dfrac{1}{2}$ tablets twice a day.

4. The *dosage ordered* is more than the *dose on hand,* so it is logical that the amount to administer is more than 1 tablet. According to the drug label, the tablets are deep-scored, making it possible for you to administer half a tablet.

> **EXAMPLE 3** Find the amount of medication to administer.

Ordered: *amoxicillin susp 250 mg po t.i.d.*

On hand:

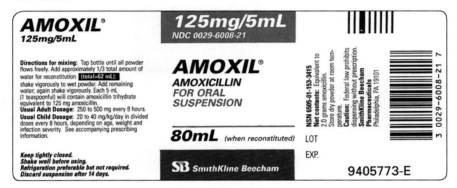

1. The *dosage ordered* and the *dose on hand* are both in mg. No further conversion is needed.

2. The *desired dose* (D) is 250 mg, the *dose on hand* (H) is 125 mg, and the *dosage unit* (Q) is 5 mL.

$$D \times \dfrac{Q}{H} = A \rightarrow 250 \text{ mg} \times \dfrac{5 \text{ mL}}{125 \text{ mg}} = A$$

3. Solve for A.

$^2\cancel{250}\text{ mg} \times \dfrac{5 \text{ mL}}{\cancel{125}\text{ mg}_1} = A$

$2 \times 5 \text{ mL} = A$

$A = \; = 10 \text{ mL}$

The amount to administer is 10 mL by mouth three times per day.

4. A quick comparison of the drug order and the drug label indicates that the *dosage ordered* (250 mg) is twice as much as the *dose on hand* (125 mg). Therefore, you estimate that you will need to administer twice the *dosage unit.*

If the patient were to take this medication at home using calibrated spoons, then you would need to convert 10 mL to tsp.

$\dfrac{10 \text{ mL}}{? \text{ tsp}} = \dfrac{5 \text{ mL}}{1 \text{ tsp}}$

$10 \times 1 = ? \times 5$

$2 = ?$

The patient would need 2 tsp three times per day to receive the proper amount of medication.

You may have already noticed from the last three examples the relationship between the dosage strength listed on the label and the values for H and Q. The drug label for

Amoxil lists the dosage strength as 125 mg/5 mL which, in fraction form, is $\frac{125 \text{ mg}}{5 \text{ mL}}$. This fraction corresponds to $\frac{H}{Q}$. Thus, $\frac{H}{Q}$ is the dosage strength.

When you solve for the *amount to administer* using the formula method, you use $\frac{Q}{H}$, the reciprocal of $\frac{H}{Q}$. Thus, $\frac{Q}{H}$ is simply the reciprocal of the dosage strength.

EXAMPLE 4 Find the amount of medication to administer.

Ordered: *Erythromycin DR 0.5 g po q12h*

On hand:

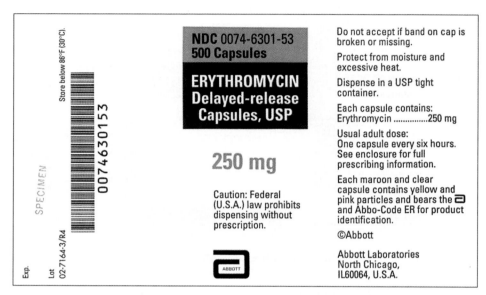

1. The *dosage ordered* and the *dose on hand* are not in the same unit. Convert the *dosage ordered* to mg to find the *desired dose.*

$$\frac{0.5 \text{ g}}{? \text{ mg}} = \frac{1 \text{ g}}{1000 \text{ mg}}$$

$$0.5 \times 1000 = ? \times 1$$

$$500 = ?$$

The *desired dose* is 500 mg.

2. Substitute the appropriate values into the $D \times \frac{Q}{H} = A$ formula. The dosage strength is 250 mg/1 capsule or $\frac{250 \text{ mg}}{1 \text{ capsule}}$. The reciprocal of the dosage strength, or $\frac{Q}{H}$, is $\frac{1 \text{ capsule}}{250 \text{mg}}$.

$$D \times \frac{Q}{H} = A \rightarrow 500 \text{ mg} \times \frac{1 \text{ capsule}}{250 \text{ mg}} = A$$

3. Solve for A.

$$^2\cancel{500} \text{ } \cancel{mg} \times \frac{1 \text{ capsule}}{1 \text{ } \cancel{250} \text{ } \cancel{mg}} = A$$

$$2 \times 1 \text{ capsule} = A$$

$$A = 2 \text{ capsules}$$

You would administer 2 tablets by mouth twice a day. Although the usual dose is one tablet every six hours, the physician has chosen to order two tablets every twelve hours.

4. You can convert from g to mg by multiplying 0.5 g by 1000, so that 0.5 g = 500 mg. Because 500 mg is twice 250 mg, you can estimate that you will administer twice the *dosage unit.*

THE FORMULA METHOD

Using the formula method, find the amount of medication to administer.

1. Ordered: *Keflex 500 mg PO q12h*
   On hand: Keflex 250 mg per 5 mL

2. Ordered: *Decadron 6 mg IM q.i.d.*
   On hand: Decadron 4 mg per mL

3. Ordered: *ketoconazole 100 mg po qd*
   On hand: ketoconazole 200 mg scored tablets

4. Ordered: *Dilaudid 2 mg IM prn for pain q6h*
   On hand: Dilaudid for injection, 4 mg per mL

5. Ordered: *Lorabid Oral Suspension 150 mg po bid*
   On hand: Refer to Label A.

6. Ordered: *furosemide 80 mg p.o. now*
   On hand: Refer to Label B.

A

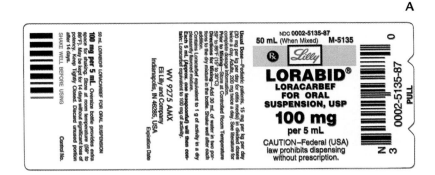

B

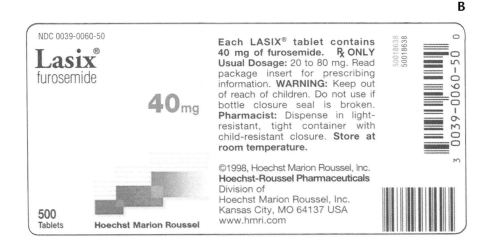

7. Ordered: *Heparin 8000 U sc stat*
   On hand: Refer to Label C.

8. Ordered: *Lente Iletin II 28 U sc stat*
   On hand: Refer to Label D.

9. Ordered: *Ritalin 15 mg po bid ac*
   On hand: Refer to Label E.

10. Ordered: *Univasc 3.75 mg po q am ac*
    On hand: Refer to Label F.

C

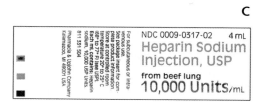

D

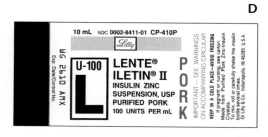

E

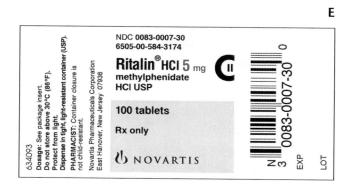

F

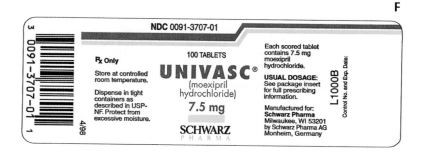

If you want more practice using the formula method, rework the Review and Practice problems from the previous section.

The formula method or either of the proportion methods (fraction proportions or ratio proportions) will lead you to the same result. Select a method for calculating the *desired dose* and a method for calculating the *amount to administer.* Choose a combination that is comfortable for you. In the next chapter, you will learn yet one more method for calculating dosages. This method, dimensional analysis, combines the two calculations (*desired dose* and *amount to administer*) into one.

CRITICAL THINKING ON THE JOB

When in Doubt, Check

Jorge was working as an emergency room nurse when a patient arrived with life-threatening internal bleeding. The physician in charge told Jorge, "Aminocaproic acid 5 grams STAT. You'd better give him the liquid. I don't think he's able to swallow pills." Jorge repeated the order, "Aminocaproic acid liquid 5 grams STAT."

On hand, Jorge had Amicar Syrup (aminocaproic acid) 25%, 250 mg/mL. Jorge first converted the 5 grams to 5000 milligrams so that the unit of the *desired dose* would match the unit of the *dose on hand.* Next, he calculated the *amount to administer,* using the ratio-proportion method.

250 mg:1 mL::5000 mg:? mL

$1 \times 5000 = 250\ ?$

$20 = ?$

He then converted 20 mL to tsp.

20 mL = 4 tsp

Think Before You Act

As he looked at his answer of 4 tsp, Jorge's initial thought was that 4 tsp was a lot of medication to give the patient. First, Jorge rechecked his calculations, which were correct. Still not sure that 4 tsp was an appropriate amount to give the patient, Jorge went to the physician in charge and confirmed the order.

In this case, Jorge heard the order correctly. The usual first dose of aminocaproic acid is large: 5 grams, which amounts to either 4 tsp of Amicar Syrup 25% or 10 of the 500-mg Amicar capsules. Because of the unusually large volume of liquid or number of tablets, Jorge was correct to reconfirm the order. Since the order was given orally in an emergency situation, it was important that he check directly with the ordering physician before administering the drug.

If Jorge's question had occurred in another circumstance, when a physician was not readily available, Jorge could consult the pharmacist or refer to the PDR (*Physicians' Desk Reference*) or another reliable reference to check the usual dose.

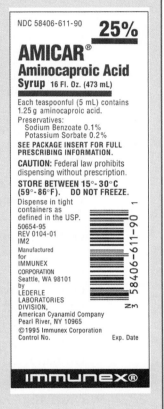

NDC 58406-611-90 **25%**

AMICAR®
Aminocaproic Acid
Syrup 16 Fl. Oz. (473 mL)

Each teaspoonful (5 mL) contains 1.25 g aminocaproic acid.
Preservatives:
 Sodium Benzoate 0.1%
 Potassium Sorbate 0.2%
SEE PACKAGE INSERT FOR FULL PRESCRIBING INFORMATION.
CAUTION: Federal law prohibits dispensing without prescription.
STORE BETWEEN 15°-30°C (59°-86°F). DO NOT FREEZE.
Dispense in tight containers as defined in the USP.
50654-95
REV 0104-01
IM2
Manufactured for
IMMUNEX CORPORATION
Seattle, WA 98101
by
LEDERLE LABORATORIES DIVISION,
American Cyanamid Company
Pearl River, NY 10965
©1995 Immunex Corporation
Control No.   Exp. Date

IMMUNEX®

CHAPTER 7 REVIEW

CHECK UP

In Exercises 1–14, calculate the *desired dose*. Then calculate the *amount to administer*.

1. Ordered: *Valium 5 mg po tid*
   On hand: Valium 2 mg scored tablets
   desired dose: _____   Amount to administer: _____

2. Ordered: *Atacand 16 mg po bid*
   On hand: Atacand 8 mg tablets
   desired dose: _____   Amount to administer: _____

3. Ordered: *cimetidine 400 mg po qid hs*
   On hand: Tagamet 200 mg tablets
   desired dose: _____   Amount to administer: _____

4. Ordered: *Noroxin 800 mg po qd ac c̄ H₂O*
   On hand: Noroxin 400 mg tablets
   desired dose: _____   Amount to administer: _____

5. Ordered: *Tenex 2 mg po qd hs*
   On hand: Tenex 1 mg tablets
   desired dose: _____   Amount to administer: _____

6. Ordered: *Tranxene 7.5 mg po qd hs*
   On hand: Tranxene 3.75 mg tablets
   desired dose: _____   Amount to administer: _____

7. Ordered: *pergolide mesylate 100 mcg po tid*
   On hand: pergolide mesylate 0.05 mg tablets
   desired dose: _____   Amount to administer: _____

8. Ordered: *Zyloprim 0.25 g p.o. b.i.d.*
   On hand: Zyloprim 100 mg scored tablets
   desired dose: _____   Amount to administer: _____

9. Ordered: *ciprofloxacin hydrochloride 500 mg po q12h*
   On hand: Refer to Label A.
   desired dose: _____   Amount to administer: _____

A

851210   NDC 0026-8512-51

CIPRO®
(ciprofloxacin hydrochloride)

Equivalent to
250 mg ciprofloxacin
100 Tablets

℞ Only

Bayer

Bayer Corporation
Pharmaceutical Division
400 Morgan Lane
West Haven, CT 06516

DESCRIPTION: Each tablet contains
ciprofloxacin hydrochloride equivalent to
250 mg of ciprofloxacin.
DOSAGE: See accompanying literature for
complete information on dosage and
administration.
RECOMMENDED STORAGE:
Store below 86°F (30°C).

Batch:
Expires:

SAMPLE
ONLY

PL500199 ©1999 Bayer Corporation 8919
6505-01-333-4155   Printed in USA

3 0026-8512-51 3

10. Ordered: *Prilosec-DR 20 mg po qd*
On hand: Refer to Label B.
desired dose: _____   Amount to administer: _____

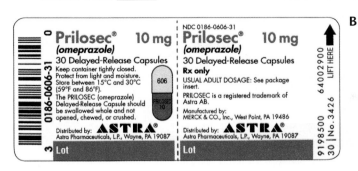

11. Ordered: *Augmentin 200 mg po q8h*
On hand: Refer to Label C.
desired dose: _____   Amount to administer: _____

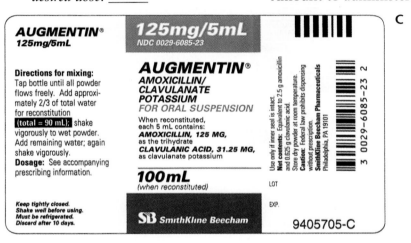

12. Ordered: *Zovirax 400 mg po bid*
On hand: Refer to Label D.
desired dose: _____   Amount to administer: _____

13. Ordered: *albuterol sulfate liquid 4 mg po tid*
   On hand: Refer to Label E.
   desired dose: _____   Amount to administer: _____

NDC 0173-0351-54
GlaxoWellcome
Ventolin®
(albuterol sulfate, USP)
Syrup

2 mg* per 5 mL

*Potency expressed as albuterol.

Each teaspoonful (5 mL) contains: 2 mg
of albuterol as the sulfate.

Usual Dose: See package insert.

Read accompanying directions carefully.

Store between 2° and 30°C (36° and 86°F).

Manufactured for Glaxo Wellcome Inc.
Research Triangle Park, NC 27709
by Schering Corporation
Kenilworth, NJ 07033

SAMPLE.
FOR EDUCATIONAL
USE ONLY.

4065646   Rev. 8/96   16194751

NDC 0173-0351-54
GlaxoWellcome
Ventolin®
(albuterol sulfate, USP)
Syrup

2 mg* per 5 mL

*Potency expressed as
albuterol.

Caution: Federal law prohibits
dispensing without prescription.

3 0173-0351-54 8

16 Fl. Oz.
(1 Pint)

E

14. Ordered: *Vistaril susp 60 mg po qid*
   On hand: Refer to Label F.
   desired dose: _____ Amount to administer: _____

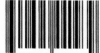

F

Vistaril®
(hydroxyzine pamoate)

ORAL SUSPENSION

*Each teaspoonful (5mL) contains
hydroxyzine pamoate equivalent
to 25 mg hydroxyzine hydrochloride.

USUAL DAILY DOSAGE
Adults: 1 to 4 teaspoonfuls 3-4 times daily
Children: 6 years and over—2 to 4 teaspoonfuls
daily in divided doses.
Under 6 years—2 teaspoonfuls daily
in divided doses.

READ ACCOMPANYING
PROFESSIONAL INFORMATION.

Store below 77°F (25°C)

Dispense in tight, light-resistant containers (USP)

SHAKE VIGOROUSLY UNTIL PRODUCT IS
COMPLETELY RESUSPENDED.

IMPORTANT: This closure is not child-resistant

DYE FREE FORMULA

CAUTION: Federal law
prohibits dispensing
without prescription.

05-0844-00-4
MADE IN USA

4387

E117A
EXP 1 MAY 02

NDC 0069-5440-93

1 Pint (473 mL)

Vistaril®
(hydroxyzine pamoate)

ORAL SUSPENSION

25 mg/5 mL*

For Oral Use Only

3 0069-5440-93 9

 Pfizer Labs
Division of Pfizer Inc, NY, NY 10017

CRITICAL THINKING

Use the following label to answer these questions.

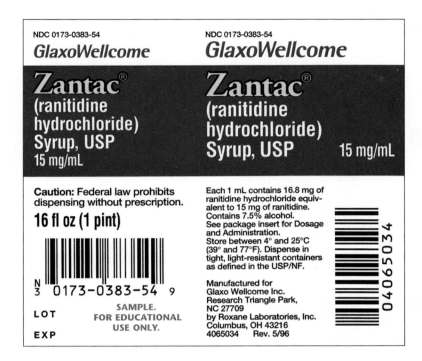

NDC 0173-0383-54

GlaxoWellcome

Zantac®
(ranitidine hydrochloride)
Syrup, USP
15 mg/mL

Caution: Federal law prohibits dispensing without prescription.

16 fl oz (1 pint)

N
3 0173-0383-54 9

LOT

EXP

SAMPLE.
FOR EDUCATIONAL
USE ONLY.

NDC 0173-0383-54

GlaxoWellcome

Zantac®
(ranitidine hydrochloride)
Syrup, USP   15 mg/mL

Each 1 mL contains 16.8 mg of ranitidine hydrochloride equivalent to 15 mg of ranitidine. Contains 7.5% alcohol. See package insert for Dosage and Administration. Store between 4° and 25°C (39° and 77°F). Dispense in tight, light-resistant containers as defined in the USP/NF.

Manufactured for
Glaxo Wellcome Inc.
Research Triangle Park,
NC 27709
by Roxane Laboratories, Inc.
Columbus, OH 43216
4065034   Rev. 5/96

1. A physician's order reads *Zantac 150 mg po b.i.d.* Calculate the *amount to administer.*

2. In some cases, the patient may receive 300 mg once a day at bedtime. Calculate the *amount to administer* for this dose.

3. In cases of severe pathologic hypersecretory conditions, a physician may order up to 6 g per day. If the patient is to be given 1.5 g per day, divided into four doses, what is the *amount to administer* per dose?

CASE STUDY

You are working in a pharmacy when the following prescription comes in: *Valium 7.5 mg po t.i.d. for 7 days*. The drug labels on page 184 represent what you have on hand for filling this prescription.

1. How would you fill this prescription?

2. What instructions should be given to the patient?

3. What changes would you make in filling the order if the prescription read *Valium 7 mg po t.i.d. for 7 days*?

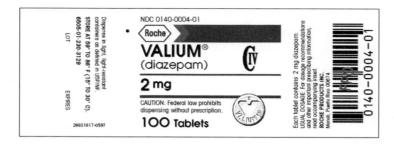

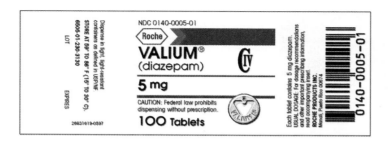

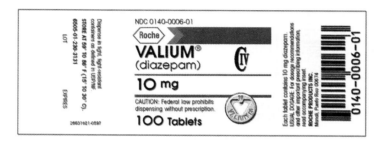

To check your answers, see page 350.

INTERNET ACTIVITY

Note: The Internet is a research tool from which to get basic information. Validate the accuracy of all Internet information.

You are working on an oncology ward. Many of the patients are confused about the amount, frequency, and duration of the chemotherapy drugs they are taking. Conduct an Internet search to find information in "plain English" to help them understand more about their medications. In addition, locate links to professional sites that will help you learn more about chemotherapy treatments.

Suggested key words: chemotherapy drugs, chemotherapy treatment, cancer therapy, cancer medication.

DIMENSIONAL ANALYSIS

8

Objectives

When you have completed Chapter 8, you will be able to:

- **Define dimensional analysis.**
- **Identify the different parts of a dimensional analysis calculation.**
- **Select the information for each factor.**
- **Solve dosage calculation problems using dimensional analysis.**
- **Recognize common errors that can occur using dimensional analysis.**

Introducing Dimensional Analysis

In Chapter 7 you learned two steps needed to calculate the amount of medication to administer to a patient. The first was to find the *desired dose.* The second was to use this quantity to find the *amount to administer.* Now you will learn to use dimensional analysis to combine these two steps into one.

Dimensional analysis (DA) allows you to convert one quantity to another using conversion factors. With DA, you analyze the dimensions (or units of measurement) in a calculation, hence the name *dimensional analysis.*

When you calculate the amount of a medication to administer, your starting point is the *dosage ordered* (the amount of medication that the physician has ordered for the patient, along with instructions about when it is to be administered). Your task is to calculate the ending point: what is the *amount to administer* to the patient at one time? When you use dimensional analysis for dosage calculations, you multiply the *dosage ordered* by one or more conversion factors. By selecting the appropriate factors, you cancel out various units of measurement. The remaining unit will be the unit of the *amount to administer.*

Finding the Dimensions

When you compute a dosage, your starting point, the *dosage ordered,* has both a quantity and a dimension (or unit of measurement). Your ending point, the *amount to administer,* also has a dimension—the same as the dimension of the *dosage unit* of the medication that you will be administering. For example, a physician orders 500 mg of an antibiotic to be administered orally every 8 hours. You have the antibiotic available in both tablet and injection form. Because the physician's order states "orally," you will administer the antibiotic that is in tablet form. Your task is to get from the starting point, 500 mg, to the ending point, the number of tablets to be administered.

Rule 8-1

The dimension of the *dosage ordered* is found on the physician's order. The *amount to administer* has the same dimension as the *dosage unit*, which is found on the drug label.

EXAMPLE 1 Find the dimensions of the *dosage ordered* and the *amount to administer.*

Ordered: *Ampicillin 500 mg po qid*

On hand: Ampicillin 250 mg capsules

The *dosage ordered* is 500 mg of Ampicillin delivered orally four times a day. An individual dose is 500 mg; its dimension is mg. The dosage strength is the *dose on hand* per *dosage unit* or 250 mg per 1 capsule. The dimension of the *amount to administer* is the same as the dimension of the *dosage unit,* in this example, capsule.

EXAMPLE 2 Find the dimensions of the *dosage ordered* and the *amount to administer.*

Ordered: *Haldol 4 mg IM stat*

On hand: Haldol Injection, 5 mg/mL

An individual dose of the *dosage ordered* is 4 mg; its dimension is mg. The dosage strength is 5 mg/mL. The *dosage unit* is 1 mL; therefore, the dimension of the *amount to administer* is mL.

EXAMPLE 3 Find the dimensions of the *dosage ordered* and the *amount to administer.*

Ordered: *Ceclor susp 375 mg po bid*

On hand: Ceclor 250 mg tablets

Ceclor 187 mg/5 mL for oral suspension

The *dosage ordered* is 375 mg of Ceclor given twice a day; its dimension is mg. The medication is available in two forms, tablets and oral suspension. The physician's order includes "susp" in it. Therefore, the oral suspension should be used. The dosage strength is 187 mg/5 mL. The *dosage unit* is 5 mL; therefore, the dimension of the *amount to administer* is mL.

In the three preceding examples, dimensional analysis can help you calculate how many capsules are needed to administer 500 mg of Ampicillin, how many mL of solution are needed to inject 4 mg of Haldol, and how many mL of oral suspension are needed to administer 375 mg of Ceclor.

Conversion Factors

Conversion factors are at the heart of dimensional analysis. They enable you to convert a quantity from one unit of measurement (or dimension) to another.

Rule 8-2

A conversion factor and its reciprocal both equal one.

Recall from Chapters 3 and 7 that a conversion factor equals one. Its numerator and denominator are equivalent. For example, $\frac{1000 \text{ mcg}}{1 \text{ mg}}$ and its reciprocal $\frac{1 \text{ mg}}{1000 \text{ mcg}}$ both equal one; therefore, they equal each other.

EXAMPLE 1 Find the reciprocal for each of the following:

a. $\frac{1 \text{ g}}{1000 \text{ mg}}$ **a.** The reciprocal of $\frac{1 \text{ g}}{1000 \text{ mg}}$ is $\frac{1000 \text{ mg}}{1 \text{ g}}$.

b. $\dfrac{5\text{ mL}}{1\text{ tsp}}$ **b.** The reciprocal of $\dfrac{5\text{ mL}}{1\text{ tsp}}$ is $\dfrac{1\text{ tsp}}{5\text{ mL}}$.

c. $\dfrac{30\text{ mg}}{\text{gr ss}}$ **c.** The reciprocal of $\dfrac{30\text{ mg}}{\text{gr ss}}$ is $\dfrac{\text{gr ss}}{30\text{ mg}}$.

Because a conversion factor has a value of one, you can multiply a quantity by a conversion factor without changing its value. For example, if you multiply 500 mcg by either $\dfrac{1000\text{ mcg}}{1\text{ mg}}$ or $\dfrac{1\text{ mg}}{1000\text{ mcg}}$, you will get a quantity equal to 500 mcg. If you use the first factor, $\dfrac{1000\text{ mcg}}{1\text{ mg}}$, the answer is not useful.

$$500\text{ mcg} \times \dfrac{1000\text{ mcg}}{1\text{ mg}} = \dfrac{500000\text{ mcg}^2}{1\text{ mg}}$$

However, if you use the second conversion factor, $\dfrac{1\text{ mg}}{1000\text{ mcg}}$, the *mcg* dimensions cancel each other, leading to a useful answer:

$$500\text{ mcg} \times \dfrac{1\text{ mg}}{1000\text{ mcg}} = \dfrac{500\ \cancel{\text{mcg}}}{1} \times \dfrac{1\text{ mg}}{1000\ \cancel{\text{mcg}}} = \dfrac{500\text{ mg}}{1000} = 0.5\text{ mg}$$

$$500\text{ mcg} = 0.5\text{ mg}$$

In this case, selecting the proper conversion factor enabled you to convert from mcg to mg.

Rule 8-3

To convert a value to an equivalent value with a different dimension, multiply the first value by a conversion factor in which

1. the denominator of the conversion factor has the same dimension as the first value.

2. the numerator of the conversion factor has the same dimension as the second value.

EXAMPLE 1   Use a conversion factor to convert 0.8 g to mg.

The conversion factors $\dfrac{1\text{ g}}{1000\text{ mg}}$ and $\dfrac{1000\text{ mg}}{1\text{ g}}$ relate *g* to *mg*. You can write the first value 0.8 g as $\dfrac{0.8\text{ g}}{1}$, with *g* in the numerator. Select the conversion factor with *g* in its denominator. The units will then cancel each other, leaving the dimension of the second value, *mg*, as the remaining unit.

$$\dfrac{0.8\text{ g}}{1} \times \dfrac{1000\text{ mg}}{1\text{ g}} = \dfrac{0.8\ \cancel{\text{g}}}{1} \times \dfrac{1000\text{ mg}}{1\ \cancel{\text{g}}} = \dfrac{800\text{ mg}}{1} = 800\text{ mg}$$

$$0.8\text{ g} = 800\text{ mg}$$

EXAMPLE 2   Use a conversion factor to convert 2 tsp to mL.

The conversion factors $\dfrac{5\text{ mL}}{1\text{ tsp}}$ and $\dfrac{1\text{ tsp}}{5\text{ mL}}$ relate *tsp* to *mL*. You can write the first value 2 tsp as $\dfrac{2\text{ tsp}}{1}$, with *tsp* in the numerator. Select the conversion factor with *tsp* in its denominator. The units will then cancel each other, leaving the dimension of the second value, *mL*, as the remaining unit.

$$\dfrac{2\text{ tsp}}{1} \times \dfrac{5\text{ mL}}{1\text{ tsp}} = \dfrac{2\ \cancel{\text{tsp}}}{1} \times \dfrac{5\text{ mL}}{1\ \cancel{\text{tsp}}} = \dfrac{10\text{ mL}}{1} = 10\text{ mL}$$

$$2\text{ tsp} = 10\text{ mL}$$

EXAMPLE 3 Use a conversion factor to convert gr ii to mg.

The conversion factors $\dfrac{60 \text{ mg}}{\text{gr i}}$ and $\dfrac{\text{gr i}}{60 \text{ mg}}$ relate *gr* to *mg*. You can write the first value gr ii as $\dfrac{\text{gr ii}}{1}$, with *gr* in the numerator. Select the conversion factor with *gr* in its denominator.

$$\frac{\text{gr ii}}{1} \times \frac{60 \text{ mg}}{\text{gr i}} = \frac{\cancel{\text{gr}} \text{ ii}}{1} \times \frac{60 \text{ mg}}{\cancel{\text{gr}} \text{ i}} = \frac{\text{ii} \times 60 \text{ mg}}{1 \times \text{i}} = \frac{120 \text{ mg}}{1} = 120 \text{ mg}$$

gr ii = 120 mg

As noted in Chapter 7, the relationship given between mg and gr is an approximate one, not an exact one. You will use $\dfrac{60 \text{ mg}}{\text{gr i}}$ or $\dfrac{\text{gr i}}{60 \text{ mg}}$ with medications such as nitroglycerin, codeine, and morphine, but $\dfrac{65 \text{ mg}}{\text{gr i}}$ or $\dfrac{\text{gr i}}{65 \text{ mg}}$ with aspirin and iron.

REVIEW and PRACTICE

INTRODUCING DIMENSIONAL ANALYSIS

In Exercises 1–12, find the dimensions of the *dosage ordered* and of the *amount to administer.*

1. Ordered: *Tegretol 200 mg po tid*
   On hand: Tegretol 100 mg chewable tablets

2. Ordered: *Danocrine 200 mg po tid*
   On hand: Danocrine 100 mg capsules

3. Ordered: *Tagamet 300 mg po qid ac hs*
   On hand: Tagamet liquid 300 mg/5 mL

4. Ordered: *Phenergan 12.5 mg deep IM prn q4h*
   On hand: Phenergan injection 25 mg/mL

5. Ordered: *Heparin 5000 U deep sc 2 h pre-op*
   On hand: Heparin Sodium Injection 10,000 units/mL

6. Ordered: *Heparin 6000 U deep sc bid*
   On hand: Heparin Sodium Injection 7500 units/mL

7. Ordered: *Zantac 50 mg IM q8h*
   On hand: Zantac injection 25 mg/mL, 6-mL multidose vial
   Zantac syrup, 15 mg/mL, 16 fl oz

8. Ordered: *Lanoxin 250 mcg deep IM stat*
   On hand: Lanoxin 125 mcg tablets
   Lanoxin injection 500 mcg/mL

9. Ordered: *Zofran 8 mg po bid*
   On hand: Refer to Label A.

10. Ordered: *Biaxin 500 mg po bid*
    On hand: Refer to Label B.

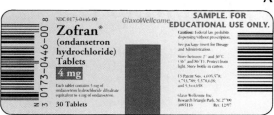

A

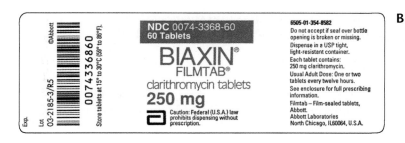

B

11. Ordered: *Atropine sulfate 0.5 mg sc q4h*
    On hand: Refer to Label C.

12. Ordered: *Dilaudid 2 mg sc prn q6h*
    On hand: Refer to Label D.

D

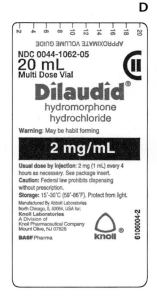

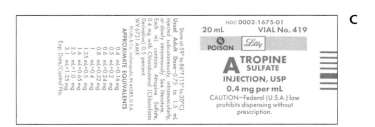

C

In Exercises 13–16, find the reciprocal of each conversion factor.

13. $\dfrac{1 \text{ oz}}{30 \text{ mL}}$

14. $\dfrac{2.2 \text{ lb}}{1 \text{ kg}}$

15. $\dfrac{1 \text{ L}}{1000 \text{ mL}}$

16. $\dfrac{\text{gr xv}}{1 \text{ g}}$

In Exercises 17–26, use a conversion factor to make each conversion.

17. 700 mg to g

18. 0.3 g to mg

19. 150 mcg to mg

20. 0.6 mg to mcg

21. 20 mL to tsp

22. 2 oz to mL

23. gr $\dfrac{1}{20}$ to mg

24. 90 mg to gr

25. 40 kg to lb

26. 121 lb to kg

To check your answers, see page 352.

Calculating the Amount to Administer

In dimensional analysis, the conversion factor that you will use most often when calculating the *amount to administer* is the reciprocal of a medication's dosage strength.

Dimensional Analysis with One Conversion Factor

Sometimes the *dosage ordered* already has the same dimension as the available medication, and no separate conversion is needed to find the *desired dose*. In these cases, the reciprocal of the dosage strength is the only conversion factor you will need to calculate the *amount to administer*.

Rule 8-4

The product of the *desired dose* and the reciprocal of the dosage strength is the *amount to administer*, or

$$\text{desired dose} \times \frac{\text{dosage unit}}{\text{dose on hand}} = \text{amount to administer}$$

Suppose you want to convert from one value, the *desired dose*, to a second value, the *amount to administer*. According to Rule 8-3, you would set up the following equation,

$$\text{desired dose} \times \text{conversion factor} = \text{amount to administer}$$

The conversion factor's denominator has the same dimension as the *desired dose*, and the numerator has the same dimension as the *amount to administer*.

Recall from Rule 7-2 that the *desired dose* has the same unit of measurement (or dimension) as the *dose on hand*. Therefore, the *dose on hand* can be the denominator of the conversion factor. From Rule 8-1, you know that the *amount to administer* has the same dimension as the *dosage unit*. Therefore, you can use the *dosage unit* as the numerator of the conversion factor.

Now you can set up your equation so that,

$$\text{desired dose} \times \frac{\text{dosage unit}}{\text{dose on hand}} = \text{amount to administer}$$

EXAMPLE 1 Find the *amount to administer*.

Desired dose: 30 mg

On hand: 15 mg tablets

The *desired dose* is 30 mg. The available medication has a dosage strength of $\frac{15mg}{1 \text{ tablet}}$. The reciprocal of the dosage strength is $\frac{1 \text{ tablet}}{15mg}$. The *amount to administer* is the number of tablets you administer so that the patient receives 30 mg of medication.

$$30 \text{ mg} \times \frac{1 \text{ tablet}}{15mg} \quad \text{amount to administer}$$

$$\overset{2}{\cancel{30}} \text{ }\cancel{mg} \times \frac{1 \text{ tablet}}{\underset{1}{\cancel{15}}\cancel{mg}} = 2 \times 1 \text{ tablet} = 2 \text{ tablets}$$

You would administer 2 tablets to the patient.

Note that the dimension of the conversion factor's denominator, mg, cancels out the dimension of the *desired dose*. The remaining dimension of the *dosage unit* becomes the dimension of the *amount to administer*.

EXAMPLE 2

Find the *amount to administer.*

Desired dose: 75 mg

On hand: 150 mg/mL injection

The *desired dose* is 75 mg. The available medication has a dosage strength of $\frac{150\ mg}{1\ mL}$. The reciprocal of the dosage strength is $\frac{1\ mL}{150\ mg}$. The *amount to administer* is the number of mL you administer so that the patient receives 75 mg of medication.

$$75\ mg \times \frac{1\ mL}{150\ mg} = amount\ to\ administer$$

$$^1\cancel{75}\ \cancel{mg} \times \frac{1\ mL}{_2\cancel{150}\ \cancel{mg}} = 1 \times \frac{1}{2}mL = \frac{1}{2}mL = 0.5\ mL$$

You would administer 0.5 mL to the patient by injection.

In this example, the dimension of the conversion factor's denominator, mg, cancels the dimension of the *desired dose*. The remaining dimension, the *dosage unit's* mL, becomes the dimension of the *amount to administer*.

If you substitute D for *desired dose,* Q for *dosage unit* (or quantity), H for *dose on hand,* and A for *amount to administer,* then you can write the general equation as

$$D \times \frac{Q}{H} = A$$

This is the same formula used in the last part of Chapter 7. This formula is commonly written in an alternate form, as

$$\frac{D}{H} \times Q = X$$

The version $D \times \frac{Q}{H} = A$ has two advantages over the alternate form. First, as the reciprocal of the dosage strength, $\frac{Q}{H}$ is easy to find on the drug label. Second, $D \times \frac{Q}{H} = A$ is an effective building block for more complex calculations.

EXAMPLE 3

Find the *amount to administer.*

Ordered: *Sandostatin 200 mcg sc tid*

On hand:

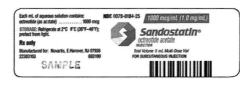

The *desired dose* is 200 mcg. The dosage strength is 1000 mcg/mL; its reciprocal is 1 mL/1000 mcg. The *dosage unit* is 1 mL; therefore, the dimension of the *amount to administer* is mL. You want to calculate how many mL to administer so that the patient receives 200 mcg of Sandostatin.

$$200\ mcg \times \frac{1\ mL}{1000\ mcg} = amount\ to\ administer$$

$$^1\cancel{200}\ \cancel{mcg} \times \frac{1\ mL}{_5\cancel{1000}\ \cancel{mcg}} = amount\ to\ administer$$

$$1 \times \frac{1\ mL}{5} = \frac{1}{5}\ mL = 0.2\ mL$$

The *amount to administer* is 0.2 mL of Sandostatin.

DIMENSIONAL ANALYSIS WITH ONE CONVERSION FACTOR

Go back to Exercises 1–12 in this chapter's first Review and Practice (Introducing Dimensional Analysis). Calculate the *amount to administer*.

Calculating the Desired Dose with the One-Step Method

The last example began with the *dosage ordered,* unlike the previous two examples which began with the *desired dose.* However, the *dosage ordered* and the *dose on hand* had the same dimension, mcg. Therefore, you did not need a conversion factor to get from the *dosage ordered* to the *desired dose.* In many cases, however, you will need to make that conversion. Building from Rule 8-3, dimensional analysis provides a one-step method for converting the *dosage ordered* to the *desired dose.*

Rule 8-5

To convert from the *dosage ordered* to the *desired dose,* multiply the *dosage ordered* by a conversion factor in which

1. the denominator has the same dimension as the *dosage ordered,* and

2. the numerator has the same dimension as the *dose on hand,* so that

dosage ordered × conversion factor = *desired dose*

EXAMPLE 1 The *dosage ordered* is 0.2 mg. The *dose on hand* is in mcg. Find the *desired dose.*

The dimension of the *dosage ordered* is mg. Therefore, the denominator of the conversion factor will also be mg. The dimension of the *desired dose* will be the same dimension as the *dose on hand,* or mcg. In turn, the numerator of the conversion factor is mcg. The conversion factor, then, should relate mcg to mg. Use the conversion factor $\dfrac{1000 \text{ mcg}}{1 \text{ mg}}$.

dosage ordered × conversion factor = *desired dose*

$$0.2 \text{ mg} \times \frac{1000 \text{ mcg}}{1 \text{ mg}} = \textit{desired dose}$$

$$0.2 \text{ m\!g} \times \frac{1000 \text{ mcg}}{1 \text{ m\!g}} = 0.2 \times 1000 \text{ mcg} = 200 \text{ mcg}$$

The *desired dose* is 200 mcg.

Notice that this example has the same problem statement as the examples that followed Rules 7-3 and 7-4 in the previous chapter. All three versions of the example reached the same answer: the *desired dose* is 200 mcg. The one-step method is an alternative method to the conversion-factor method and the ratio-proportion method, both shown in Chapter 7 for finding the *desired dose.*

EXAMPLE 2 The *dosage ordered* is 0.8 g. The *dose on hand* is in mg. Find the *desired dose.*

The dimension of the *dosage ordered* is g. Therefore, the denominator of the conversion factor will also be g. The dimension of the *desired dose* will be the same dimension as the *dose on hand,* or mg. In turn, the numerator of the conversion factor is mg. The conversion factor, then, should relate mg to g. Use the conversion factor $\dfrac{1000 \text{ mg}}{1 \text{ g}}$.

dosage ordered × conversion factor = *desired dose*

$$0.8 \text{ g} \times \frac{1000 \text{ mg}}{1 \text{ g}} = \textit{desired dose}$$

$$0.8 \text{ \!g} \times \frac{1000 \text{ mg}}{1 \text{ \!g}} = 0.8 \times 1000 \text{ mg} = 800 \text{ mg}$$

The *desired dose* is 800 mg.

EXAMPLE 3 The order reads: *ASA gr v po qd.* The drug label indicates 325 mg tablets. Find the *desired dose.*

The dimension of the *dosage ordered,* gr, will be the dimension of the conversion factor's denominator. The *dose on hand* is 325 mg. The *desired dose* will have the same dimension, mg, as the *dose on hand.* Use the conversion factor $\dfrac{65 \text{ mg}}{\text{gr i}}$.

dosage ordered × conversion factor = *desired dose*

$$\text{gr v} \times \frac{65 \text{ mg}}{\text{gr i}} = \text{desired dose}$$

$$\cancel{\text{gr}} \text{ v} \times \frac{65 \text{ mg}}{\cancel{\text{gr}} \text{ i}} = 5 \times \frac{65 \text{ mg}}{1} = 325 \text{ mg}$$

This example is one you have seen before: Example 2, following both Rules 7-3 and 7-4. Once again, the desired dose is 325 mg. Only the method for finding the desired dose is different.

REVIEW and PRACTICE

CALCULATING THE DESIRED DOSE WITH THE ONE-STEP METHOD

In each of the following exercises, use dimensional analysis to find the *desired dose.*

1. Ordered: 0.4 mg
   On hand: 200 mcg caplets

2. Ordered: 250 mg
   On hand: 0.5 g scored tablets

3. Ordered: 200 mcg
   On hand: 0.1 mg/mL elixir

4. Ordered: 0.15 g
   On hand: 300 mg/2 mL for injection

5. Ordered: *Ampicillin 0.5 g po q.i.d.*
   On hand: Principen 250 mg ampicillin capsules

6. Ordered: *Decadron 750 mcg p.o. q.d.*
   On hand: Decadron 1.5 mg scored tablets

7. Ordered: *Vistaril susp 50 mg po q8h*
   On hand: Vistaril 25 mg/5 mL oral suspension

8. Ordered: *Ancef 250 mg IM q6h*
   On hand: Ancef 1 gram for I.V. or I.M. use

9. Ordered: *Depo-Provera 0.6 g IM*
   On hand: Refer to Label A.

10. Ordered: *morphine sulfate gr ss po q6h*
    On hand: Refer to Label B.

A

B

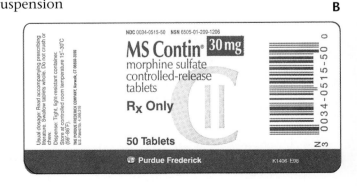

Dimensional Analysis with Two Conversion Factors

Thus far, you have used dimensional analysis to calculate the *amount to administer* from the *desired dose* as well as the *desired dose* from the *dosage ordered*. Now you can combine these steps into one calculation that takes you from the *dosage ordered* to the *amount to administer*.

Earlier in the chapter, you learned that

$$desired\ dose \times \frac{dosage\ unit}{dose\ on\ hand} = amount\ to\ administer$$

and that

$$dosage\ ordered \times conversion\ factor = desired\ dose$$

Now you can substitute the left side of this last equation for *desired dose* in the previous one, so that

$$dosage\ ordered \times conversion\ factor \times \frac{dosage\ unit}{dose\ on\ hand} = amount\ to\ administer$$

At first glance, this formula may seem complicated. It is not. The first two factors are the ones you use in the one-step method. The third factor is the reciprocal of the dosage strength.

Rule 8-6

To find A, the *amount to administer,* multiply the *dosage ordered,* a conversion factor, and the reciprocal of the dosage strength, so that

$$dosage\ ordered \times conversion\ factor \times \frac{dosage\ unit}{dose\ on\ hand} = A$$

The key to making this formula work for you is to select the correct conversion factor. Dimensional analysis provides that step so that you can easily calculate the amount of medication to administer to a patient. In later chapters you will learn expanded versions of this formula that take into account a patient's weight or the rate at which intravenous medication flows into a patient's bloodstream. However, for many routine calculations for adult patients, the above formula will help you find the *amount to administer.*

> **EXAMPLE 1** Find the *amount to administer.*
>
> Ordered: *Erythromycin 0.5 g po bid*
>
> On hand: Erythromycin 250 mg delayed-release capsules
>
> The dimension of the *dosage ordered* is g. The dimension of the *amount to administer,* which is the same as the *dosage unit,* is capsules. You need to determine how many capsules to administer so that the patient receives 0.5 g of medication.
>
> The dosage strength is 250 mg per capsule; therefore, the reciprocal of the dosage strength is $\frac{1\ capsule}{250\ mg}$. Developing your calculation, you can now see that
>
> $$0.5\ g \times conversion\ factor \times \frac{1\ capsule}{250\ mg} = A$$
>
> The conversion factor should have g in its denominator to cancel the g of the *dosage ordered.* It should have mg in its numerator to cancel the mg of the *dose on hand.* The correct conversion factor, then, is $\frac{1000\ mg}{1\ g}$. By canceling the g and mg dimensions, the remaining dimension will be the capsule of the *dosage unit.* This is the dimension you want for the *amount to administer.*
>
> $$0.5\ g \times \frac{1000\ mg}{1\ g} \times \frac{1\ capsule}{250\ mg} = A$$
>
> $$0.5\ \cancel{g} \times \frac{1000\ \cancel{mg}}{1\ \cancel{g}} \times \frac{1\ capsule}{250\ \cancel{mg}} = A$$

$$0.5 \times \frac{1000}{1} \times \frac{1 \text{ capsule}}{250} = A$$

$$0.5 \times \frac{^4\cancel{1000}}{1} \times \frac{1 \text{ capsule}}{\cancel{250}_1} = A$$

$$0.5 \times 4 \times 1 \text{ capsule} = A$$

$$2 \text{ capsules} = A$$

The amount to administer is 2 capsules. Please note that this example is the same as Example 4 following Rule 7-7. When you saw this example earlier, you first calculated the d*esired dose.* You then calculated the *amount to administer.* Here, you combined the two calculations into one.

EXAMPLE 2   Find the *amount to administer.*

Ordered: *Augmentin 0.4 g susp po q12h*

On hand: Refer to the label below.

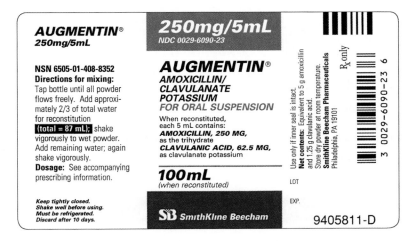

The dimension of the *dosage ordered* is g. The dimension of the *amount to administer* is mL. You need to determine how many mL to administer so that the patient receives 0.4 g of medication.

The *dosage ordered* is 0.4 g. The reciprocal of the dosage strength is $\frac{5 \text{ mL}}{250 \text{ mg}}$. You can now see that

$$0.4 \text{ g} \times \text{conversion factor} \times \frac{5 \text{ mL}}{250 \text{ mg}} = A$$

The conversion factor should have g in its denominator to cancel the g of the *dosage ordered.* It should also have mg in its numerator to cancel the mg of the *dose on hand.* The remaining dimension will be the mL of the *dosage unit.* This is the dimension you want for the amount to administer.

$$0.4 \text{ g} \times \frac{1000 \text{ mg}}{1 \text{ g}} \times \frac{5 \text{ mL}}{250 \text{ mg}} = A$$

$$0.4 \text{ } \cancel{g} \times \frac{^4\cancel{1000} \text{ } \cancel{mg}}{1 \text{ } \cancel{g}} \times \frac{5 \text{ mL}}{_1\cancel{250} \text{ } \cancel{mg}} = A$$

$$0.4 \times 4 \times 5 \text{ mL} = A$$

$$8 \text{ mL} = A$$

The *amount to administer* is 8 mL of Augmentin.

EXAMPLE 3 Find the *amount to administer.*

Ordered: *Armour Thyroid 150 mg po qd*

On hand: Armour Thyroid gr v scored tablets

The dimension of the *dosage ordered* is mg. The dimension of the *amount to administer* is tablets. You need to determine how many tablets to administer so that the patient receives 150 mg of medication.

The *dosage ordered* is 150 mg. The reciprocal of the dosage strength is $\frac{1 \text{ tablet}}{\text{gr v}}$. You can see that

$$150 \text{ mg} \times \text{conversion factor} \times \frac{1 \text{ tablet}}{\text{gr v}} = A$$

The conversion factor should have mg in its denominator to cancel the mg of the *dosage ordered.* It should also have gr in its numerator to cancel the gr of the *dose on hand.* The correct conversion factor, then, is $\frac{\text{gr i}}{60 \text{ mg}}$. The remaining dimension will be the tablet of the *dosage unit.* This is the dimension you want for the *amount to administer.*

$$150 \text{ mg} \times \frac{\text{gr i}}{60 \text{ mg}} \times \frac{1 \text{ tablet}}{\text{gr v}} = A$$

$$^{30}\cancel{150} \,\cancel{mg} \times \frac{\cancel{gr}\text{ i}}{60 \,\cancel{mg}} \times \frac{1 \text{ tablet}}{\cancel{gr\ v}_1} = A$$

$$^1\cancel{30} \times \frac{\text{i}}{\cancel{60}_2} \times 1 \text{ tablet} = A$$

$$\frac{1}{2} \times 1 \text{ tablet} = A$$

The *amount to administer* is $\frac{1}{2}$ tablet of the gr v scored tablet. Because the tablet is scored, you may break it in half.

CRITICAL THINKING ON THE JOB

Applying Dimensional Analysis

As a visiting nurse at an extended-care health facility, Charlene receives an order to give one of her patients a usual dose of the fiber supplement Metamucil. According to the drug label, the usual dose is 1 rounded teaspoon mixed with 8 oz of liquid. However, the only available measuring device is calibrated in mL. Furthermore, the conversion chart available to her does not relate oz to mL. It does, however, note that 1 oz = 30 cc and 1 cc = 1 mL.

Think Before You Act

While Charlene is fairly sure how much liquid to measure, she decides to check her work by using dimensional analysis. She must convert 8 oz to mL.

She uses one conversion factor, $\frac{30 \text{ cc}}{1 \text{ oz}}$, to cancel the oz unit of measurement. Her second conversion factor must now relate cc to mL, and cancel cc. She selects $\frac{1 \text{ mL}}{1 \text{ cc}}$. Thus, Charlene sets up her calculation as follows:

$$8 \text{ oz} \times \frac{30 \text{ cc}}{1 \text{ oz}} \times \frac{1 \text{ mL}}{1 \text{ cc}} = A$$

$$8 \,\cancel{oz} \times \frac{30 \,\cancel{cc}}{1 \,\cancel{oz}} \times \frac{1 \text{ mL}}{1 \,\cancel{cc}} = A$$

$$8 \times 30 \times 1 \text{ mL} = A$$

$$240 \text{ mL} = A$$

She mixes the Metamucil with 240 mL of liquid. Because 1 cc = 1 mL, Charlene is fairly confident she can substitute mL for cc when calculating the amount of liquid.

By taking the moment to check her work, Charlene increases the likelihood that her calculation is accurate. Had she confused conversion factors, and substituted 1 mL for 1 oz, she would have mixed the Metamucil with too small an amount of liquid. This error could have resulted in the patient choking. Her careful work ensures the patient's safety.

Check the factors in your calculations.

Whenever you calculate with dimensional analysis and conversion factors, you should include the units of measurement in your work. Be sure that the units correctly cancel each other so that the remaining unit of measurement has the same dosage unit as the *dose on hand*. Also be certain that you have used the correct quantities.

Suppose a drug order reads *250 mg PO q8h* and that you have 0.5 g scored tablets available. Knowing that there are 1000 mg per 1 g, you multiply

$$0.5 \times \frac{1000}{1} \times \frac{1}{250} = \frac{0.5 \times 1000}{250} = 2$$

You administer 2 tablets to the patient. This amount is four times as much as was ordered.

If you include the units of measurement with your calculation, you will find such errors more quickly:

$$0.5 \text{ g} \times \frac{1000 \text{ mg}}{1 \text{ g}} \times \frac{1 \text{ tablet}}{250 \text{ mg}}$$

At first glance, this formula seems correct because the conversion factor cancels the units g and mg, leaving tablets as the unit of measurement for the answer.

However, with a closer look, you can see that 0.5 g is the *dose on hand*, not the *dosage ordered*. Reviewing the drug order, you realize that 250 mg is the *dosage ordered*. In addition, the dosage strength is $\frac{0.5 \text{ g}}{1 \text{ tablet}}$, making its reciprocal $\frac{1 \text{ tablet}}{0.5 \text{ g}}$, not $\frac{1 \text{ tablet}}{250 \text{ mg}}$. After correcting these factors, your calculation reads

$$250 \text{ mg} \times \frac{1000 \text{ mg}}{1 \text{ g}} \times \frac{1 \text{ tablet}}{0.5 \text{ g}}$$

Now you can see that your conversion factor is incorrect. It does not help you cancel any units of measurement. The correct conversion factor has g as the numerator and mg as the denominator, $\frac{1 \text{ g}}{1000 \text{ mg}}$, so that the formula reads

$$250 \text{ mg} \times \frac{1 \text{ g}}{1000 \text{ mg}} \times \frac{1 \text{ tablet}}{0.5 \text{ g}} = A$$

$$\frac{1}{2} \text{ tablet} = A$$

In this case, you should administer $\frac{1}{2}$ tablet to the patient, not 2 tablets. Including the units of measurement and checking that each factor is correct will help you avoid errors.

REVIEW and PRACTICE

CALCULATING THE AMOUNT TO ADMINISTER

In Exercises 1–24, find the *amount to administer*.

1. Ordered: *300 mcg po q6h ac hs*
   On hand: 0.15 mg tablets

2. Ordered: *750 mg po q8h*
   On hand: 0.5 g scored tablets

3. Ordered: *0.2 mg po bid*
   On hand: 100 mcg/5 mL

4. Ordered: *0.3 g IM q8h*
   On hand: 200 mg/mL

5. Ordered: *gr iss IM q12h*
   On hand: 300 mg/10 mL

6. Ordered: *gr $\frac{1}{60}$ sc stat*
   On hand: 2 mg/5 mL

7. Ordered: *1200 mcg tid*
   On hand: 0.6 mg per inhalation

8. Ordered: *0.2 mg qid*
   On hand: 100 mcg per inhalation

9. Ordered: *240,000 U IM qid*
   On hand: 300,000 Units per mL

10. Ordered: *250,000 U po tid*
    On hand: 100,000 Units per 5 mL

11. Ordered: *Diabinese 0.5 g po qd*
    On hand: Diabinese 250 mg tablets

12. Ordered: *Coumadin 2.5 mg po bid*
    On hand: Coumadin 5 mg scored tablets

13. Ordered: *Flumadine 0.1 g po bid*
    On hand: Flumadine syrup 50 mg/5 mL

14. Ordered: *Keflex 0.5 g by nasogastric tube q12h*
    On hand: Keflex oral suspension 250 mg/5 mL

15. Ordered: *Diazepam 7.5 mg IM stat*
    On hand: Diazepam 5 mg/mL, 10 mL multidose vial

16. Ordered: *Codeine gr $\frac{1}{4}$ IM q4h prn for pain*
    On hand: Codeine phosphate injection, 30 mg/mL

17. Ordered: *pirbuterol acetate 400 mcg q6h*
    On hand: Maxair Inhaler 0.2 mg per puff

18. Ordered: *Bicillin C-R 1,200,000 Units deep IM qod*
    On hand: Bicillin C-R 600,000 Units/mL

19. Ordered: *Felbatol 1.2 g po tid*
    On hand: Refer to Label A.

A

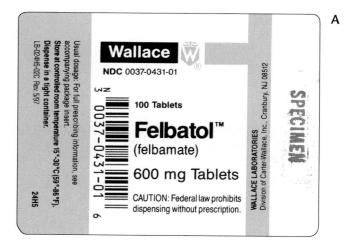

20. Ordered: *Azulfidine 1 g po tid*
    On hand: Refer to Label B.

B

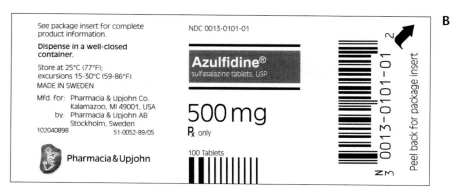

21. Ordered: *ritonavir 600 mg po bid*
On hand: Refer to Label C.

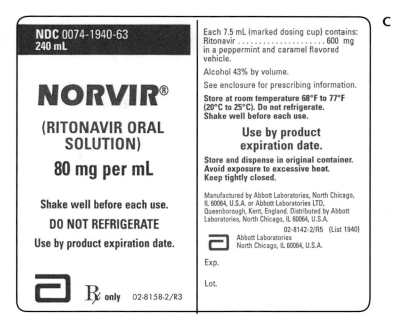

C

NDC 0074-1940-63
240 mL

NORVIR®

(RITONAVIR ORAL SOLUTION)

80 mg per mL

Shake well before each use.

DO NOT REFRIGERATE

Use by product expiration date.

Rx only   02-8158-2/R3

Each 7.5 mL (marked dosing cup) contains:
Ritonavir . . . . 600 mg
in a peppermint and caramel flavored vehicle.

Alcohol 43% by volume.

See enclosure for prescribing information.

Store at room temperature 68°F to 77°F (20°C to 25°C). Do not refrigerate. Shake well before each use.

Use by product expiration date.

Store and dispense in original container. Avoid exposure to excessive heat. Keep tightly closed.

Manufactured by Abbott Laboratories, North Chicago, IL 60064, U.S.A. or Abbott Laboratories LTD, Queenborough, Kent, England. Distributed by Abbott Laboratories, North Chicago, IL 60064, U.S.A.

02-8142-2/R5   (List 1940)

Abbott Laboratories
North Chicago, IL 60064, U.S.A.

Exp.

Lot.

22. Ordered: *Ceftin 0.25 g po bid*
On hand: Refer to Label D.

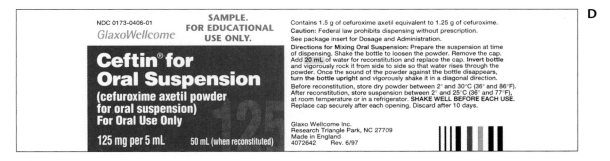

D

NDC 0173-0406-01
GlaxoWellcome

SAMPLE. FOR EDUCATIONAL USE ONLY.

Ceftin® for Oral Suspension

(cefuroxime axetil powder for oral suspension)
For Oral Use Only

125 mg per 5 mL   50 mL (when reconstituted)

Contains 1.5 g of cefuroxime axetil equivalent to 1.25 g of cefuroxime.
Caution: Federal law prohibits dispensing without prescription.
See package insert for Dosage and Administration.
Directions for Mixing Oral Suspension: Prepare the suspension at time of dispensing. Shake the bottle to loosen the powder. Remove the cap. Add 20 mL of water for reconstitution and replace the cap. Invert bottle and vigorously rock it from side to side so that water rises through the powder. Once the sound of the powder against the bottle disappears, turn the bottle upright and vigorously shake it in a diagonal direction.
Before reconstitution, store dry powder between 2° and 30°C (36° and 86°F). After reconstitution, store suspension between 2° and 25°C (36° and 77°F), at room temperature or in a refrigerator. SHAKE WELL BEFORE EACH USE. Replace cap securely after each opening. Discard after 10 days.

Glaxo Wellcome Inc.
Research Triangle Park, NC 27709
Made in England
4072642   Rev. 6/97

23. Ordered: *isoniazid 0.3 g IM qd*
On hand: Refer to Label E.

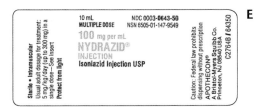

E

10 mL
MULTIPLE DOSE   NDC 0003-0643-50
NSN 6505-01-147-9549

100 mg per mL
NYDRAZID®
INJECTION
Isoniazid Injection USP

Sterile • Intramuscular
Usual adult dosage for treatment: 5 mg/kg/day (up to 300 mg) in a single dose—See insert
Protect from light

Caution: Federal law prohibits dispensing without prescription
APOTHECON®
A Bristol-Myers Squibb Co.
Princeton, NJ 08540 USA

C2764B I 64350

24. Ordered: *Antilirium 500 mcg IM stat*
On hand: Refer to Label F.

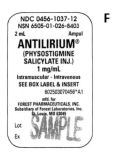

F

NDC 0456-1037-12
NSN 6505-01-026-8403
2 mL   Ampul
ANTILIRIUM®
(PHYSOSTIGMINE SALICYLATE INJ.)
1 mg/mL
Intramuscular - Intravenous
SEE BOX LABEL & INSERT
602503070456*A1
mfd. for
FOREST PHARMACEUTICALS, INC.
Subsidiary of Forest Laboratories, Inc.
St. Louis, MO 63045
Lot
Ex   SAMPLE

To check your answers, see page 353.

CHAPTER 8 REVIEW

CHECK UP

In Exercises 1–22, use dimensional analysis to find the *amount to administer*.

1. Ordered: 1.5 mg
   On hand: 750 mcg capsules

2. Ordered: 1 g
   On hand: 400 mg scored tablets

3. Ordered: 0.9 g
   On hand: 225 mg/5 mL elixir

4. Ordered: 0.9 mg
   On hand: 125 mcg/mL oral suspension

5. Ordered: 500,000 Units
   On hand: 125,000 U/mL

6. Ordered: 1,500,000 Units
   On hand: 300,000 U/2 mL

7. Ordered: 90 mEq
   On hand: 15 mEq/mL

8. Ordered: 50 mEq
   On hand: 25 mEq/5 mL

9. Ordered: *Excedrin Extra Strength 0.5 g po q6h prn for pain*
   On hand: Extra Strength Excedrin 250 mg tablets

10. Ordered: *Lopid 0.6 g po bid 30 minutes ac*
    On hand: Lopid 600 mg tablets

11. Ordered: *phenobarbital gr i elix po bid*
    On hand: Phenobarbital Elixir 0.4 g/ 100 mL

12. Ordered: *penicillin V potassium 0.4 g po q8h*
    On hand: Pen Vee K 125 mg/5 mL for oral solution

13. Ordered: *morphine sulfate gr $\frac{1}{8}$ IM q4h prn for pain*
    On hand: Morphine sulfate 15 mg/mL, 20 mL multiple dose vial

14. Ordered: *Robinul 100 mcg IM qid*
    On hand: Robinul 0.2 mg/mL single dose vials

15. Ordered: *Oxycontin 40 mg po q12h prn for pain*
On hand: Refer to Label A.

A

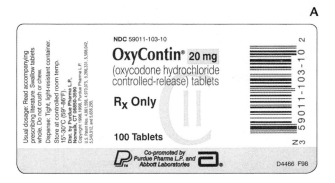

NDC 59011-103-10

OxyContin® 20 mg
(oxycodone hydrochloride
controlled-release) tablets

R_X Only

100 Tablets

Usual dosage: Read accompanying prescribing literature. Swallow tablets whole. Do not crush or chew.
Dispense: Tight, light-resistant container.
Store at controlled room temp.
15°-30°C (59°-86°F).
Dist. by Purdue Pharma L.P.,
Norwalk, CT 06850-3590
Copyright 1996, Purdue Pharma L.P.
U.S. Patent Nos. 4,861,598, 4,970,075, 5,266,331, 5,508,042, 5,549,912, and 5,656,295.

Co-promoted by
Purdue Pharma L.P. and
Abbott Laboratories

D4466 F98

16. Ordered: *Zyloprim 0.2 g po bid*
On hand: Refer to Label B.

B

SAMPLE FOR EDUCATIONAL USE ONLY.

100 Tablets   NDC 0173-0996-55

ZYLOPRIM®
(allopurinol)
Each scored tablet contains
100 mg

CAUTION: Federal law prohibits dispensing
without prescription.
Manufactured by Catalytica Pharmaceuticals, Inc.
Greenville, NC 27834
for Glaxo Wellcome Inc.
Research Triangle
Park, NC 27709   650337

LOT
EXP

for indications, dosage, precautions, etc., see
accompanying package insert.
Store at 15° to 25°C (59° to 77°F) in a dry place.
Dispense in tight container as defined in the USP.
Made in U.S.A.   NSN 6505-00-998-4381   4097572   Rev. 11/97

17. Ordered: *Claritin syrup 10 mg po qd*
On hand: Refer to Label C.

C

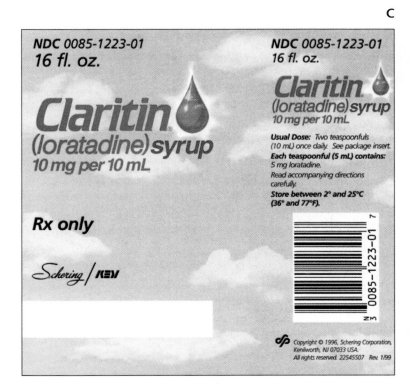

NDC 0085-1223-01
16 fl. oz.

Claritin
(loratadine) syrup
10 mg per 10 mL

Rx only

Schering / KEY

NDC 0085-1223-01
16 fl. oz.

Claritin
(loratadine) syrup
10 mg per 10 mL

Usual Dose: Two teaspoonfuls
(10 mL) once daily. See package insert.
Each teaspoonful (5 mL) contains:
5 mg loratadine.
Read accompanying directions
carefully.
**Store between 2° and 25°C
(36° and 77°F).**

Copyright © 1996, Schering Corporation,
Kenilworth, NJ 07033 USA.
All rights reserved. 22545507 Rev. 1/99

18. Ordered: *lactulose 20 g po qd*
    On hand: Refer to Label D.

D

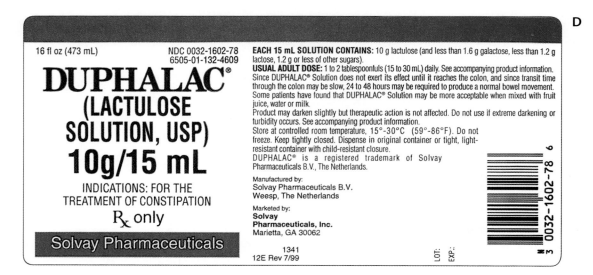

16 fl oz (473 mL)   NDC 0032-1602-78
6505-01-132-4609

DUPHALAC®
(LACTULOSE SOLUTION, USP)
10g/15 mL
INDICATIONS: FOR THE
TREATMENT OF CONSTIPATION
Rx only
Solvay Pharmaceuticals

EACH 15 mL SOLUTION CONTAINS: 10 g lactulose (and less than 1.6 g galactose, less than 1.2 g lactose, 1.2 g or less of other sugars).
USUAL ADULT DOSE: 1 to 2 tablespoonfuls (15 to 30 mL) daily. See accompanying product information. Since DUPHALAC® Solution does not exert its effect until it reaches the colon, and since transit time through the colon may be slow, 24 to 48 hours may be required to produce a normal bowel movement. Some patients have found that DUPHALAC® Solution may be more acceptable when mixed with fruit juice, water or milk.
Product may darken slightly but therapeutic action is not affected. Do not use if extreme darkening or turbidity occurs. See accompanying product information.
Store at controlled room temperature, 15°-30°C (59°-86°F). Do not freeze. Keep tightly closed. Dispense in original container or tight, light-resistant container with child-resistant closure.
DUPHALAC® is a registered trademark of Solvay Pharmaceuticals B.V., The Netherlands.

Manufactured by:
Solvay Pharmaceuticals B.V.
Weesp, The Netherlands

Marketed by:
Solvay
Pharmaceuticals, Inc.
Marietta, GA 30062

1341
12E Rev 7/99

LOT: EXP:

19. Ordered: *Augmentin 0.5 g po q8h*
    On hand: Refer to Label E.

E

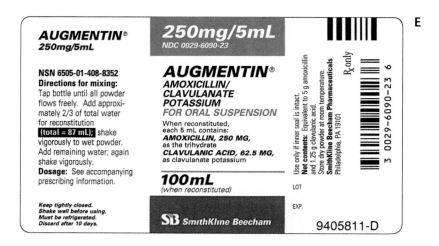

AUGMENTIN®
250mg/5mL

250mg/5mL
NDC 0029-6090-23

NSN 6505-01-408-8352
Directions for mixing:
Tap bottle until all powder flows freely. Add approximately 2/3 of total water for reconstitution **(total = 87 mL);** shake vigorously to wet powder. Add remaining water; again shake vigorously.
Dosage: See accompanying prescribing information.

Keep tightly closed.
Shake well before using.
Must be refrigerated.
Discard after 10 days.

AUGMENTIN®
AMOXICILLIN/
CLAVULANATE
POTASSIUM
FOR ORAL SUSPENSION
When reconstituted,
each 5 mL contains:
AMOXICILLIN, 250 MG,
as the trihydrate
CLAVULANIC ACID, 62.5 MG,
as clavulanate potassium

100mL
(when reconstituted)

Use only if inner seal is intact.
Net contents: Equivalent to 5 g amoxicillin and 1.25 g clavulanic acid.
Store dry powder at room temperature.
SmithKline Beecham Pharmaceuticals
Philadelphia, PA 19101

Rx only

3 0029-6090-23 6

LOT

EXP.

SB SmithKline Beecham   9405811-D

20. Ordered: E.E.S. susp 0.8 g po tid 3 7 days
    On hand: Refer to Label F.

F

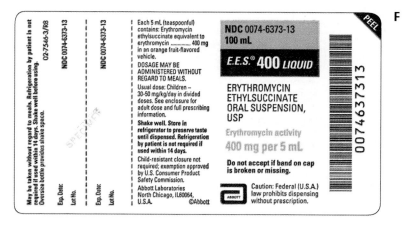

May be taken without regard to meals. Refrigeration by patient is not required if used within 14 days. Shake well before using. Oversize bottle provides shake space.

02-7546-3/R8

NDC 0074-6373-13

NDC 0074-6373-13

Exp. Date: Lot No.

Exp. Date: Lot No.

Each 5 mL (teaspoonful) contains: Erythromycin ethylsuccinate equivalent to erythromycin .... 400 mg in an orange fruit-flavored vehicle.
DOSAGE MAY BE ADMINISTERED WITHOUT REGARD TO MEALS.
Usual dose: Children – 30-50 mg/kg/day in divided doses. See enclosure for adult dose and full prescribing information.
Shake well. Store in refrigerator to preserve taste until dispensed. Refrigeration by patient is not required if used within 14 days.
Child-resistant closure not required; exemption approved by U.S. Consumer Product Safety Commission.
Abbott Laboratories
North Chicago, IL 60064, U.S.A.   ©Abbott

NDC 0074-6373-13
100 mL

E.E.S.® 400 LIQUID

ERYTHROMYCIN
ETHYLSUCCINATE
ORAL SUSPENSION,
USP

Erythromycin activity
400 mg per 5 mL

Do not accept if band on cap is broken or missing.

ABBOTT   Caution: Federal (U.S.A.) law prohibits dispensing without prescription.

21. Ordered: clindamycin phosphate 0.6 g IM bid
On hand: Refer to Label G.

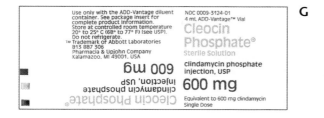

22. Ordered: Thorazine 12.5 mg IM 1h pre-op
On hand: Refer to Label H.

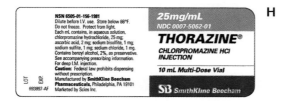

CRITICAL THINKING

You are working at an emergency shelter set up following a hurricane in your community. A man at the shelter has been taking a maintenance dose of Moban. His drug order reads

Moban 25 mg po tid

The supply of 25 mg tablets has run out and you have no other tablets available. You do have access to the liquid (concentrate) form. The label on the bottle indicates a dosage strength of 20 mg/mL. All that is available to you for measuring the dose is a set of baking spoons calibrated for $\frac{1}{4}$ tsp, $\frac{1}{2}$ tsp, 1 tsp, $\frac{1}{2}$ tbs, and 1 tbs.

Assuming the liquid form is acceptable, how do you measure the amount to administer?

CASE STUDY

Three different patients under your care are being prescribed different dosages of alprazolam. The first patient is to receive 1.25 mg per day, divided into two doses. The second patient is to receive 3 mg per day, divided into two doses. The third patient is to receive 3.75 mg per day, divided into three doses.

Alprazolam is available in the following four ways:

a. 250 mcg scored tablets

b. 500 mcg scored tablets

c. 1 mg scored tablets

d. 2 mg scored tablets

Given the above information, answer each of the following questions:

1. How would you measure the amount to administer to each patient?

2. If all the tablets *except* the 500 mcg tablets were available, what adjustments would you make?

3. If all the tablets *except* the 1 mg tablets were available, what adjustments would you make?

To check your answers, see page 353.

INTERNET ACTIVITY

Note: The Internet is a research tool from which to get basic information. Validate the accuracy of all Internet information.

Medications for thyroid therapy, such as Levothroid and Synthroid, come in numerous levels of dosage strength. For example, Levothroid tablets are available in twelve different dosage strengths. Synthroid tablets are available in eleven different dosage strengths; they are also scored.

The many dosage strengths provide the opportunity to individualize thyroid therapy for patients. You may decide to learn more about thyroid disorders and therapies.

Assignment: Search the Internet for information about thyroid disorders. Suggested key words: thyroid; thyroid + disorder; thyroid + therapy. You can also look up specific thyroid medications such as Levothroid and Synthroid.

ORAL DOSAGES

Objectives

When you have completed Chapter 9, you will be able to:

- Distinguish different types of oral medications.
- Recognize the types of solid oral medications that may not be altered by crushing or opening them.
- List appropriate techniques for administering medication to patients with difficulty swallowing or with feeding tubes.
- Accurately calculate the amount of solid or liquid oral medication to administer to a patient.
- Identify common errors that occur in calculating and preparing dosages for oral administration or via a feeding tube.

In Chapter 7, you learned several ways to calculate dosages. You learned fraction and ratio proportions as well as a basic formula for simple calculations. Then in Chapter 8, you learned how to calculate dosages by using dimensional analysis. In this chapter, you will apply these methods to oral dosages.

Tablets and Capsules

Solid oral medications come in several forms, including tablets, caplets, capsules, and gelcaps (see Figure 9-1).

The *tablet* is the most common form of solid oral medication. It combines an amount of drug with inactive ingredients such as starch or talc to form a solid disk or cylinder that is convenient for swallowing. Certain tablets are specially designed to be administered sublingually (under the tongue) or buccally (between the cheek and gum). Sublingual and buccal tablets release medication into an area rich in blood vessels, where it can be quickly absorbed for rapid action. Some tablets are designed to be chewed; others dissolve in water to make a liquid that the patient can drink. Always check the drug label to determine how a tablet is meant to be administered.

Caplets are similar to tablets. Oval-shaped, they have a special coating that makes them easy to swallow. *Capsules* are usually oval-shaped gelatin shells that contain medication in powder or granule form. The gelatin shell usually has two pieces that fit together. These pieces often may be separated to remove the medication when the patient cannot swallow a pill. *Gelcaps* consist of medication, usually liquid, in gelatin shells that are not designed to be opened.

Figure 9-1

Solid oral medications, including tablets, capsules, and gelcaps.

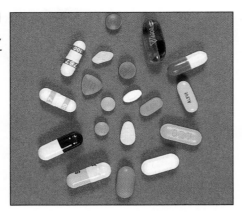

Figure 9-2

Scored tablets.

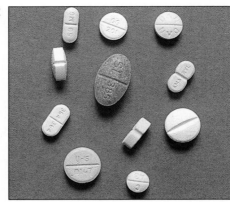

Calculating Dosages for Tablets and Capsules

Tablets are often scored so that they can be divided when smaller doses are ordered. Most often, scored tablets divide into halves, but some are scored to divide into thirds or quarters (see Figure 9-2). The medication in scored tablets is evenly distributed throughout the tablet, allowing the dose to be divided evenly when the tablet is broken.

Rule 9-1

Tablets may be broken into parts *only if they are scored,* and they must be broken only along the line of the scoring. Unscored tablets **must not** be broken into parts.

Rule 9-2

Question your calculation if it indicates that you should give a part of a tablet that you cannot obtain by breaking the tablet along its scored lines.

EXAMPLE 1 Do not administer $\frac{1}{2}$ of an unscored tablet.

EXAMPLE 2 Do not administer $\frac{1}{3}$ or $\frac{1}{4}$ of a tablet scored for division in two.

Rule 9-3

Any calculation that indicates that you should administer more than three tablets or capsules should be questioned.

If the situations in Rules 9-2 and 9-3 arise, recheck your calculations. If you are confident that your calculations are correct, then check with the physician or pharmacist, or your drug reference book to be sure there is no error in the order or the dosage strength you are using.

Before administering medication to a patient, you need to determine how many tablets or capsules will deliver the *desired dose.* This process has the following steps:

1. If necessary, convert the *dosage ordered* to the *desired dose,* using the same unit of measurement as the *dose on hand.*

2. Calculate the *amount to administer.* Use
   a. the fraction proportion method (Rule 7-5),

$$\frac{dose\ on\ hand}{dosage\ unit} = \frac{desired\ dose}{amount\ to\ administer}$$

b. the ratio proportion method (Rule 7-6), or

dose on hand:dosage unit::desired dose:amount to administer

c. the formula method (Rule 7-7)

$$desired\ dose \times \frac{dosage\ unit}{dose\ on\ hand} = amount\ to\ administer$$

(If you use dimensional analysis, you will combine Steps 1 and 2 into one step. See Rules 8-4 and 8-6.)

3. Apply critical thinking skills to determine whether the amount you have calculated is reasonable.

Recall from Chapter 7 that to calculate the *amount to administer,* you must know the *desired dose,* the *dose on hand,* and the *dosage unit.* The *desired dose* and the *dose on hand* must be in the same unit of measurement. Generally, the *dosage unit* for solid oral medications will be 1, such as 1 tablet, 1 caplet, 1 capsule, or 1 geltab.

EXAMPLE 1 The *dosage ordered* is 15 mg. The *dose on hand* is 30 mg and the *dosage unit* is 1 tablet. Because the *dosage ordered* and the *dose on hand* already have the same unit, mg, no conversion is necessary to find the *desired dose* of 15 mg.

Using the fraction proportion method,

$$\frac{30\ mg}{1\ tablet} = \frac{15\ mg}{?\ tablets}$$

$$30 \times ? = 1 \times 15$$

$$? = \frac{1}{2}$$

The amount to administer is $\frac{1}{2}$ tablet.

Using the ratio proportion method,

30 mg:1 tablet::15 mg:? tablets

$$1 \times 15 = 30 \times ?$$

$$\frac{1}{2} = ?$$

The amount to administer is $\frac{1}{2}$ tablet.

Using the formula method,

$$15\ mg \times \frac{1\ tablet}{30\ mg} = amount\ to\ administer$$

$$^{1}\cancel{15}\ \cancel{mg} \times \frac{1\ tablet}{_{2}\cancel{30}\ \cancel{mg}} = 1 \times \frac{1}{2}\ tablet = \frac{1}{2}\ tablet$$

The *amount to administer* is $\frac{1}{2}$ tablet.

Think critically about the result. Because 15 mg is half of 30 mg, $\frac{1}{2}$ tablet is an appropriate answer. Before you administer this dose, however, be sure the available tablets are scored so that they can be broken in half.

EXAMPLE 2 Ordered: *Inderal 80 mg PO QID.*

On hand: Inderal 40 mg tablets

The *dosage ordered* is 80 mg, the *dose on hand* is 40 mg, and the *dosage unit* is 1 tablet. The units of the *dosage ordered* and the *dose on hand* are the same, so no conversion is necessary. The *desired dose* is 80 mg. Using the $D \times \frac{Q}{H} = A$ formula,

$$80\ mg \times \frac{1\ tablet}{40\ mg} = A$$

$$^{2}\cancel{80}\ \cancel{mg} \times \frac{1\ tablet}{40\ \cancel{mg}_{1}} = 2 \times 1\ tablet = 2\ tablets$$

Think critically about this result. Because 80 is twice 40, this dose requires twice 1 tablet. The calculated dosage does not call for more than 3 tablets. This answer seems reasonable.

If you reverse the *desired dose* and the *dose on hand,* then the result is $\frac{1}{2}$ tablet. Thinking critically, you realize that 80 mg is larger than 40 mg; it does not make sense to give less than one 40-mg tablet. You then review the calculation and recognize the error.

EXAMPLE 3   Ordered: See Figure 9-3.

On hand: See Figure 9-4.

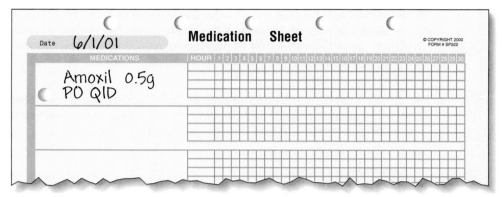

Figure 9-3

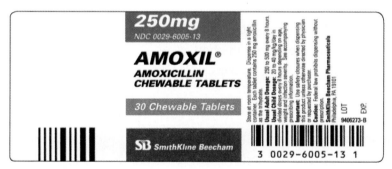

Figure 9-4

The *dosage ordered* is in g, but the *dose on hand* is in mg. You need to convert the *dosage ordered* to mg. The appropriate conversion factors are $\frac{1\ g}{1000\ mg}$ and $\frac{1000\ mg}{1\ g}$. Using the conversion factor method,

$$\frac{0.5\ g}{?\ mg} = \frac{1\ g}{1000\ mg}$$

$$0.5 \times 1000 = 1 \times ?$$

$$500\ mg = ?$$

Using the ratio proportion method,

$$0.5\ g : ?\ mg :: 1\ g : 1000\ mg$$

$$? \times 1 = 0.5 \times 1000$$

$$? = 500\ mg$$

Using the one-step method,

$$0.5\ g \times \frac{1000\ mg}{1\ g} = 0.5\ \cancel{g} \times \frac{1000\ mg}{1\ \cancel{g}} = 0.5 \times 1000\ mg = 500\ mg$$

Now you can apply the $D \times \frac{Q}{H} = A$ formula, using 500 mg as the *desired dose*:

$$500\ mg \times \frac{1\ tablet}{250\ mg} = A$$

$$^2\cancel{500} \text{ mg} \times \frac{1 \text{ tablet}}{\cancel{250} \text{ mg}_1} = 2 \times 1 \text{ tablet} = 2 \text{ tablets}$$

Thinking critically, you recognize that 500 mg is larger than 250 mg. It is logical to give more than 1 tablet. The calculation does not call for more than 3 tablets. The answer of 2 tablets is reasonable.

You can also use dimensional analysis to solve this problem. Recall from Chapter 8 that to find A, the *amount to administer,* you multiply the *dosage ordered,* a conversion factor, and the reciprocal of the dosage strength, $\frac{Q}{H}$, so that

$$dosage \ ordered \times conversion \ factor \times \frac{dosage \ unit}{dose \ on \ hand} = A$$

The factors are arranged so that all units cancel each other except for the dosage unit.

EXAMPLE 4   Use dimensional analysis to calculate the *amount to administer* from the previous example.

The *amount to administer* should be in tablets, the same unit as the *dosage unit.* Use 0.5 g as the *desired dose* (from the MAR). Use 250 mg as the *dose on hand* and 1 tablet as the *dosage unit* (from the drug label).

$$0.5 \text{ g} \times conversion \ factor \times \frac{1 \text{ tablet}}{250 \text{ mg}} = A$$

The conversion factor should have g in its denominator and mg in its numerator to cancel out those units. Use $\frac{1000 \text{ mg}}{1 \text{ g}}$.

$$0.5 \ \cancel{g} \times \frac{^4 \cancel{1000} \text{ mg}}{1 \text{ g}} \times \frac{1 \text{ tablet}}{_1 \cancel{250} \text{ mg}}$$

$$= 0.5 \times 4 \times 1 \text{ tablet} = 2 \text{ tablets}$$

CRITICAL THINKING ON THE JOB

Calculating Factors Incorrectly

A nurse caring for a patient with chest pain is instructed to give $\frac{1}{200}$ gr of nitroglycerin stat. She takes the first bottle of nitroglycerin available; It contains $\frac{1}{100}$ gr tablets. She calculates that $\frac{1}{200}$ gr is two $\frac{1}{100}$ gr tablets.

Think Before You Act

If the nurse administers two $\frac{1}{100}$ gr tablets, the patient will receive $\frac{2}{100}$ gr, or $\frac{1}{50}$ gr, *four times the ordered dose of nitroglycerin.* As a result, the patient is likely to have a severe decrease in blood pressure.

If the nurse thinks critically, she will realize that when an object is divided into 200 parts, each part is smaller than when the object is broken into 100 parts. Therefore, $\frac{1}{200}$ gr must be smaller than $\frac{1}{100}$ gr. This conclusion should alert her to rework the calculation as follows:

$$\frac{1}{200} \cancel{gr} \times \frac{1 \text{ tablet}}{\frac{1}{100} \cancel{gr}} = A$$

$$\frac{1}{200} \times 1 \text{ tablet} \div \frac{1}{100} = A$$

$$\frac{1}{\cancel{200}_2} \times 1 \text{ tablet} \times \frac{^1\cancel{100}}{1} = A$$

$$\frac{1}{2} \times 1 \text{ tablet} = \frac{1}{2} \text{ tablet} = A$$

Working with complex fractions can be tricky (see Chapter 1). When you divide a number by a fraction, multiply that number by the reciprocal of the fraction. Instead of dividing 1 tablet by $\frac{1}{100}$, multiply 1 tablet by $\frac{100}{1}$. The *amount to administer* is $\frac{1}{2}$ tablet. Because nitroglycerin tablets are not scored, the nurse must look for a bottle of $\frac{1}{200}$ gr tablets. The nurse **must not** administer one-half of an unscored tablet.

Calculation errors often involve fractions and decimals. Take extra care when working with decimals and fractions.

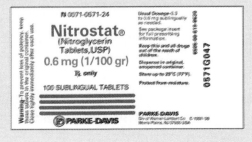

Crushing Tablets or Opening Capsules

For patients who have difficulty swallowing pills, you may crush certain tablets and open certain capsules. However, in many settings such as nursing homes, you must first get a physician's order. Check with your facility about these policies before crushing tablets.

Sometimes you can mix a crushed tablet or an opened capsule with soft food or liquid. First check for interactions between the medication and the food or fluid being mixed with it (see Table 9-1). For example, tetracycline is inactivated by milk. It must not be dissolved in foods that contain milk. In addition, it should not be given with either antacids or vitamin and mineral supplements.

Oral forms of medication are also ordered for patients with nasogastric, gastrostomy, or jejunostomy tubes. Before administering medication through the tube, you first dissolve the contents from a crushed tablet or opened capsule in a small amount of warm water.

Some medications cannot be crushed. If these medications are ordered for a patient with a feeding tube or one who cannot swallow pills, determine whether an alternative form of the medication exists (e.g., consult a drug reference or the pharmacist). Then ask the physician whether the medication should be ordered in one of these forms.

Table 9-1 Some Common Food and Drug Interactions

This list illustrates common examples; it is not complete.

Drug	Food	Interaction
Antipsychotics	coffee and tea	reduced effectiveness of drug
Bronchodilators	caffeine	stimulation of the nervous system
Central nervous system (CNS) depressants	black cohosh, ginseng kava kava, St. John's Wort, valerian	intensified sedative effects of CNS depressant
Erythromycin	acidic fruits or juices, carbonated beverages	decreased antimicrobial activity
Ferrous sulfate	tea	decreased absorption
Haloperidol	coffee and tea	decreased absorption
Insulin	coffee	stimulated excretion
Monoamine oxidase inhibitors	foods containing tyramine, such as hard cheeses, chocolate, red wine, and beef or chicken liver	headache, nosebleed, chest pain, severe hypertension
Tetracyclines	dairy products	reduced effectiveness of drug

Rule 9-4

Do not crush or otherwise alter any of the following:

- Enteric-coated tablets.
- Sustained-release forms of medication.
- Any tablet with a hard shell or coating.
- Any tablet with layers or speckles of different colors.
- Tablets for sublingual or buccal use.
- Capsules with seals that prevent separating the two parts.

Enteric-coated tablets have a coating that dissolves only in an alkaline environment, such as the small intestine. These tablets deliver medication that would be destroyed by stomach acid or that could injure the stomach lining. Enteric-coated tablets often look like candies that have a soft center and a hard shell. Some aspirins are enteric-coated, as are certain iron tablets such as ferrous gluconate. Enteric-coated tablets must *never* be crushed, broken, or chewed. A patient must swallow them with their coating intact (see Figure 9-5).

Some medications are available in *sustained-release* forms. They allow the drug to be released slowly into the bloodstream over a period of several hours. If the medication is scored, you may break it at the scored line. Otherwise you must not break it. Crushing or dissolving sustained-release tablets would allow more than the intended amount of medication to be absorbed at one time, causing overdose or toxicity of the drug.

Special capsules, often called *spansules,* contain granules of medication with different coatings that delay release of some of the medication. You may open spansules and gently mix the granules in soft food, but you must not crush or dissolve the granules. (See Figure 9-6.)

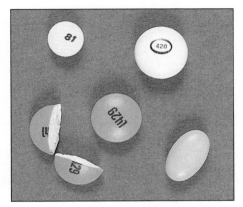

Figure 9-5   *Enteric-coated tablets.*

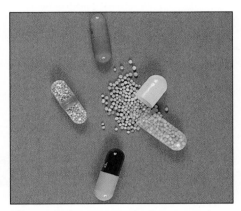

Figure 9-6   *Sustained-release capsules.*

Table 9-2 Medications That *Must Not* Be Crushed or Dissolved

This table lists examples. Your pharmacy can provide you with an updated "do not crush" list for easy reference.

Names that indicate *sustained-release* medications:

-Bid	LA	Tempule
-Dur	CR	Chronotab
Plateau Cap	XL	Repetab
Span	Sequel	Tembid
SA	Spansule	
SR	Extentab	

Names that indicate *enteric-coated* medications:

EC

Enseal

Review with patients the following guidelines for taking tablets and capsules:

1. Perform all necessary calculations, so that you can tell patients how many pills to take.

2. Tell patients whether or not they need to take a medication with food. Encourage them to drink at least 8 ounces of water with any medication.

3. Tell patients who need to divide tablets that pharmacists can provide this service on request. If the patients will be dividing the tablets, demonstrate and advise them as follows:
   a. Wash hands before handling tablets.
   b. Grasp the tablet with the scored line between your fingers. Exert pressure in the same direction—downward or upward—with both hands, until the tablet breaks along the scored line.

c. You may use a knife or pill cutter to break the tablet. Place the tablet on a clean surface, place the blade in the scored line, and press directly downward until the tablet breaks.

4. For patients who have difficulty swallowing, offer the following suggestions:
   a. Drink water before taking pills, so your mouth is moist.
   b. Place whole tablets or capsules in a small amount of food, such as applesauce or pudding. The pill will go down when the food is swallowed. *Note: Also tell patients which foods should **not** be used.*
   c. Crush tablets by placing them on a spoon and pressing another spoon down on top of them. *Note: Warn patients not to crush any medication without first checking with the pharmacist or physician.*

REVIEW and PRACTICE

TABLETS AND CAPSULES

In Exercises 1–16, calculate the *amount to administer.* Unless otherwise noted, all scored tablets are scored in half.

1. Ordered: *Tegretol 400 mg po bid*
   On hand: Tegretol 200 mg unscored tablets
   Administer:_____

2. Ordered: *Luvox 75 mg po qd*
   On hand: Luvox 50 mg scored tablets
   Administer:_____

3. Ordered: *Seroquel 75 mg po tid*
   On hand: Seroquel 25 mg unscored tablets
   Administer:_____

4. Ordered: *Tolectin 300 mg tid*
   On hand: Tolectin 200 mg scored tablets
   Administer:_____

5. Ordered: *Isordil Titradose 15 mg*
   On hand: Isordil Titradose 10 mg deep-scored tablets
   Administer:_____

6. Ordered: *Felbatol 600 mg po qid*
   On hand: Felbatol 400 mg scored tablets
   Administer:_____

7. Ordered: *Decadron 1.5 mg po qd*
   On hand: Decadron 0.75 mg unscored tablets
   Administer:_____

8. Ordered: *Coumadin 5 mg po qd*
   On hand: Coumadin 2 mg scored tablets
   Administer:_____

9. Ordered: *Cardizem 90 mg po tid*   Administer:_____
    On hand: Cardizem 60 mg scored tablets

10. Ordered: *Tambocor 150 mg po q12h*   Administer:_____
    On hand: Tambocor 100 mg scored tablets

11. Ordered: *Clozaril 50 mg po qd*   Administer:_____
    On hand: Refer to label A. Tablets are unscored.

12. Ordered: *Alprazolam 0.5 mg po tid*   Administer:_____
    On hand: Refer to label B. Tablets are scored into fourths.

13. Ordered: *Isoptin SR 240 mg po q12h*   Administer:_____
    On hand: Refer to label C. Tablets are scored.

14. Ordered: *Famvir 250 mg po bid*   Administer:_____
    On hand: Refer to label D. Tablets are unscored.

A

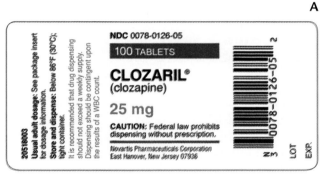

NDC 0078-0126-05

100 TABLETS

CLOZARIL®
(clozapine)

25 mg

CAUTION: Federal law prohibits
dispensing without prescription.

Novartis Pharmaceuticals Corporation
East Hanover, New Jersey 07936

Usual adult dosage: See package insert
for dosage information.
Store and dispense: Below 86°F (30°C);
tight container.
It is recommended that drug dispensing
should not exceed a weekly supply.
Dispensing should be contingent upon
the results of a WBC count.

20518003

Used with the express permission of the Novartis Pharmaceuticals Corporation.

B

NDC 0009-0094-03
6505-01-336-6198

Xanax®
Tablets

C IV

alprazolam tablets, USP

2 mg

500 Tablets

Caution: Federal law
prohibits dispensing
without prescription.
See package insert for
complete product
information.
Keep container tightly
closed.
Dispense in tight, light-
resistant container.
Store at controlled room
temperature 20° to 25° C
(68° to 77° F) (see USP).
813 156 205
Pharmacia & Upjohn
Company
Kalamazoo, MI
49001, USA

C

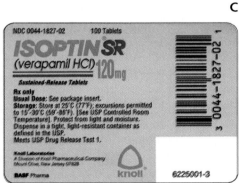

NDC 0044-1827-02   100 Tablets

ISOPTIN SR
(verapamil HCl) **120 mg**

Sustained-Release Tablets

Rx only
Usual Dose: See package insert.
Storage: Store at 25°C (77°F); excursions permitted
to 15°-30°C (59°-86°F). [See USP Controlled Room
Temperature]. Protect from light and moisture.
Dispense in a tight, light-resistant container as
defined in the USP.
Meets USP Drug Release Test 1.

Knoll Laboratories
A Division of Knoll Pharmaceutical Company
Mount Olive, New Jersey 07828

BASF Pharma   knoll   6225001-3

D

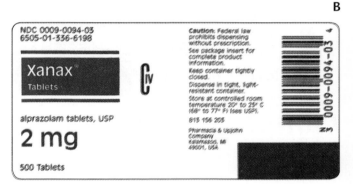

49147US1
40147US1
40147US1
40147US1

Product No. 411567   NOT FOR SALE
Store between 15° and 30°C (59° and 86°F).
Each tablet contains famciclovir, 125 mg.
Physician: See prescribing information for
complete dosing information.
Caution: Federal law prohibits dispensing without
prescription.
For _____
Dose _____ Dr. _____
Manufactured by **SmithKline Beecham**
Pharmaceuticals, Crawley, UK, for
SmithKline Beecham Pharmaceuticals
Philadelphia, PA 19101   670809-A

125 mg

FAMVIR®
famciclovir
TABLETS

125mg 10 TABLETS
NOT FOR SALE

15. Ordered: *Aricept 10 mg po qd*   Administer:_____
On hand: Refer to label E. Tablets are unscored.

16. Ordered: *Lasix 120 mg po bid*   Administer:_____
On hand: Refer to label F. Tablets are scored.

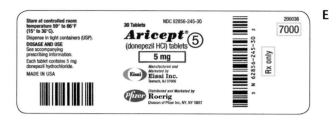

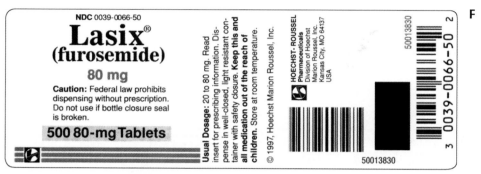

To check your answers, see page 354.

Liquid Medications

Many medications are available in liquid form. Liquids can be measured in small units of volume; thus, a greater range of dosages can be ordered and administered. Because they are easier to swallow than tablets and capsules, they are often used for children and elderly patients. Liquids can also be administered easily through feeding tubes.

Liquids may be less stable than solid forms of drugs. Many medications that are intended to be administered as liquids are provided as powders which must be reconstituted. Many liquids, especially antibiotics, require refrigeration.

Rule 9-5

To reconstitute a liquid medication, check the drug label for the correct amount of liquid to add to the container. Add only the specified amount and type of liquid.

EXAMPLE 1 How would you reconstitute the following medication? Find the *amount to administer.*
Ordered: *EES susp 400 mg po q6h x 10*
On hand: Refer to the label below.

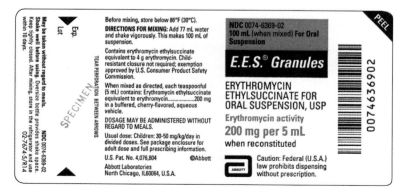

According to the label, you add 77 mL of water to the bottle of granules and shake. You then have a total of 100 mL of oral suspension that could be stored for up to 10 days.

You can use dimensional analysis to find the *amount to administer*. The *dosage ordered* is 400 mg. The dosage strength is 200 mg/5 mL; 200 mg is the *dose on hand* and 5 mL is the *dosage unit*. No conversion is needed to find the *desired dose*.

$$400 \text{ mg} \times \frac{5 \text{ mL}}{200 \text{ mg}} = A$$

$$^{2}\cancel{400} \text{ } \cancel{mg} \times \frac{5 \text{ mL}}{_{1}\cancel{200} \text{ } \cancel{mg}} = 2 \times 5 \text{ mL} = 10 \text{ mL}$$

The *amount to administer* is 10 mL.

You can extend dimensional analysis to find how many bottles of EES granules you need to provide the complete ten-day dosage. Conversion factors cancel all units but bottles.

$$10 \text{ days} \times \frac{4 \text{ doses}}{\text{day}} \times \frac{400 \text{ mg}}{\text{dose}} \times \frac{5 \text{ mL}}{200 \text{ mg}} \times \frac{1 \text{ bottle}}{100 \text{ mL}} = ? \text{ bottles}$$

Canceling the units leads to

$$10 \text{ \cancel{days}} \times \frac{4 \text{ doses}}{\cancel{day}} \times \frac{400 \text{ \cancel{mg}}}{\cancel{dose}} \times \frac{5 \text{ \cancel{mL}}}{200 \text{ \cancel{mg}}} \times \frac{1 \text{ bottle}}{100 \text{ \cancel{mL}}}$$

$$= 10 \times 4 \times 400 \times \frac{5}{200} \times \frac{1 \text{ bottle}}{100} = 4 \text{ bottles}$$

You need four bottles to provide the full ten-day dosage.

Table 9-3 Reconstituting Liquid Medications

1. Use only the liquid specified on the drug label.

2. Use the exact amount of liquid specified on the drug label.

3. Check the label to determine whether the medication should be shaken before administering.

4. Check the label to determine whether the reconstituted medication must be refrigerated.

5. Write on the label the date and time you reconstitute the medication. Also, write your initials. Check the label to determine how long the reconstituted medication may be stored. Discard any medication left after this time period has passed.

6. When medication can be reconstituted in different strengths, write on the label the strength that you choose.

7. When medication can be reconstituted in different strengths, select the strength that will allow the desired dose to be administered in the smallest volume.

The physician usually orders the dose in units of drug, not volume of liquid. The person administering the medication calculates the volume needed to administer the desired dose.

Rule 9-6

To calculate the volume of liquid oral medication to administer, use the same methods that you use for solid oral medications: fraction proportions, ratio proportions, $D \times \frac{Q}{H} = A$, or dimensional analysis.

EXAMPLE 1 Ordered: *Depakene syrup 500 mg PO BID*

On hand: Refer to the label below.

Do not accept if band on cap is broken or missing.

Each 5 mL contains equivalent of 250 mg valproic acid as the sodium salt.

See enclosure for prescribing information.

©Abbott

Abbott Laboratories
North Chicago,
IL60064, U.S.A.

Exp.

Lot

NDC 0074-5682-16
16 fl oz Syrup

DEPAKENE®

VALPROIC ACID
SYRUP, USP

**250 mg
per 5 mL**

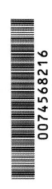
Caution: Federal (U.S.A.) law prohibits dispensing without prescription.

6505-01-094-9241

Dispense in the original container or a glass, USP tight container.

Store below 86°F (30°C).

0074568216

02-7538-2/R12

In this example, the *desired dose* is 500 mg, the *dose on hand* is 250 mg, and the *dosage unit* is 5 mL.

$$D \times \frac{Q}{H} = A$$

$$500 \text{ mg} \times \frac{5 \text{ mL}}{250 \text{ mg}} = A$$

$$^2\cancel{500 \text{ mg}} \times \frac{5 \text{ mL}}{_1\cancel{250 \text{ mg}}} = 2 \times 5 \text{ mL} = 10 \text{ mL}$$

If your calculations result in a decimal, round the answer to units that can be measured by the device you are using.

PATIENT EDUCATION

Review with patients who are taking medications in a home environment the steps in Table 9-3 for reconstituting liquid medications. If necessary, copy the table for them. Then discuss all the steps. If you are dispensing medications, give the patients the same information that the pharmacist would, if you are allowed to do so. Give patients the following information about handling liquid medication:

1. Read the label to learn how to store the medication.

2. Use the measuring device provided or a device purchased specifically to measure medications.

Household teaspoons and tablespoons do not measure liquid accurately.

3. Do not store medication longer than the label indicates. Medication used after its expiration date may have lost potency or its chemical composition may have changed.

4. Wash the measuring device with hot water and a dishwashing detergent after each use. Dry it thoroughly. Store it in a clean container such as a plastic sandwich bag.

5. Keep liquid medication in its original container. Do not transfer it to other containers.

CRITICAL THINKING ON THE JOB

Reconstituting Powders

A pharmacy technician is preparing a bottle of Amoxil suspension for this order: *Amoxil 500 mg po q8h x 5.* The pharmacy has available 100-mL bottles and 150-mL bottles containing 250 mg/5 mL (see Figures 9-7 and 9-8.)

After calculating as follows,

$$500 \text{ mg} \times \frac{5 \text{ mL}}{250 \text{ mg}} = A$$

$$^2\cancel{500} \text{ mg} \times \frac{5 \text{ mL}}{\cancel{1}\cancel{250} \text{ mg}} = 2 \times 5 \text{ mL} = 10 \text{ mL}$$

the technician determines that the patient will receive 10 mL for each dose and three doses each day. This will require 30 mL of suspension each day for five days, or a total of 150 mL. The reconstituted medication can be refrigerated for 14 days.

The technician selects the 150 mL bottle and adds 150 mL of water to it. However, the liquid overflows from the bottle.

Think Before You Act

Checking the label, the technician realizes that 111 mL of water, *not* 150 mL, should have been used. Furthermore, only $\frac{1}{3}$ of the water, or 37 mL, should have been added at first to wet the powder, followed by the remaining 74 mL.

The powder's volume must be considered when calculating the final volume of solution. The manufacturer has performed this calculation and listed the correct amount of water to add to the powder. The label calls for 111 mL of water to be added. When the technician added 150 mL of water instead of 111 mL, a volume of 189 mL of suspension was produced, instead of 150 mL.

During the week, the patient will be administered 150 mL of liquid medication, yet 189 mL has been prepared. The patient will receive $\frac{150}{189}$ of the total solution and, in turn, only $\frac{150}{189}$ of the

drug itself. Thus, instead of receiving 250 mg/5 mL, the patient will receive ($\frac{150}{189} \times 250$ mg) or 198 mg in each 5 mL.

This lesser amount of medication may be ineffective in treating the patient's infection. If the patient does not improve, the physician may order a different antibiotic. The technician's error, if not corrected, could cause the patient to suffer symptoms for a longer time period, to be exposed to side effects from an unnecessary medication, and to spend additional money to purchase a drug that would not otherwise have been needed.

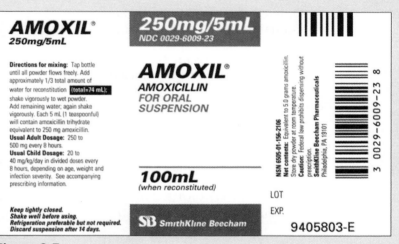

Figure 9-7

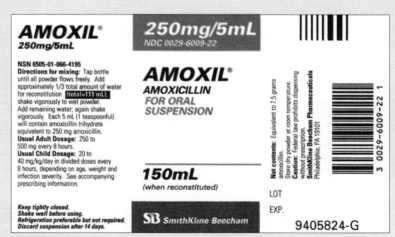

Figure 9-8

LIQUID MEDICATIONS

In Exercises 1–10, calculate the *amount to administer.*

1. Ordered: *Trilisate 400 mg po tid*
   On hand: Trilisate liquid labeled 500 mg/5 mL

   Administer:_____

2. Ordered: *MSIR sol 15 mg po q4h*
   On hand: MSIR solution labeled 10 mg/5 mL

   Administer:_____

3. Ordered: *Megace 200 mg po qid*
   On hand: Megace solution labeled 40 mg/mL

   Administer:_____

4. Ordered: *Norvir 62.5 mg po bid*
   On hand: Norvir solution labeled 80 mg/mL

   Administer:_____

5. Ordered: *Zofran 8 mg po q12h*
   On hand: Zofran liquid labeled 4 mg/5 mL

   Administer:_____

6. Ordered: *Motrin 600 mg po tid*
   On hand: Motrin liquid labeled 100 mg/5mL

   Administer:_____

7. Ordered: *Ceftin liq 500 mg po bid*
   On hand: Refer to label A.

   Administer:_____

8. Ordered: *Cedax susp 270 mg po qd*
   On hand: Refer to label B.

   Administer:_____

A

SAMPLE. FOR EDUCATIONAL USE ONLY.

NDC 0173-0406-01

GlaxoWellcome

Ceftin® for Oral Suspension
(cefuroxime axetil powder for oral suspension)
For Oral Use Only

125 mg per 5 mL   50 mL (when reconstituted)

Contains 1.5 g of cefuroxime axetil equivalent to 1.25 g of cefuroxime.

Caution: Federal law prohibits dispensing without prescription.

See package insert for Dosage and Administration.

Directions for Mixing Oral Suspension: Prepare the suspension at time of dispensing. Shake the bottle to loosen the powder. Remove the cap. Add 20 mL of water for reconstitution and replace the cap. Invert bottle and vigorously rock it from side to side so that water rises through the powder. Once the sound of the powder against the bottle disappears, turn the bottle upright and vigorously shake it in a diagonal direction.

Before reconstitution, store dry powder between 2° and 30°C (36° and 86°F). After reconstitution, store suspension between 2° and 25°C (36° and 77°F), at room temperature or in a refrigerator. SHAKE WELL BEFORE EACH USE. Replace cap securely after each opening. Discard after 10 days.

Glaxo Wellcome Inc.
Research Triangle Park, NC 27709
Made in England
4072642   Rev. 6/97

B

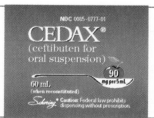

9. Ordered: *Zithromax 250 mg po qd*   Administer:_____
   On hand: Refer to label C.

10. Ordered: *Zovirax 800 mg po q4h*   Administer:_____
    On hand: Refer to label D.

C

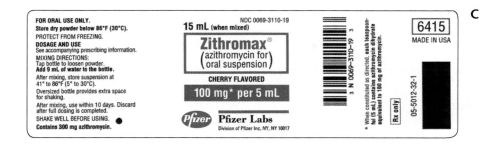

D

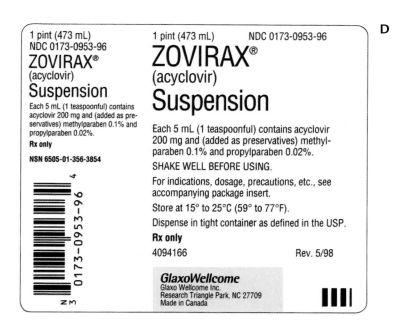

To check your answers, see page 354.

CHAPTER 9 REVIEW

CHECK UP

In Exercises 1–18, calculate the *amount to administer*. Unless otherwise noted, tablets are scored in half.

1. Ordered: *Dilaudid 4 mg po q6h*   Administer:_____
    On hand: Dilaudid 8 mg scored tablets

2. Ordered: *DiaBeta 2.5 mg po qam ac*   Administer:_____
    On hand: DiaBeta 1.25 mg scored tablets

3. Ordered: *Biltricide 450 mg po q8h*   Administer:_____
    On hand: Biltricide 600 mg tablets scored in quarters

4. Ordered: *Amoxicillin 300 mg po q12h*   Administer:_____
    On hand: Amoxicillin suspension labeled 50 mg/mL

5. Ordered: *Artane 3 mg po qd*   Administer:_____
    On hand: Artane solution labeled 2 mg/5 mL

6. Ordered: *Fosamax 10 mg po qam 30 min ac with water*   Administer:_____
    On hand: Fosamax 5 mg unscored tablets

7. Ordered: *Biaxin liquid 62.5 mg po q12h*   Administer:_____
    On hand: Biaxin liquid labeled 125 mg/5 mL

8. Ordered: *Isoptin 270 mg po qam*   Administer:_____
    On hand: Isoptin 180 mg scored tablets

9. Ordered: *Duricef 0.5 g po bid*   Administer:_____
    On hand: Duricef suspension labeled 250 mg/5 mL

10. Ordered: *Levoxyl 0.45 mg po qd*   Administer:_____
    On hand: Levoxyl 300 mcg scored tablets

11. Ordered: *Hivid 750 mcg po q8h*   Administer:_____
    On hand: Hivid 0.375 mg unscored tablets

12. Ordered: *Duricef 500 mg po bid*   Administer:_____
    On hand: Duricef 1 g scored tablets

13. Ordered: *MSIR $\frac{1}{8}$ gr po q4h*   Administer:_____
    On hand: MSIR 15 mg scored tablets

14. *Ordered: Felbatol 400 mg po tid*   Administer:_____
    On hand: Felbatol liquid labeled 600 mg/5 mL

15. *Ordered: Synthroid 0.175 mg po qd*   Administer:_____
    On hand: Refer to label A. Tablets are unscored.

16. Ordered: *Tonocard 800 mg po bid*   Administer:_____
    On hand: Refer to label B. Tablets are scored.

17. Ordered: *Prilosec 40 mg po qd*   Administer:_____
    On hand: Refer to label C.

18. Ordered: *Megace 200 mg po qid*   Administer:_____
    On hand: Refer to label D.

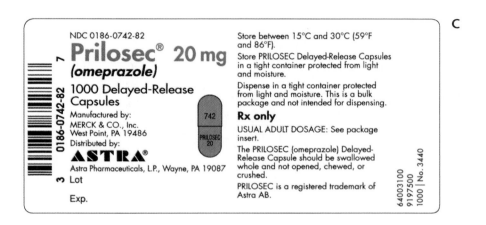

A

NDC 0048-1100-03
Code 3P1153

SYNTHROID®
(Levothyroxine Sodium
Tablets, USP)

175 mcg   (0.175 mg)

100 TABLETS

Caution: Federal (USA) law
prohibits dispensing without
prescription.

See full prescribing
information for dosage
and administration.

Dispense in a tight,
light-resistant container
as described in USP.

Store at controlled room
temperature, 15°-30°C
(59°-86°F).

**Knoll Pharmaceutical
Company**
Mount Olive, NJ 07828
USA

BASF Pharma   knoll   7893-02

B

NDC 0186-0707-68

Tonocard® 400 mg
(tocainide HCl)

100 Tablets

Manufactured by:
MERCK & CO., Inc.
West Point, PA 19486
Distributed by:
ASTRA®

TONOCARD

Astra Pharmaceuticals, L.P., Wayne, PA 19087

Lot

Store below 40°C (104°F),
preferably between 15°C and
30°C (59°F and 86°F). Store in a
well-closed container. Dispense in
a well-closed container.

Rx only

USUAL ADULT DOSAGE: See
package insert.

This is a bulk package and not
intended for dispensing.

TONOCARD is a registered trademark
of Astra Pharmaceuticals, L.P.

65000100   9175600   100 | No. 3409

C

NDC 0186-0742-82

Prilosec® 20 mg
(omeprazole)

1000 Delayed-Release
Capsules

Manufactured by:
MERCK & CO., Inc.
West Point, PA 19486
Distributed by:
ASTRA®

Astra Pharmaceuticals, L.P., Wayne, PA 19087

Lot

Exp.

742
PRILOSEC 20

Store between 15°C and 30°C (59°F
and 86°F).
Store PRILOSEC Delayed-Release Capsules
in a tight container protected from light
and moisture.

Dispense in a tight container protected
from light and moisture. This is a bulk
package and not intended for dispensing.

Rx only

USUAL ADULT DOSAGE: See package
insert.

The PRILOSEC (omeprazole) Delayed-
Release Capsule should be swallowed
whole and not opened, chewed, or
crushed.

PRILOSEC is a registered trademark of
Astra AB.

64003100   9197500   1000 | No. 3440

D

See package
insert for
indications and
dosage
schedule.
Store the oral
suspension at or
below 25°C and
dispense in a
tight container.
Protect
from heat.
Shake well
immediately
before dosing.

240 mL (8 fl. oz.)   NDC 0015-0508-42

Megace® *Oral Suspension*
(megestrol acetate)

Each mL contains 40 mg of
micronized megestrol acetate in
a lemon-lime flavored oral suspension. Alcohol: max. 0.06% v/v.

**CAUTION: FEDERAL LAW PROHIBITS
DISPENSING WITHOUT PRESCRIPTION**

40 mg/mL   **Mead Johnson**
ONCOLOGY PRODUCTS

Mead Johnson
ONCOLOGY PRODUCTS
A Bristol-Myers Squibb Co.
Princeton, New Jersey 08543
U.S.A.

P5744-00   P5744-00

0015-0508-42

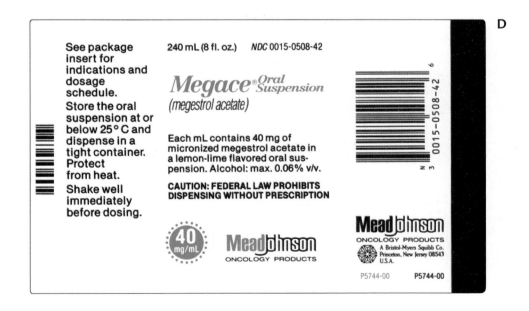

19. What combination will provide the *desired dose* with the fewest tablets?
    Ordered: *Hytrin 5 mg po qpm*
    On hand: Hytrin 1 mg unscored tablets and Hytrin 2 mg unscored tablets

20. A patient receives 15 mL of Lortab elixir every 6 hours. Lortab elixir contains 7.5 mg hydro-
    codone and 500 mg acetaminophen in each 15 mL. How much acetaminophen will this patient
    receive in 24 hours?

Each of the following sets of exercises provides a medication administration record (MAR) listing several medication orders and a variety of drug labels. Select the correct label for each medication order. Then calculate the *amount to administer.*

Set 1:

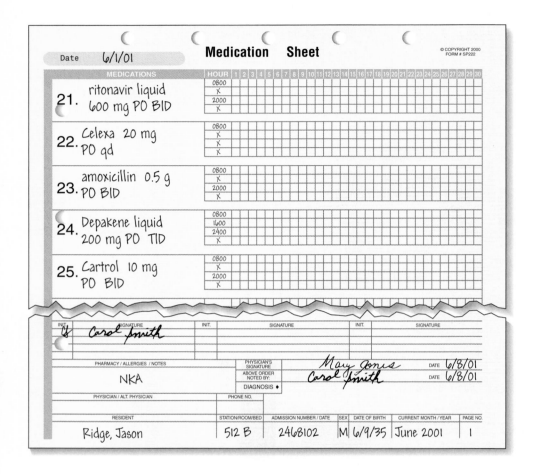

	MEDICATIONS	HOUR																													
			1	2	3	4	5	6	7	8	9	10	11	12	13	14	15	16	17	18	19	20	21	22	23	24	25	26	27	28	29	30

Medication Sheet

Date 6/1/01

© COPYRIGHT 2000
FORM # SP222

21. ritonavir liquid 600 mg PO BID — 0800 X / 2000 X

22. Celexa 20 mg PO qd — 0800 X / X / X

23. amoxicillin 0.5 g PO BID — 0800 X / 2000 X

24. Depakene liquid 200 mg PO TID — 0800 / 1600 / 2400 X

25. Cartrol 10 mg PO BID — 0800 X / 2000 X

INIT. SIGNATURE — Carol Smith

PHARMACY / ALLERGIES / NOTES
NKA

PHYSICIAN'S SIGNATURE — Mary Jones — DATE 6/8/01
ABOVE ORDER NOTED BY: Carol Smith — DATE 6/8/01
DIAGNOSIS ♦

PHYSICIAN / ALT. PHYSICIAN — PHONE NO.

RESIDENT	STATION/ROOM/BED	ADMISSION NUMBER / DATE	SEX	DATE OF BIRTH	CURRENT MONTH / YEAR	PAGE NO.
Ridge, Jason	512 B	2468102	M	6/9/35	June 2001	1

Keep this and all drugs out of the reach of children.
Dispense in tight container as described in the USP.
Rev. Date— 7/98

LOT NO.

EXP. DATE

NDC 0456-4040-01

Celexa
citalopram HBr ™

Tablets—40 mg
Equivalent to **40 mg** citalopram
100 Tablets

Marketed by:
FOREST PHARMACEUTICALS, INC.
Subsidiary of Forest Laboratories, Inc.
St. Louis, Missouri 63045

PARKE-DAVIS
Division of Warner-Lambert Company

N 3 0456404001 5

Store at 25°C (77°F)—Excursions permitted to 15° to 30°C (59° to 86°F)
Rx only—See package insert for full prescribing information
MANUFACTURED BY:
Forest Laboratories Ireland Ltd.
Clonshaugh Industrial Estate
Dublin 17 Ireland
Made in Ireland
DISTRIBUTED BY:
Forest Pharmaceuticals, Inc.
Subsidiary of Forest Laboratories, Inc.
St. Louis, Missouri 63045 USA
Licensed from H. Lundbeck A/S

E

scored

21. Use:_____ Administer:_____

22. Use:_____ Administer:_____

23. Use:_____ Administer:_____

24. Use:_____ Administer:_____

25. Use:_____ Administer:_____

Do not accept if band on cap is broken or missing.

Each 5 mL contains equivalent of 250 mg valproic acid as the sodium salt.

See enclosure for prescribing information.

©Abbott

Abbott Laboratories
North Chicago,
IL60064, U.S.A.

Exp.

Lot

NDC 0074-5682-16
16 fl oz Syrup

DEPAKENE®

VALPROIC ACID
SYRUP, USP

250 mg
per 5 mL

Caution: Federal (U.S.A.) law prohibits dispensing without prescription.

6505-01-094-9241

Dispense in the original container or a glass, USP tight container.

Store below 86°F (30°C).

0074568216

02-7538-2/R12

F

liquid

250mg
NDC 0029-6006-30

AMOXIL®
AMOXICILLIN
CAPSULES

100 Capsules

 SmithKline Beecham

NSN 6505-01-010-7953

Store at room temperature. Dispense in a tight container.
Each capsule contains 250 mg amoxicillin as the trihydrate.
See accompanying prescribing information.
Usual Adult Dosage: 250 to 500 mg every 8 hours.
Important: Use safety closures when dispensing this product unless otherwise directed by physician or requested by purchaser.
Caution: Federal law prohibits dispensing without prescription.
SmithKline Beecham Pharmaceuticals
Philadelphia, PA 19101

3 0029-6006-30 5

LOT   EXP.
9406680-D

G

capsules

SPECIMEN

NDC 0074-1665-13
100 Filmtab® Tablets

Cartrol®

CARTEOLOL
HYDROCHLORIDE
TABLETS

5 mg

Caution: Federal (U.S.A.) law prohibits dispensing without prescription.

Store at controlled room temperature 59°–86°F (15°–30° C).

02-7181-2/R3

Exp.   Lot

Do not accept if break-away ring on cap is broken or missing.
Dispense in a USP tight container.
Each tablet contains:
Carteolol Hydrochloride ....5 mg
Each white tablet bears the 🄰 and the Abbo-Code IC for product identification.
See enclosure for prescribing information.
Filmtab–Film-sealed tablets, Abbott.   ©Abbott
Abbott Laboratories
North Chicago, IL60064, U.S.A.

H

unscored

SPECIMEN

NDC 0074-1664-13
100 Filmtab® Tablets

Cartrol®

CARTEOLOL
HYDROCHLORIDE
TABLETS

2.5 mg

Caution: Federal (U.S.A.) law prohibits dispensing without prescription.

Store at controlled room temperature 59°–86°F (15°–30°C).

02-7179-2/R5

Exp.   Lot

Do not accept if break-away ring on cap is broken or missing.
Dispense in a USP tight container.
Each tablet contains:
Carteolol Hydrochloride ....2.5 mg
Each gray tablet bears the 🄰 and Abbo-Code IA for product identification.
See enclosure for prescribing information.
Filmtab–Film-sealed tablets, Abbott.   ©Abbott
Abbott Laboratories
North Chicago, IL60064, U.S.A.

I

unscored

NDC 0074-1940-63
240 mL

NORVIR®

(RITONAVIR ORAL
SOLUTION)

80 mg per mL

Shake well before each use.

DO NOT REFRIGERATE

Use by product expiration date.

 Rx only   02-8158-2/R3

Each 7.5 mL (marked dosing cup) contains:
Ritonavir .... 600 mg
in a peppermint and caramel flavored vehicle.

Alcohol 43% by volume.

See enclosure for prescribing information.

Store at room temperature 68°F to 77°F (20°C to 25°C). Do not refrigerate. Shake well before each use.

Use by product expiration date.

Store and dispense in original container. Avoid exposure to excessive heat. Keep tightly closed.

Manufactured by Abbott Laboratories, North Chicago, IL 60064, U.S.A. or Abbott Laboratories LTD, Queenborough, Kent, England. Distributed by Abbott Laboratories, North Chicago, IL 60064, U.S.A.

02-8142-2/R5   (List 1940)

Abbott Laboratories
North Chicago, IL 60064, U.S.A.

Exp.

Lot.

J

liquid

SET 2:

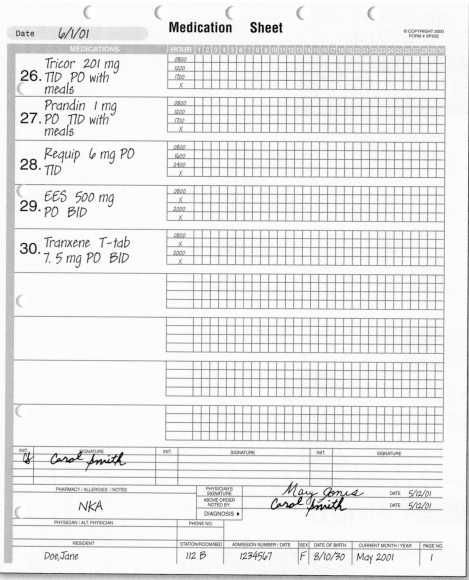

Medication Sheet

Date 6/1/01

© COPYRIGHT 2000
FORM # SP222

MEDICATIONS	HOUR	1	2	3	4	5	6	7	8	9	10	11	12	13	14	15	16	17	18	19	20	21	22	23	24	25	26	27	28	29	30
26. Tricor 201 mg TID PO with meals	0800 1200 1700 X																														
27. Prandin 1 mg PO TID with meals	0800 1200 1700 X																														
28. Requip 6 mg PO TID	0800 1600 2400 X																														
29. EES 500 mg PO BID	0800 X 2000 X																														
30. Tranxene T-tab 7.5 mg PO BID	0800 X 2000 X																														

INIT.	SIGNATURE	INIT.	SIGNATURE	INIT.	SIGNATURE
CS	Carol Smith				

PHARMACY / ALLERGIES / NOTES	PHYSICIAN'S SIGNATURE	Mary Jones	DATE 5/12/01
NKA	ABOVE ORDER NOTED BY:	Carol Smith	DATE 5/12/01
	DIAGNOSIS ♦		

PHYSICIAN / ALT. PHYSICIAN		PHONE NO.				
RESIDENT	STATION/ROOM/BED	ADMISSION NUMBER / DATE	SEX	DATE OF BIRTH	CURRENT MONTH / YEAR	PAGE NO.
Doe, Jane	112 B	1234567	F	8/10/30	May 2001	1

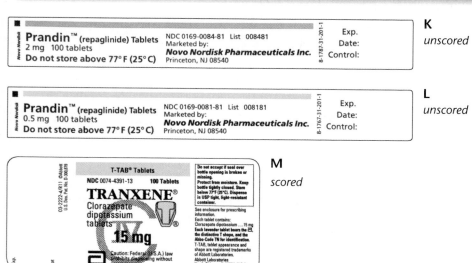

K *unscored*

Prandin™ (repaglinide) Tablets NDC 0169-0084-81 List 008481
2 mg 100 tablets Marketed by:
Novo Nordisk Pharmaceuticals Inc.
Do not store above 77° F (25° C) Princeton, NJ 08540
8-1787-31-201-1 Exp. Date: Control:

L *unscored*

Prandin™ (repaglinide) Tablets NDC 0169-0081-81 List 008181
0.5 mg 100 tablets Marketed by:
Novo Nordisk Pharmaceuticals Inc.
Do not store above 77° F (25° C) Princeton, NJ 08540
8-1767-31-201-1 Exp. Date: Control:

M *scored*

T-TAB® Tablets
NDC 0074-4391-13 100 Tablets
TRANXENE®
Clorazepate dipotassium tablets
15 mg
Caution: Federal (U.S.A.) law prohibits dispensing without prescription.

Do not accept if seal over bottle opening is broken or missing.
Protect from moisture. Keep bottle tightly closed. Store below 77°F (25°C). Dispense in USP tight, light-resistant container.
See enclosure for prescribing information.
Each tablet contains:
Clorazepate dipotassium ....15 mg
Each lavender tablet bears the ☐, the distinctive T-shape, and the Abbo-Code TN for identification.
T-TAB, tablet appearance and shape are registered trademarks of Abbott Laboratories.
Abbott Laboratories
North Chicago, IL 60064, U.S.A.

liquid

Do not accept if band on cap is broken or missing.

Child-resistant closure not required on containers of 200 mL (8 g erythromycin) or less; exemption approved by U.S. Consumer Product Safety Commission.

Each 5 mL (teaspoonful) contains: Erythromycin ethylsuccinate equivalent to erythromycin ....200 mg in a fruit-flavored vehicle.

DOSAGE MAY BE ADMINISTERED WITHOUT REGARD TO MEALS.

Usual dose: Children– 30-50 mg/kg/day in divided doses.

See package enclosure for adult dose and full prescribing information.

Exp.

Lot

NDC 0074-6306-16
ONE PINT (473 mL)

E.E.S.® 200 LIQUID

ERYTHROMYCIN ETHYLSUCCINATE ORAL SUSPENSION, USP

Erythromycin Activity
200 mg per 5 mL

Caution: Federal (U.S.A.) law prohibits dispensing without prescription.

Abbott Laboratories
North Chicago, IL 60064

SHAKE WELL BEFORE USING. Oversize bottle provides shake space.
Store in refrigerator to preserve taste until dispensed. Refrigeration by patient is not required if used within 14 days.
Dispense in a USP tight, light-resistant container.

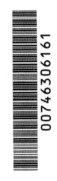

©Abbott
02-7544-4/R8

---

unscored

40145US1
40145US1
40145US1

2mg
NDC 0007-4893-20

REQUIP™
ROPINIROLE HYDROCHLORIDE TABLETS

100 Tablets

SB SmithKline Beecham

Store at controlled room temperature 20° to 25°C (68° to 77°F) [see USP]. Protect from light. Each tablet contains ropinirole hydrochloride, 2 mg.
Dosage: See accompanying prescribing information.
Important: Use safety closures when dispensing this product unless otherwise directed by physician or requested by purchaser.
Caution: Federal law prohibits dispensing without prescription.
Manufactured by
SmithKline Beecham Pharmaceuticals Crawley, UK, for
SmithKline Beecham Pharmaceuticals Philadelphia, PA 19101   670806-A

LOT   EXP.
3 0007-4893-20 2

40146US1
40146US1
40146US1

5mg
NDC 0007-4894-20

REQUIP™
ROPINIROLE HYDROCHLORIDE TABLETS

100 Tablets

SB SmithKline Beecham

Store at controlled room temperature 20° to 25°C (68° to 77°F) [see USP]. Protect from light. Each tablet contains ropinirole hydrochloride, 5 mg.
Dosage: See accompanying prescribing information.
Important: Use safety closures when dispensing this product unless otherwise directed by physician or requested by purchaser.
Caution: Federal law prohibits dispensing without prescription.
Manufactured by
SmithKline Beecham Pharmaceuticals Crawley, UK, for
SmithKline Beecham Pharmaceuticals Philadelphia, PA 19101   670807-A

LOT   EXP.
3 0007-4894-20 9

unscored

26. Use:_____   Administer:_____

27. Use:_____   Administer:_____

28. Use:_____   Administer:_____

29. Use:_____   Administer:_____

30. Use:_____   Administer:_____

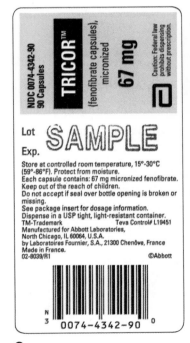

NDC 0074-4342-90
90 Capsules

TRICOR™
(fenofibrate capsules), micronized

67 mg

Caution: Federal law prohibits dispensing without prescription.

Lot
Exp.   SAMPLE

Store at controlled room temperature, 15°-30°C (59°-86°F). Protect from moisture.
Each capsule contains: 67 mg micronized fenofibrate.
Keep out of the reach of children.
Do not accept if seal over bottle opening is broken or missing.
See package insert for dosage information.
Dispense in a USP tight, light-resistant container.
TM-Trademark   Teva Control# L19451
Manufactured for Abbott Laboratories,
North Chicago, IL 60064, U.S.A.
by Laboratoires Fournier, S.A., 21300 Chenôve, France
Made in France.
02-8039/R1   ©Abbott

3 0074-4342-90 0

unscored

CRITICAL THINKING

The following medications are ordered for a patient with a gastrostomy tube who cannot swallow and must receive all medications through the tube:

a. *Isoptin SR 180 mg q12h*

b. *Valium 4 mg qid*

c. *Dilaudid 3 mg prn for pain*

d. *Keflex 500 mg*

On hand: Refer to labels R, S, T, and U. The Isoptin SR and Valium tablets are scored.

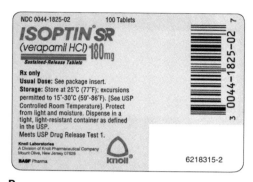

R

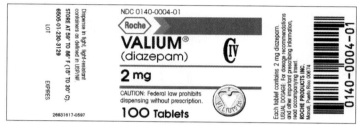

S

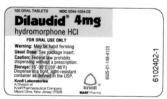

T

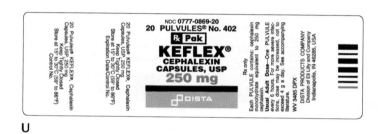

U

1. For each medication, calculate the *amount to administer.*

2. Are there any medications on the list that cannot be given as ordered?

3. How would you administer these medications?

4. What action would you take if you could not give a medication as ordered?

CASE STUDY

Ordered: *Biaxin liquid 187.5 mg PO*
On hand: Refer to label V.

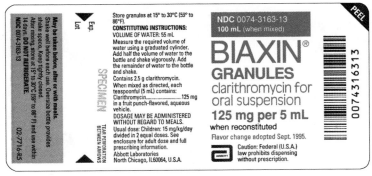

V

1. Describe how you would reconstitute this medication.

2. Calculate the *amount to administer.*

3. What measuring device would you use to give this dose?

To check your answers, see page 354.

INTERNET ACTIVITY

Note: The Internet is a research tool from which to get basic information. Validate the accuracy of all Internet information.

You are working in a physician's office where a patient with diabetes is having difficulty with blood glucose control. The physician discovers that the patient, who has trouble swallowing, has been crushing Glucotrol XL tablets. Because this sustained-release medication should not be crushed, the patient has been receiving too much medication at one time. You realize that this problem could occur with any patient who is taking a sustained-release medication.

Assignment: Search the Internet for patient-education materials warning patients about crushing medications.

Suggested key words: medication + crushing; medication + swallowing; pills + swallowing

PARENTERAL DOSAGES 10

Objectives

When you have completed Chapter 10, you will be able to:

- Calculate the amount of a parenteral medication to administer.
- Select the appropriate syringe.
- Correctly reconstitute powdered medications.
- Measure insulin doses correctly.
- Accurately calculate doses of inhalant, rectal, and transdermal medications.
- Identify errors that occur when calculating and preparing parenteral doses.

Recall from Chapter 4 that parenteral medications bypass the digestive tract. In many cases, they are administered by injection. This chapter focuses primarily on intramuscular (IM), subcutaneous (SC), and intradermal (ID) injections. Chapter 11 then looks at intravenous (IV) injections. Parenteral medications include inhalants, as well as rectal and transdermal medications, also discussed in this chapter.

Calculating Parenteral Dosages

Injections are usually administered as solutions or suspensions in which the drug itself (solute) is dissolved in an appropriate liquid (solvent or diluent). You calculate the amount of solution that delivers the *desired dose* of medication. You also choose the proper syringe. The dosage or solution strength on an injectable medication's label indicates the amount of drug contained within a volume of solution (see Table 10-1). Dosage strength may also be expressed as a percent or a ratio.

Table 10-1 Sample Solution Strengths

Label Description	Interpretation
Compazine 5 mg/mL	1 mL contains 5 mg of Compazine
Epogen 3000 units/mL	1 mL contains 3000 units of Epogen
lidocaine 1%	100 mL contains 1 g lidocaine
epinephrine 1:1000	1000 mL contains 1 g epinephrine

As with oral medications, calculate the *amount to administer* starting with the *dosage ordered, dose on hand,* and *dosage unit.* If the *dosage ordered* and the *dose on hand* have different units, then convert the *dosage ordered* to the *desired dose*. If you use dimensional analysis, calculate directly from the *dosage ordered*. Ways to calculate the *amount to administer* include 1) the fraction proportion method, 2) the ratio proportion method, 3) the formula method (D $\times \frac{Q}{H}$ = A), and 4) dimensional analysis. You learned these calculations in Chapters 7 and 8.

To avoid errors, the physician's order should specify the amount of medication, not the quantity of solution, to administer. Some solutions are available in more than one strength. Therefore, the same quantity of solution could provide different amounts of medication.

Rule 10-1

When selecting a syringe,

1. If the amount of medication to administer is 1 mL or more, use a standard syringe.

2. If the amount of medication to administer is less than 1 mL, use a 1-mL tuberculin syringe.

3. If the amount of medication to administer is less than 0.5 mL, use a 0.5-mL tuberculin syringe.

In addition to selecting the correct syringe, you may have to select the correct needle. See Chapter 4 and Table 4-1 for a discussion of needle lengths and gauges.

EXAMPLE 1 Find the *amount to administer* and select the proper syringe.

Ordered: *Compazine 7.5 mg deep IM on call*

On hand: Refer to the label below:

The *dosage ordered* and the *dose on hand* are already expressed in the same units. No conversion is necessary. Using the formula method, D $\times \frac{Q}{H}$ = A, and restating 7.5 as $\frac{15}{2}$ (to avoid combining fractions and decimals),

$$\frac{15}{2} \text{ mg} \times \frac{1 \text{ mL}}{5 \text{ mg}} = A$$

$$\frac{3\cancel{15}}{2 \cancel{mg}} \times \frac{1 \text{ mL}}{\cancel{5} \cancel{mg}1} = \frac{3}{2} \times 1 \text{ mL} = \frac{3}{2} \text{ mL} = 1.5 \text{ mL}$$

Administer 1.5 mL of solution so that the patient receives 7.5 mg of Compazine. Now select the proper syringe. Insulin syringes should be used only for insulin. Tuberculin syringes hold 1 mL of solution or less. However, standard syringes hold up to 3 mL of solution and are calibrated in tenths of a mL. You would use a standard syringe for this dose.

EXAMPLE 2 Find the *amount to administer* and select the proper syringe.

Ordered: *Epogen 1200 Units sc tiw*

On hand: Refer to the label below:

Using the D $\times \frac{Q}{H}$ = A formula,

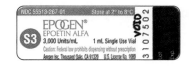

$$1200 \text{ Units} \times \frac{1 \text{ mL}}{3000 \text{ Units}} = A$$

$$^2\cancel{1200} \cancel{Units} \times \frac{1 \text{ mL}}{_5\cancel{3000} \cancel{Units}} = 2 \times \frac{1}{5} \text{ mL} = \frac{2}{5} \text{ mL} = 0.4 \text{ mL}$$

Administer 0.4 mL of solution so that the patient receives 1200 Units of Epogen. Because the amount is less than 0.5 mL, use a 0.5-mL tuberculin syringe (see Figure 10-1).

Figure 10-1

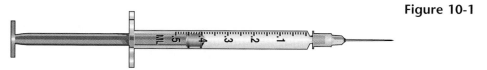

Epogen is one of many medications for which the *dosage ordered* may be based on a person's body weight. Sometimes, Epogen ordered is at the rate of 50 Units/kg: for every kilogram that the patient weighs, the patient receives 50 Units. Physicians usually factor this conversion into their orders. Body weight calculations are discussed further in Chapters 11 and 12.

Calculations often lead to a fractional volume which is rounded to match the calibrations of the syringe.

Rule 10-2

When rounding the amount of medication to administer,
1. Round volumes greater than 1 mL to the nearest tenth.
2. Round volumes less than 1 mL to the nearest hundredth.

EXAMPLE 1 Find the *amount to administer* and select the proper syringe.

Ordered: *Actimmune 65 mcg sc tiw*

On hand: Refer to the label below:

This label indicates that 3 million Units are in a single dose vial. It does not indicate the amount of drug (in mcg) or the volume of solution in the vial. The package insert and the PDR specify that each vial contains 100 mcg of Actimmune in 0.5 mL of solution. Using fraction proportions,

NDC 64116-011-01	SINGLE DOSE VIAL
Interferon gamma-1b injection	DOSAGE AND ADMINISTRATION: See package insert.
ACTIMMUNE (3 million U)	DO NOT SHAKE. STORAGE:
US License No.: 1267 Manufactured by: InterMune Pharmaceuticals, Inc. Palo Alto, CA 94303	Refrigerate at 2–8°C/36–46°F. DO NOT FREEZE
LB-0161 4817900	**Rx only**

$$\frac{100 \text{ mcg}}{0.5 \text{ mL}} = \frac{65 \text{ mcg}}{? \text{ mL}}$$

$$100 \text{ mcg} \times ? \text{ mL} = 0.5 \text{ mL} \times 65 \text{ mcg}$$

$$100 \times ? = 32.5$$

$$? = 0.325$$

Because 0.325 mL is less than 1 mL, round to the nearest hundredth, or 0.33 mL, and select a 0.5-mL tuberculin syringe.

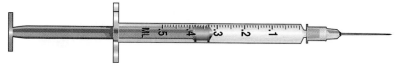

Actimmune is one of many medications for which the *dosage ordered* is based on the patient's body surface area (BSA). The physician usually factors in the patient's BSA when preparing the drug order (see Chapter 12).

When medications are available with different dosage strengths, you will need to determine which form to use.

Rule 10-3

When multiple solution strengths are available, select the form that requires you to administer the smallest volume.

EXAMPLE 1 Find the *amount to administer* and select the proper syringe.

Ordered: *Synthroid 50 mcg IM QD*

On hand: Refer to Labels A and B below:

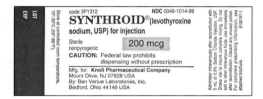

A

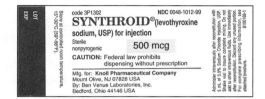

B

Both containers are reconstituted with 5 mL of solution. The package inserts indicate that, in certain cases, Synthroid may be injected intramuscularly. Using the formula method,

Vial A: $50 \text{ mcg} \times \dfrac{5 \text{ mL}}{200 \text{ mcg}} = A$

$^1\cancel{50} \text{ mcg} \times \dfrac{5 \text{ mL}}{\cancel{200}_4 \text{ mcg}} = 1 \times \dfrac{5}{4} \text{ mL} = 1.25 \text{ mL}$

Vial B: $50 \text{ mcg} \times \dfrac{5 \text{ mL}}{500 \text{ mcg}} = A$

$^1\cancel{50} \text{ mcg} \times \dfrac{^1\cancel{5}/ \text{ mL}}{_2{}^{10}\cancel{500} \text{ mcg}} = 1 \times \dfrac{1}{2} \text{ mL} = 0.5 \text{ mL}$

Because 0.5 mL is the smaller volume, select Vial B. Administer 0.5 mL of the 500 mcg/5 mL Synthroid, using either a standard or 0.5-mL tuberculin syringe. In general, *medications that have greater dosage strengths or concentrations are administered in smaller amounts.*

You must also decide whether the amount to be administered can be safely injected in a single site.

Rule 10-4

For intramuscular injections, the maximum amount that may be administered in one site is:

Adult (average 150 lbs)	3 mL
Child (6-12 years old)	2 mL
Child (0-5 years old)	1 mL
Infant (premature)	0.5 mL

For subcutaneous injections, no more than 1 mL should be administered in a single site.

When the *amount to administer* exceeds the amount that can safely be given in one site, divide the amount into equal (or nearly equal) parts. Then administer them in separate sites. For example, to administer 4.5 mL to an adult, draw up 2 mL in one syringe and 2.5 mL in another. Inject the contents of each syringe into a different site.

> **EXAMPLE 1** Find the *amount to administer* and select the proper syringe for an adult patient who weighs 180 lbs.
>
> Ordered: *Lasix 40 mg IM stat*
>
> On hand: 4-mL ampule of Lasix 10 mg/mL for injection
>
> Using the formula method,
>
> $$40 \text{ mg} \times \frac{1 \text{ mL}}{10 \text{ mg}} = A$$
>
> $$\overset{4}{\cancel{40}} \text{ } \cancel{mg} \times \frac{1 \text{ mL}}{\underset{1}{\cancel{10} \text{ } \cancel{mg}}} = 4 \times 1 \text{ mL} = 4 \text{ mL}$$
>
> This dose must be divided into two parts. Draw up 2 mL in each of two standard syringes and administer them into different sites.

CRITICAL THINKING ON THE JOB

Confirming the Physician's Order

A patient in an agitated state is brought to the emergency department. The physician verbally orders 2 mL of Vistaril. The nurse draws up 2 mL from a vial labeled 50 mg/mL. She then notices another vial labeled 25 mg/mL.

Think Before You Act

The nurse realizes that the physician has ordered a quantity of solution rather than a quantity of drug. She checks with the physician, who clarifies that the intended dose is 50 mg. If the nurse administers the injection without thinking, the patient receives 100 mg, twice the intended dose, and may experience excessive sedation or even a seizure. The nurse calculates that 1 mL of 50 mg/mL solution contains the 50-mg dose. She discards 1 mL of the original dose and administers the remaining 1 mL.

Medications Expressed in Percent or Ratio Format

When a medication's dosage or solution strength is expressed as a percent or a ratio, you must convert it before calculating the amount to administer. Recall from Chapter 2 that the percent of a solution indicates the number of grams of pure drug in 100 mL of solution. For example, *lidocaine 1%* contains 1 g lidocaine in 100 mL of solution. When solution strength is expressed as a ratio, it indicates how much solution contains 1 g of pure drug. For example, *epinephrine 1:2000* contains 1 g of epinephrine in 2000 mL of solution.

Rule 10-5

When a solution strength is expressed as a percent or ratio,

1. Convert the percent or ratio to a dosage strength of g/mL or mg/mL.

2. Calculate the *amount to administer.*

> **EXAMPLE 1** Find the *amount to administer* and select the proper syringe.
>
> Ordered: *magnesium sulfate 500 mg IM stat*
>
> On hand: vial of magnesium sulfate 10% solution

First convert the percent to g/mL:

$$10\% \text{ solution} = \frac{10 \text{ g}}{100 \text{ mL}}$$

Now use dimensional analysis to find the *amount to administer*. The *dosage ordered* is 500 mg, the *dose on hand* is 10 g, and the *dosage unit* is 100 mL.

$$500 \text{ mg} \times \text{conversion factor} \times \frac{100 \text{ mL}}{10 \text{ g}} = A$$

A conversion factor relating g to mg cancels these units, leaving mL. Using the factor $\frac{1 \text{ g}}{1000 \text{ mg}}$,

$$500 \text{ mg} \times \frac{1 \text{ g}}{1000 \text{ mg}} \times \frac{100 \text{ mL}}{10 \text{ g}} = A$$

$$\overset{1}{500} \text{ mg} \times \frac{1 \text{ g}}{\underset{2}{\underset{1}{1000}} \text{ mg}} \times \frac{\overset{5}{\overset{10}{100}} \text{ mL}}{\underset{1}{10} \text{ g}} = 1 \times 1 \times 5 \text{ mL} = 5 \text{ mL}$$

Administer 5 mL of magnesium sulfate intramuscularly. Use two standard syringes to inject 2.5 mL each into different sites.

When lidocaine is ordered for use as a local anesthetic, the physician often specifies both the solution strength and the amount to inject. For example, the physician may ask for 5 mL of 0.5% lidocaine. This order is an exception to the rule that the physician orders a dose, not an amount. Here, the physician has specified both the dosage strength (0.5%) and the amount (5 mL).

EXAMPLE 2 Find the *amount to administer* and select the proper syringe.

Ordered: *epinephrine 0.2 mg sc stat*

On hand: vial of epinephrine 1:2000 solution for injection

First convert the ratio to g/mL:

$$1:2000 \text{ solution} = \frac{1 \text{ g}}{2000 \text{ mL}}$$

Now use dimensional analysis to find the *amount to administer*. The *dosage ordered* is 0.2 mg, the *dose on hand* is 1 g, and the *dosage unit* is 2000 mL.

$$0.2 \text{ mg} \times \text{conversion factor} \times \frac{2000 \text{ mL}}{1 \text{ g}} = A$$

The factor $\frac{1 \text{ g}}{1000 \text{ mg}}$ cancels g and mg, leaving mL,

$$0.2 \text{ mg} \times \frac{1 \text{ g}}{1000 \text{ mg}} \times \frac{2000 \text{ mL}}{1 \text{ g}} = A$$

$$0.2 \text{ mg} \times \frac{1 \text{ g}}{\underset{1}{1000} \text{ mg}} \times \frac{\overset{2}{2000} \text{ mL}}{\underset{1}{1} \text{ g}} = 0.2 \times 1 \times 2 \text{ mL} = 0.4 \text{ mL}$$

Administer 0.4 mL of epinephrine. Because this amount is less than 0.5 mL, you can use a 0.5-mL tuberculin syringe.

Some drugs, such as heparin, are measured in units, and may have their solution strength expressed in ratio format. The ratio indicates the number of *Units* contained in 1 mL. For example, heparin sodium 1:10,000 contains 10,000 units in 1 mL.

EXAMPLE 3 Find the *amount to administer* and select the proper syringe.

Ordered: *heparin sodium 5,000 Units deep sc q8h*

On hand: Refer to the label below.

Using the formula method,

$$5000 \text{ Units} \times \frac{1 \text{ mL}}{10{,}000 \text{ Units}} = A$$

$${}^1\cancel{5000} \text{ Units} \times \frac{1 \text{ mL}}{\cancel{10{,}000} \text{ Units}_{\,2}} = 1 \times \frac{1}{2} \text{ mL} = 0.5 \text{ mL}$$

The *amount to administer* is 0.5 mL. Select a 0.5-mL tuberculin syringe to administer this amount of heparin.

	NDC 0009-0317-02 4 mL
	Heparin Sodium Injection, USP
	from beef lung **10,000 Units**/mL

Pharmacia & Upjohn Company
Kalamazoo, MI 49001 USA
811 351 904

For subcutaneous or intravenous use.
See package insert for complete product information.
Store at controlled room temperature 20° to 25°C
(68° to 77°F) [see USP].
Each mL contains: Heparin sodium, 10,000 USP Units

CRITICAL THINKING ON THE JOB

Confusing the Amount of Solution with the Dosage Unit

A patient is brought to the physician's office with severe vomiting. The physician orders *Compazine 5 mg IM stat*. The medical assistant obtains a vial labeled 5 mg/mL. The label also lists the total quantity of medication as 5 mL. The medical assistant misinterprets the solution strength as 5 mg/5 mL, and injects a total of 5 mL of Compazine.

Think Before You Act

The actual solution strength is 5 mg/1 mL, not 5 mg/ 5 mL. When 5 mL is administered, the patient receives 25 mg of Compazine, five times the desired dose. He develops respiratory depression and is admitted to the hospital for close observation.

This error can be avoided if the medical assistant reads the label three times. The medical assistant must take extra care not to confuse the total volume in the vial (5 mL) with the dosage unit (1 mL), as indicated by the dosage strength (5 mg/mL).

REVIEW and PRACTICE

CALCULATING PARENTERAL DOSAGES

Find the *amount to administer* for each of the following orders. Then select the proper syringe.

1. Ordered: *magnesium sulfate 750 mg stat*
   On hand: magnesium sulfate 20% solution
   Administer: _____   Syringe: _____

2. Ordered: *lidocaine 200 mg IM stat*
   On hand: lidocaine 10% solution
   Administer: _____   Syringe: _____

3. Ordered: *epinephrine 0.3 mg sc stat*
   On hand: epinephrine 1:1000 solution
   Administer: _____   Syringe: _____

4. Ordered: *Adrenalin 0.5 mg sc stat*
   On hand: Adrenalin 1:1000 solution
   Administer: _____   Syringe: _____

5. Ordered: *Prostigmin 0.25 mg post-op q6h*
   On hand: Prostigmin 1:4000 solution
   Administer: _____   Syringe: _____

6. Ordered: *Prostigmin 0.5 mg IM stat*
   On hand: Prostigmin 1:2000 solution
   Administer: _____   Syringe: _____

7. Ordered: *heparin sodium 8000 Units deep sc q8h*
   On hand: heparin sodium 1:5000 solution
   Administer: _____   Syringe: _____

8. Ordered: *heparin sodium 5000 Units sc q12h × 7*
   On hand: heparin sodium 1:10,000 solution
   Administer: _____   Syringe: _____

9. Ordered: *Depo Provera 1000 mg IM qw*
   On hand: Refer to Label A.
   Administer: _____   Syringe: _____

10. Ordered: *Zantac 50 mg IM q6h*
    On hand: Refer to Label B.
    Administer: _____   Syringe: _____

A

| See package insert for complete product information. | NDC 0009-0626-02 | 10 mL Vial |

Shake vigorously immediately before each use. Store at controlled room temperature 20° to 25°C (68° to 77°F) (see USP).

Each mL contains: Medroxyprogesterone acetate, 400 mg. Also, polyethylene glycol 3350, 20.5 mg; sodium sulfate anhydrous, 11 mg; myristyl-gamma-picolinium chloride, 1.69 mg added as preservative. When necessary, pH was adjusted with sodium hydroxide and/or hydrochloric acid.

Depo-Provera®
medroxyprogesterone acetate injectable suspension, USP

400 mg/mL

For intramuscular use only

Rx only

813 275 405
Pharmacia & Upjohn Company
Kalamazoo, Michigan 49001, USA

B

SAMPLE. FOR EDUCATIONAL USE ONLY.

NDC 0173-0363-01

GlaxoWellcome

Zantac®
(ranitidine hydrochloride) Injection

25 mg/mL*
Sterile
6-mL Multidose Vial

Caution: Federal law prohibits dispensing without prescription.
* Each mL contains ranitidine 25 mg (as the hydrochloride) in a buffered aqueous solution with phenol 5 mg as preservative.
Usual Adult Dosage: 50 mg (2 mL) every 6 to 8 hours or 150 mg (6 mL) over 24 hours.
For IV or IM injection, or IV infusion.
See package insert for full prescribing information.
Store between 4° and 30°C (39° and 86°F). Protect from light. Zantac® Injection tends to exhibit a yellow color that may intensify over time without adversely affecting potency.
U.S. Patent No. 4,585,790

Glaxo Wellcome Inc.
Research Triangle Park,
NC 27709
Made in England
Rev. 4/97

4 0 7 6 7 8 8

11. Ordered: *Tigan 200 mg IM TID*
    On hand: Refer to Label C.
    Administer: _____   Syringe: _____

12. Ordered: *Sandostatin 200 mcg sc q12h*
    On hand: Refer to Label D.
    Administer: _____   Syringe: _____

C

NDC 61570-541-20

100mg/mL

Tigan®
(trimethobenzamide HCl)
Injection

20mL Multi-Dose Vial

Rx Only

Monarch Pharmaceuticals®

NOT FOR USE IN CHILDREN.
For IM USE ONLY.
Store from 15° to 30° C (59° to 86°F).
Each mL of solution contains 100 mg trimethobenzamide hydrochloride compounded with 0.45% phenol as preservative, 0.5 mg sodium citrate and 0.2 mg citric acid as buffers, and sodium hydroxide to adjust pH to approximately 5.0.
Dosage: See accompanying prescribing information. For use only (preferably by deep IM Injection).
Distributed by: Monarch Pharmaceuticals, Inc., Bristol, TN 37620
Manufactured by: King Pharmaceuticals, Inc., Bristol, TN 37620
0934063 Rev. 11/99

Reprinted with permission of King Pharmaceuticals, Inc.

D

Each mL of aqueous solution contains:
octreotide (as acetate) .... 1000 mcg
STORAGE: Refrigerate at 2°C 8°C (36°F–46°F);
protect from light.

Rx only

Manufactured for: Novartis, E.Hanover, NJ 07936
22383103   692190

SAMPLE

NDC 0078-0184-25   1000 mcg/mL (1.0 mg/mL)

Sandostatin®
octreotide acetate
INJECTION

Total Volume 5 mL Multi-Dose Vial
FOR SUBCUTANEOUS INJECTION

13. Ordered: *Neupogen 180 mcg sc qd*
    On hand: Refer to Label E.
    Administer: _____   Syringe: _____

14. Ordered: *Neupogen 240 mcg sc qd*
    On hand: Refer to label F.
    Administer: _____   Syringe: _____

E

NDC 55513-530-01   Refrigerate at 36° to 46°F

Neupogen®
Filgrastim

300 mcg

300 mcg/1.0 mL   1.0 mL Single Use Vial
Caution: Federal law prohibits dispensing without prescription
Amgen Inc. Thousand Oaks, CA 91320   U.S. License No. 1080

F

NDC 55513-546-01   Refrigerate at 36° to 46°F

Neupogen®
Filgrastim

480 mcg

480 mcg/1.6 mL   (300 mcg/1.0 mL) 1.6 mL Single Use Vial
Caution: Federal law prohibits dispensing without prescription
Amgen Inc. Thousand Oaks, CA 91320   U.S. License No. 1080

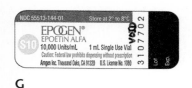

G — NDC 55513-144-01   Store at 2° to 8°C   **EPOGEN®** EPOETIN ALFA   S10   10,000 Units/mL   1 mL Single Use Vial   Caution: Federal law prohibits dispensing without prescription   Amgen Inc. Thousand Oaks, CA 91320   U.S. License No. 1080

H — NDC 55513-478-01   Store at 2° to 8°C   **EPOGEN®** EPOETIN ALFA   M20   20,000 Units/mL   1 mL Multidose Vial   Caution: Federal law prohibits dispensing without prescription   Dosage - See Package Insert   Amgen Inc. Thousand Oaks, CA 91320   U.S. License No. 1080

I — 1 mL   NDC 0091-1150-05   Rx Only   **CALCIFEROL™** In Oil Injection (ergocalciferol)   12.5 mg (500,000 Units) per mL   Distributed by: **SCHWARZ PHARMA** Milwaukee, WI 53201

J — 0.2 mL   **Fragmin®** dalteparin sodium injection   2500 IU (anti-Xa) per 0.2 mL   Manufactured for: Pharmacia & Upjohn Company   132050198   KV0307-02

15. Ordered: *Epogen 3500 Units sc tiw*
    On hand: Refer to label G.
    Administer: _____   Syringe: _____

16. Ordered: *Epogen 6000 Units sc tiw*
    On hand: Refer to label H.
    Administer: _____   Syringe: _____

17. Ordered: *Calciferol 100,000 IU IM qd*
    On hand: Refer to label I.
    Administer: _____   Syringe: _____

18. Ordered: *Fragmin 5000 IU sc qd post-op × 5*
    On hand: Refer to label J.
    Administer: _____   Syringe: _____

19. Ordered: *Compazine 7.5 mg deep IM QID*
    On hand: Refer to label K.
    Administer: _____   Syringe: _____

20. Ordered: *DDAVP (desmopressin acetate) 1.5 mcg sc bid*
    On hand: Refer to label L.
    Administer: _____   Syringe: _____

21. Ordered: *Stelazine 1.5 mg deep IM q6h prn*
    On hand: Refer to label M.
    Administer: _____   Syringe: _____

22. Ordered: *Lanoxin 300 mcg deep IM massage stat*
    On hand: Refer to label N.
    Administer: _____   Syringe: _____

To check your answers, see page 355.

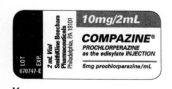

K — 2 mL Vial   SmithKline Beecham Pharmaceuticals, Philadelphia, PA 19101   **10mg/2mL**   **COMPAZINE®** PROCHLORPERAZINE as the edisylate INJECTION   5mg prochlorperazine/mL   670747-E

L — **DDAVP®** 4 μg in 1 mL (desmopressin acetate) Injection 4 μg/mL   Manufactured for **RHÔNE-POULENC RORER PHARMACEUTICALS INC.** COLLEGEVILLE, PA 19426

M — NSN 6505-01-220-1479   Store below 30°C (86°F). Do not freeze. Protect from light. Each mL contains, in aqueous solution, trifluoperazine, 2 mg, as the hydrochloride; sodium tartrate, 4.75 mg; sodium biphosphate, 11.6 mg; sodium saccharin, 0.3 mg. Contains benzyl alcohol, 0.75%, as preservative. **Dosage:** See accompanying prescribing information. For deep intramuscular injection   Manufactured by SmithKline Beecham **Pharmaceuticals**, Philadelphia, PA 19101   Marketed by Scios Inc.   670774-AG   **10mL Multi-Dose Vial** **2mg/mL** NDC 0108-4902-01   **STELAZINE®** TRIFLUOPERAZINE HCl INJECTION   **SB** SmithKline Beecham   Rx only

N — **LANOXIN®** (digoxin) Injection   **2 mL** Rx only   500 mcg (0.5 mg) in 2 mL (250 mcg [0.25 mg] per mL)   Store at 15° to 25°C (59° to 77°F). PROTECT FROM LIGHT. Dist.: Glaxo Wellcome Inc. Research Triangle Park, NC 27709   4097033   Rev. 5/98   542567   **SAMPLE. FOR EDUCATIONAL USE ONLY.**

Reconstituting Powdered Medications

Medications which lose potency quickly in solution may be supplied in powdered form. When needed, they are reconstituted by dissolving them in an appropriate solvent (or diluent). The drug label, package insert, and PDR provide instructions for reconstituting a medication. Be sure to use the directions specific to the medication you plan to administer.

First, determine what solvent should be used to dilute the medication. Common solvents include sterile water, saline, or a bacteriostatic solution containing a preservative that prevents the growth of microorganisms. Some medications are packaged with a separate container of the appropriate solvent.

Many medications, especially antibiotics, cause severe pain when injected. They may be mixed with lidocaine, a local anesthetic, to reduce this pain. The label or package insert indicates when lidocaine can be used. Because lidocaine is itself a medication, you need a physician's order to use it. Therefore, check whether the physician has ordered lidocaine. Do not confuse it with the combination of lidocaine and epinephrine, because epinephrine causes vasoconstriction, a tightening of the blood vessels which delays medication absorption.

The label or package insert lists how much solvent to combine with the medication. Read the directions carefully. Sometimes different amounts of solvent are used, based on whether the medication is for IM or IV use.

Rule 10-6

To reconstitute a powdered medication:

1. Find the directions on the medication label or package insert.

2. Use a sterile syringe and aseptic (germ-free) technique to draw up the correct amount of the appropriate diluent.

3. Inject the diluent into the medication vial.

4. Agitate the mixture by rolling, inverting, or shaking the vial. Check the directions on the label or package insert for which of these methods to use.

5. Make sure the powdered medication is completely dissolved and that the solution is free of visible particles before using it.

You must use the exact amount of solvent indicated in the directions to produce a solution with the correct dosage strength. Powder takes up volume even when dissolved. The volume of the reconstituted medication includes the volume of the solvent and the volume of the powder.

If less than the recommended amount of solvent is used, the powder may not dissolve completely, making the solution unsafe to administer. If too much solvent is used, then the patient will not receive the desired dose. When you prepare a suspension, remember that the particles will not dissolve completely. Your goal is to distribute them evenly.

Some vials contain a single dose of medication. Many must be reconstituted immediately before administering them, because they quickly lose potency. Other such medications can be stored for a short time after reconstitution. In some facilities, medications are reconstituted in the pharmacy and delivered ready to use.

Rule 10-7

When you store a medication after reconstituting it,

1. You must record the date, the time of expiration, and your name or initials.

2. For multiple-dose medications, also record the solution strength.

Check the drug label or package insert for the length of time a reconstituted medication may be stored. Storage time may depend on whether or not the medication is refrigerated.

EXAMPLE 1 How would you reconstitute and label the following medication?

Ordered: *glucagon 1 mg IM stat*

On hand: Refer to the label on the right.

A 1-mL vial of diluting solution is provided. Once mixed, the solution must either be used immediately or be discarded. Because the mixed solution will not be stored, you do not need to label the vial.

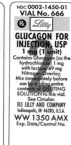

EXAMPLE 2 How would you reconstitute and label the following medication? Find the *amount to administer.*

Ordered: *Maxipime 500 mg IM q12h*

On hand: Refer to the label and portion of package insert below.

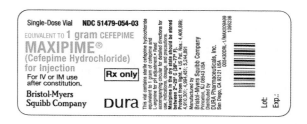

TABLE 14
Preparation of Solutions of Maxipime

Single-Dose Vials for Intravenous/Intramuscular Administration	Amount of Diluent to be added (mL)	Approximate Available Volume (mL)	Approximate Cefepime Concentration (mg/mL)
cefepime vial content			
500 mg (IV)	5.0	5.6	100
500 mg (IM)	1.3	1.8	280
1 g (IV)	10.0	11.3	100
1 g (IM)	2.4	3.6	280
2 g (IV)	10.0	12.5	160
Piggyback (100 mL)			
1 g bottle	50	50	20
1 g bottle	100	100	10
2 g bottle	50	50	40
2 g bottle	100	100	20
ADD-Vantage®			
1 g vial	50	50	20
1 g vial	100	100	10
2 g vial	50	50	40
2 g vial	100	100	20

Compatibility and Stability:
Intravenous: MAXIPIME is compatible at concentrations between 1 and 40 mg/mL with the following IV infusion fluids: 0.9% Sodium Chloride Injection, 5% and 10% Dextrose Injection, M/6 Sodium Lactate Injection, 5% Dextrose and 0.9% Sodium Chloride Injection, Lactated Ringers and 5% Dextrose Injection, Normosol-R®, and Normosol-M® in 5% Dextrose Injection. These solutions may be stored up to 24 hours at controlled room temperature 20°–25° C (68°–77° F) or 7 days in a refrigerator 2°–8° C (36°–46° F). MAXIPIME in ADD-Vantage® vials is stable at concentrations of 10–40 mg/mL in 5% Dextrose Injection or 0.9% Sodium Chloride Injection for 24 hours at controlled room temperature 20°–25° C or 7 days in a refrigerator 2°–8° C.

The amount of diluent used to reconstitute this medication is based on the amount of active drug and whether the route is IV or IM. For the 1-g vial, and IM use, use 2.4 mL of one of the several listed diluents. Once the medication is reconstituted, you will have 3.6 mL available with a dosage strength of 280 mg/mL.

Once mixed, the medication is stable for 24 hours if stored at room temperature (and for seven days if refrigerated). If you mix the medication at 1000 on 6/17/2002, and store it at room temperature, then label the vial "Exp 6/18/2002 1000. 280 mg/mL," adding your initials. (If you plan to refrigerate the vial, label it Exp "6/24/2002 1000.")

To administer 500 mg of drug, calculate the amount of solution to administer:

$$500 \text{ mg} \times \frac{1 \text{ mL}}{280 \text{ mg}} = A$$

$$25\cancel{500} \text{ mg} \times \frac{1 \text{ mL}}{\cancel{280} \text{ mg}_{14}} = 25 \times \frac{1}{14} \text{ mL} = \frac{25}{14} = 1.786 \text{ mL}$$

Round 1.786 mL to the nearest tenth. Administer 1.8 mL of solution, using a standard syringe.

ERROR ALERT!

Select the correct instructions for the strength and route ordered.

The package insert for the last example specifies that a 500-mg vial of Maxipime can be reconstituted for both IM and IV use. Suppose a nurse mistakenly reconstitutes Maxipime 500 mg IM for 500 mg IV instead. The IV instructions indicate that the nurse use 5 mL of diluent, producing a solution strength of 100 mg/mL. Calculating the *amount to administer,*

$$500 \text{ mg} \times \frac{1 \text{ mL}}{100 \text{ mg}} = A$$

$$5\cancel{500} \text{ mg} \times \frac{1 \text{ mL}}{\cancel{100} \text{ mg}_1} = 5 \times 1 \text{ mL} = 5 \text{ mL}$$

The nurse administers two injections of 2.5 mL each. The patient's discomfort increases, and the number of injection sites available for future injections are reduced. Costs increase because more diluent and syringes than necessary are used. The risk of injection complications is doubled. Correctly reconstituted for IM use, 1.3 mL of diluent will be used to produce a solution with a dosage strength of 280 mg/mL. As the previous example showed, the IM injection will require only 1.8 mL of solution, not 5 mL.

CRITICAL THINKING ON THE JOB

Recording Accurate Information

A medical assistant receives the following order: *Humatrope 2 mg IM TIW*

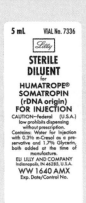

At 0800 on 10/15/01, the medical assistant prepares the medication to administer later that day. After reading the label, she draws up all of the diluent supplied with the medication and injects it into the vial. According to the drug label the remaining medication may be refrigerated for 14 days if protected from light. She labels the vial "Exp: 0800 10/29/01. Refrigerate. 5 mg/mL" and signs it with her initials. The vial will not be exposed to light in the refrigerator. Otherwise, the medical assistant might wrap it in foil or place it inside a paper bag.

Later that day, the medical assistant calculates the amount to administer, based on the label,

$$2 \text{ mg} \times \frac{1 \text{ mL}}{5 \text{ mg}} = A$$

$$2 \text{ mg} \times \frac{1 \text{ mL}}{5 \text{ mg}} = 2 \times \frac{1}{5} \text{ mL} = \frac{2}{5} \text{ mL} = 0.4 \text{ mL}$$

She uses a LoDose tuberculin syringe to administer the medication.

Think Before You Act

While the medical assistant has followed instructions carefully, she has mislabeled the vial. She used 5 mL of sterile diluent, not 1 mL. Her label should indicate 5 mg/5 mL so that her calculation is

$$2 \text{ mg} \times \frac{5 \text{ mL}}{5 \text{ mg}} = A$$

$$2 \text{ mg} \times \frac{1\cancel{5} \text{ mL}}{\cancel{5} \text{ mg}_1} = 2 \times 1 \text{ mL} = 2 \text{ mL}$$

She would administer this amount using a standard syringe. Because of her labeling error, the patient receives only $\frac{1}{5}$ the amount of medication ordered.

RECONSTITUTING POWDERED MEDICATION

In Exercises 1–4, refer to the following label and package insert:

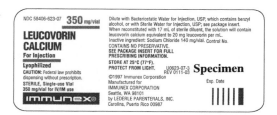

Each 350 mg vial of Leucovorin Calcium for Injection when reconstituted with 17 mL of sterile diluent yields a leucovorin concentration of 20 mg leucovorin per mL. Leucovorin Calcium for Injection contains no preservative. Reconstitute with Bacteriostatic Water for Injection, USP, which contains benzyl alcohol, or with Sterile Water for Injection, USP. When reconstituted with Bacteriostatic Water for Injection, USP, the resulting solution must be used within 7 days. If the product is reconstituted with Sterile Water for Injection, USP, it must be used immediately.

Because of the benzyl alcohol contained in Bacteriostatic Water for Injection, USP, when doses greater than 10 mg/m² are administered Leucovorin Calcium for Injection should be reconstituted with Sterile Water for Injection, USP, and used immediately. (See **WARNINGS**.) Because of the calcium content of the leucovorin solution, no more than 160 mg of leucovorin should be injected intravenously per minute (16 mL of a 10 mg/mL, or 8 mL of a 20 mg/mL solution per minute).

Parenteral drug products should be inspected visually for particulate matter and discoloration prior to administration, whenever solution and container permit. Leucovorin should not be mixed in the same infusion as 5-fluorouracil, since this may lead to the formation of a precipitate.

HOW SUPPLIED

Leucovorin Calcium for Injection is supplied in sterile, single-use vials

NDC 58406-623-07 - 350 mg Vial

STORE AT 25°C (77°F); EXCURSIONS PERMITTED TO 15-30°C (59-86°F).
PROTECT FROM LIGHT.

1. How much diluent should you add to the 350-mg vial?

2. What solution strength should you print on the label?

3. If Leucovorin is reconstituted with bacteriostatic water, how long will it retain its potency?

4. How should reconstituted Leucovorin be stored?

In Exercises 5–8, refer to the following order, label, and package insert:
Ordered: *Kefzol 250 mg IM Q8H*

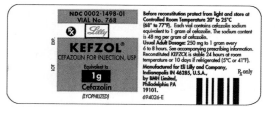

DOSAGE AND ADMINISTRATION

Kefzol may be administered intramuscularly or intravenously after reconstitution. Total daily dosages are the same for either route of administration.

Intramuscular Administration—Reconstitute 1-g vial as directed by Table 3 with Sterile Water for Injection. Shake well until dissolved. Kefzol should be injected into a large muscle mass. Pain on injection is infrequent with Kefzol.

TABLE 3. DILUTION TABLE

Vial Size	Diluent to Be Added	Approximate Available Volume	Approximate Average Concentration
1 g	2.5 mL	3 mL	330 mg/mL

Intravenous Administration—Kefzol may be administered by intravenous injection or by continuous or intermittent infusion.

STABILITY

In those situations in which the drug and diluent have been mixed, but not immediately administered to the patient, the admixture may be stored under the following conditions:

Vials—Reconstituted Kefzol diluted in Sterile Water for Injection, 5% Dextrose Injection, or 0.9% Sodium Chloride Injection is stable for 24 hours at room temperature and for 10 days if stored under refrigeration, 2° to 8°C (36° to 46°F).

Solutions of Kefzol in Sterile Water for Injection, 5% Dextrose Injection, or 0.9% Sodium Chloride Injection that are frozen immediately after reconstitution in the original vials are stable for as long as 12 weeks if stored at -20°C. Once thawed, these solutions are stable for 24 hours at room temperature or for 10 days if stored under refrigeration, 2° to 8°C (36° to 46°F). If the product is warmed, care should be taken to avoid heating it after the thawing is complete. Once thawed, the solution should not be refrozen.

5. What diluent should you use to reconstitute Kefzol?

6. How much diluent should you add to this vial?

7. If Kefzol is reconstituted at 1000 on January 3, 2002, and will be stored in the refrigerator, what should you write on the label?

8. How much solution should you administer?

In Exercises 9–14, refer to the following order, label, and package insert:
Ordered: *Follistim 150 IU IM QD*

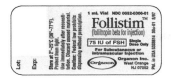

Directions for using Follistim®
1. Wash hands thoroughly with soap and water.
2. Before injections, the septum tops of the vials should be wiped with an aseptic solution to prevent contamination of the contents.
3. To prepare the Follistim® solution, inject 1 mL of Sterile Water for Injection, USP into the vial of Follistim®. **DO NOT SHAKE**, but gently swirl until the solution is clear. Generally, the Follistim® dissolves immediately. Check the liquid in the container. If it is not clear or has particles in it, **DO NOT USE IT.**
4. For patients requiring a single injection from multiple vials of Follistim®, up to 4 vials can be reconstituted with 1 mL of Sterile Water for Injection, USP. This can be accomplished by reconstituting a single vial as described above (see step 3). Then draw the entire contents of the first vial into a syringe, and inject the contents into a second vial of lyophilized Follistim®. Gently swirl the second vial, as described above, once again checking to make sure the solution is clear and free of particles. This step can be repeated with 2 additional vials for a total of up to 4 vials of lyophilized Follistim® into 1 mL of diluent.
5. Immediately **ADMINISTER** the reconstituted Follistim® either **SUBCUTANEOUSLY** or **INTRAMUSCULARLY.** Any unused reconstituted material should be discarded.
6. Draw the reconstituted Follistim® into an empty, sterile syringe.

9. What diluents can you use to reconstitute Follistim for IM administration?

10. How many vials should you administer?

11. How much diluent do you need to reconstitute the total amount of Follister that you will administer?

12. If the order was for 225 IU instead of 150 IU, how much diluent would you need?

13. If Follistim is reconstituted at 1400 on May 4, 2002, what expiration date does it have?

14. How many injections would you need to administer a 150-IU dose to a 150-lb adult?

In Exercises 15–20, refer to the following order and label:
Ordered: *Zinacef 0.8 g IM q8h × 7*

15. What diluent should you use to reconstitute this medication?

16. How much diluent should you add to the vial?

17. What solution strength should you write on the label?

18. If the Zinacef is reconstituted at 2400 on 6/5/2002, and will be stored at room temperature, what expiration date and time should you write on the label?

19. If the reconstituted Zinacef is refrigerated instead of being stored at room temperature, what expiration date should you write on the label?

20. How much solution should you administer?

In Exercises 21–24, refer to the following order, label, and package insert:
Ordered: *Penicillin G potassium 1 million U IM q2h*

21. To make a solution of 500,000 units/mL, how much diluent should you add to the vial?

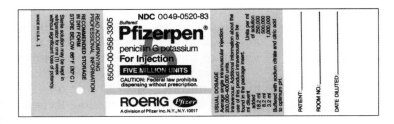

22. If the medication in the vial is reconstituted with 4.8 mL of diluent, what solution strength should you write on the label?

23. If the penicillin is reconstituted at 1200 on 11/20/02 and will be stored in the refrigerator, what expiration date and time should you write on the label?

Reconstitution
The following table shows the amount of solvent required for solution of various concentrations:

Approx. Desired Concentration (units/mL)	Approx. Volume (mL) 1,000,000 units	Solvent for Vial of 5,000,000 units	Infusion Only 20,000,000 units
50,000	20.0	–	–
100,000	10.0	–	–
250,000	4.0	18.2	75.0
500,000	1.8	8.2	33.0
750,000	–	4.8	–
1,000,000	–	3.2	11.5

When the required volume of solvent is greater than the capacity of the vial, the penicillin can be dissolved by first injecting only a portion of the solvent into the vial, then withdrawing the resultant solution and combining it with the remainder of the solvent in a larger sterile container.

Buffered Pfizerpen (penicillin G potassium) for Injection is highly water soluble. It may be dissolved in small amounts of Water for Injection, or Sterile Isotonic Sodium Chloride Solution for Parenteral Use. All solutions should be stored in a refrigerator. When refrigerated, penicillin solutions may be stored for seven days without significant loss of potency.

Buffered Pfizerpen for Injection may be given intramuscularly or by continuous intravenous drip for dosages of 500,000, 1,000,000, or 5,000,000 units. It is also suitable for intrapleural, intraarticular, and other local instillations.

THE 20,000,000 UNIT DOSAGE MAY BE ADMINISTERED BY INTRAVENOUS INFUSION ONLY.

(1) Intramuscular Injection: Keep total volume of injection small. The intramuscular route is the preferred route of administration. Solutions containing up to 100,000 units of penicillin per mL of diluent may be used with a minimum of discomfort. Greater concentration of penicillin G per mL is physically possible and may be employed where therapy demands. When large dosages are required, it may be advisable to administer aqueous solutions of penicillin by means of continuous intravenous drip.

(2) Continuous Intravenous Drip: Determine the volume of fluid and rate of its administration required by the patient in a 24 hour period in the usual manner for fluid therapy, and add the appropriate daily dosage of penicillin to this fluid. For example, if an adult patient requires 2 liters of fluid in 24 hours and a daily dosage of 10 million units of penicillin, add 5 million units to 1 liter and adjust the rate of flow so the liter will be infused in 12 hours.

(3) Intrapleural or Other Local Infusion: If fluid is aspirated, give infusion in a volume equal to $\frac{1}{4}$ or $\frac{1}{2}$ the amount of fluid aspirated, otherwise, prepare as for intramuscular injection.

(4) Intrathecal Use: The intrathecal use of penicillin in meningitis must be highly individualized. It should be employed only with full consideration of the possible irritating effects of penicillin when used by this route. The preferred route of therapy in bacterial meningitides is intravenous, supplemented by intramuscular injection.

Parenteral drug products should be inspected visually for particulate matter and discoloration prior to administration, whenever solution and container permit. Sterile solution may be left in refrigerator for one week without significant loss of potency.

24. How much solution should you administer?

To check your answers, see page 356.

Insulin

Insulin is a pancreatic hormone that stimulates glucose metabolism. People who have low or no insulin production may have insulin-dependent diabetes. They often need regular injections of insulin to keep their glucose (blood sugar) from rising to levels that could be life-threatening.

Types of Insulin

Many types of injectable insulin exist. The oldest types are beef insulin and pork insulin, extracted from cattle or pig pancreas. In the United States, animal-based insulin is being replaced by human insulin, including those produced by using genetically-engineered bacteria. A synthetic form, insulin lispro, is also available. Regular insulin is clear. Lente, NPH, and Ultralente insulins are cloudy.

Timing of Action

Insulins are classified by the timing of their action. Rapid-acting insulins include regular (R) and Semilente (S) insulins. Insulin lispro is an even more rapid-acting insulin that is generally administered 15 minutes before a meal. Other rapid-acting insulins are usually administered 30 to 60 minutes before eating. Intermediate-acting insulins include Lente (L), NPH (or N), and Protamine Zinc (P). Ultralente (U) is a long-acting insulin.

In order for insulin to be effective, it must be given at a specific time relative to food intake. Therefore, before you administer insulin, you must know the onset, peak, and duration of action of each type. The *onset* is the time when the insulin begins to lower the glucose level. The *peak* is the time at which the insulin's effect is strongest. Both onset and peak are measured from the time the insulin is administered. The *duration* is the length of time the effect of the insulin lasts. It is measured from the time of the onset.

For example, a regular dose of insulin administered at 0700 will begin to take effect after 30 minutes, at 0730 (the onset). Its peak will be 2.5 to 5 hours after it is administered, between 0930 and 1200. Its effect will last until 1530 (the duration), about 8 hours after the onset. Table 10-2 summarizes the action times of many types of insulin, including mixed insulins which are described later.

Table 10-2 Timing of Insulin Action

Insulin	Examples	Onset	Peak	Duration
rapid-acting	Humulin R	30 min	2.5-5 hrs	8 hrs
	Novolin R			
	Velosulin BR	30 min	1-3 hrs	8 hrs
	Humalog	15 min	30-90 min	6-8 hrs
intermediate	Novolin L	2.5 hrs	7-15 hrs	22 hrs
	Humulin N	1.5 hrs	4-12 hrs	24 hrs
	Novolin N			
long-acting	Humulin U	4-8 hrs	10-30 hrs	28 hrs
mixed	Humulin 70/30	30 min	2.5-12 hrs	24 hrs
	Humulin 50/50			
	Novolin 70/30			

Insulin Labels

Like other drug labels, insulin labels identify the manufacturer, the brand name, storage information, and the expiration date (Figures 10-2 and 10-3). The concentration is usually listed twice, as the traditional dosage strength (e.g., 100 Units per mL) and as the concentration. In most cases, the concentration is U-100, meaning that 100 units of insulin are contained in 1 mL of solution. Occasionally, the concentration is U-500, with 500 units per 1 mL. Insulin labels also list the type (e.g., L or Lente) and the origin (beef, pork, human, or other).

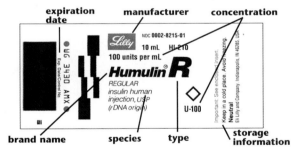

Figure 10-2

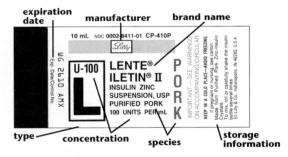

Figure 10-3

CRITICAL THINKING ON THE JOB

Clarifying the Order

An order reads: *Iletin II 20 units sc stat.* The nurse was unaware that Iletin II is available in Lente and regular forms. He administered Iletin II regular insulin. When the patient experienced symptoms of hypoglycemia, she was given 4 oz of orange juice and 6 graham crackers.

Regular insulin has a shorter duration of action than Lente insulin. As a result, the patient's morning glucose level was elevated. Based on this elevated reading, the physician increased the dose. In turn, the patient again experienced hypoglycemia the next day and required another dosage adjustment.

Think Before You Act

The physician's initial order was incomplete. The nurse should have realized that a correct order would include the type of insulin. The nurse should have checked with the physician before administering the dose.

Insulin Syringes

Recall from Chapter 4 that insulin is administered with special insulin syringes marked in units. A standard U-100 insulin syringe holds up to 100 Units or 1 mL of solution. Most of these syringes are calibrated for every two units, though some are marked for each unit.

Smaller insulin syringes, holding up to 50 units (0.5 mL of solution) or 30 units (0.3 mL), are usually calibrated for each Unit. Their larger numbers make them easier to use for visually-impaired patients.

EXAMPLE 1 ⟩ Ordered: *Novolin N 66 Units*

Because this order is for more than 50 Units, use a 100-Unit insulin syringe. Find the mark for 66 Units and fill the syringe to that calibration (Figure 10-4).

Figure 10-4

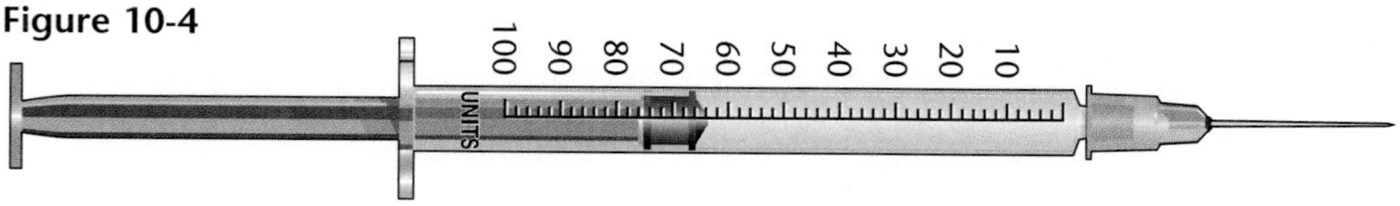

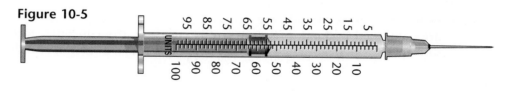

EXAMPLE 2 ⟩ Ordered: *Humulin R 55 Units*

Because this order is for more than 50 Units, you will need a 100-Unit syringe. Your best choice would be a syringe calibrated for each Unit (Figure 10-5). If you use a syringe calibrated for every 2 Units, then fill it to the imaginary line between 54 and 56 units.

Figure 10-5

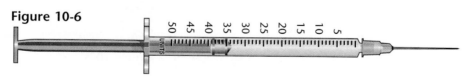

EXAMPLE 3 ⟩ Ordered: *Velosulin BR 35 Units*

Because this order is for less than 50 Units, you may use a smaller syringe in which each Unit is calibrated (Figure 10-6).

Figure 10-6

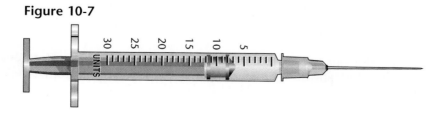

EXAMPLE 4 ⟩ Ordered: *Novolin R 8 Units*

Because this order is for less than 30 Units, you may use either a 30-Unit or 50-Unit insulin syringe in which each Unit is calibrated (Figure 10-7).

Figure 10-7

If the order is for U-500 insulin (which contains 500 units in each mL), use a tuberculin syringe. Calculate the amount to administer in mL.

EXAMPLE 5 Ordered: *Humulin R U-500 insulin 80 Units*

$$80 \text{ Units} \times \frac{1 \text{ mL}}{500 \text{ Units}} = A$$

$$^{4}\cancel{80} \cancel{\text{Units}} \times \frac{1 \text{ mL}}{\cancel{500} \cancel{\text{Units}}_{25}} = 4 \times \frac{1}{25} \text{ mL} = \frac{4}{25} \text{ mL} = 0.16 \text{ mL}$$

Administer 0.16 mL drawn up in a tuberculin syringe. (See Figure 10-8.)

Figure 10-8

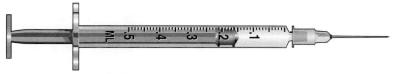

PATIENT EDUCATION

Measuring A Single Insulin Dose

Give the following information to patients:

1. Always wash your hands before handling insulin and syringes.

2. If you are using an intermediate- or long-acting insulin (Lente, NPH, UltraLente, 70/30, or 50/50), roll the vial between your palms to mix the insulin, until all of the insulin looks cloudy.

3. Cleanse the rubber stopper of the vial with an alcohol wipe, using a circular motion. Start at the center of the circle and work outward.

4. Draw up an amount of air equal to your insulin dose in the syringe. Pull back the plunger until the leading ring is aligned with the correct marking on the syringe (Figure 10-9a).

5. Inject the air into the insulin vial (Figure 10-9b).

6. Keeping the needle inserted through the stopper, turn the vial upside down. Draw up your ordered dose of insulin (Figure 10-9c).

7. Avoid touching the needle during the procedure.

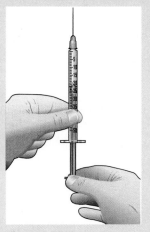

Figure 10-9a

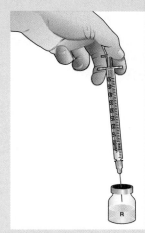

Figure 10-9b

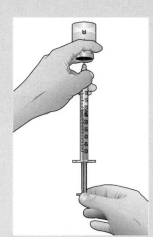

Figure 10-9c

Insulin Combinations

In some cases, in order to have more control over glucose levels, the physician will prescribe two types of insulin for a patient. For example, the combination of a rapid-acting insulin and an intermediate-acting insulin provides the patient with the rapid onset of the first and the lengthy duration of the second. The two types of insulin can be combined in one syringe so that the patient only needs to receive one injection. Two types of insulin may be combined by the drug manufacturer. For example, Novolin 70/30 is 70% intermediate-acting NPH insulin and 30% rapid-acting regular insulin (Figure 10-10). Humulin 50/50 has 50% intermediate-acting NPH (or isophane) insulin and 50% rapid-acting regular insulin (Figure 10-11). In some cases, you will need to prepare the insulin combination yourself.

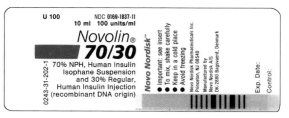

Figure 10-10

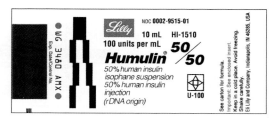

Figure 10-11

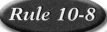 **Rule 10-8**

When preparing a combined insulin dose, always draw up the rapid-acting insulin first. Remember: the insulin which will act first is drawn up first.

Another way to remember Rule 10-8 is to draw up the clear insulin (rapid-acting) before the cloudy insulin (intermediate-acting).

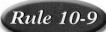 **Rule 10-9**

To prepare a combined insulin dose,

1. Calculate the total dose of insulin:

dose of rapid-acting insulin + dose of intermediate-acting insulin = total dose insulin

2. Draw up an amount of air equal to the dose of intermediate-acting insulin. Inject it into the intermediate insulin vial, but do not draw up the dose. Withdraw the needle from this vial.

3. Draw up an amount of air equal to the dose of rapid acting insulin. Inject it into the rapid-acting insulin vial.

4. Without withdrawing the needle from the stopper, invert the vial. Draw up the dose of rapid-acting insulin.

5. Carefully insert the needle through the stopper of the intermediate-acting insulin vial. Invert the vial, without injecting any of the rapid acting insulin into the vial.

6. Draw up intermediate-acting insulin until the leading ring reaches the calibration indicating the total dose.

EXAMPLE 1 Ordered: *Humulin N 42 units and Humulin R 10 units sc qd*

First calculate the total dose of insulin:

10 Units of Humulin R + 42 Units of Humulin N = 52 Units total

Next draw up 42 units of air and inject them into the vial of Humulin N. Withdraw the needle from Humulin N without drawing up the dose. Then draw up 10 units of air and inject them into the vial of Humulin R. Without withdrawing the needle, invert the vial of Humulin R and draw up 10 units of insulin (Figure 10-12a). Finally, insert the needle into the vial of Humulin N and invert the vial. Withdraw 42 units of Humulin N, until the leading ring of the syringe is at the calibration of 52 units, the total dose (Figure 10-12b).

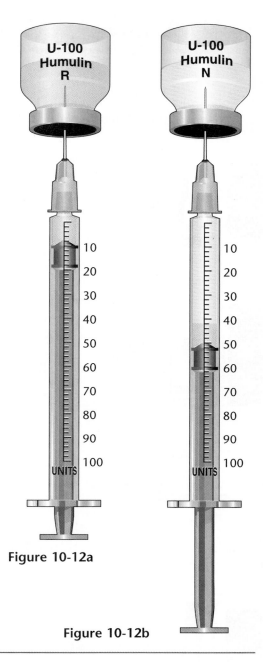

Figure 10-12a

In Figure 10-12b, the pink shading represents the Humulin R and the yellow shading represents the Humulin N. (These are not the actual colors of the insulin.)

Figure 10-12b

ERROR ALERT! *When two types of insulins are combined, measure the correct amount of each.*

An order reads: *Novolin N 37 Units and Novolin R 5 units sc stat.* Suppose you draw up 37 units from the Novolin R vial and 5 units from the Novolin N vial. Although the patient receives 42 units of insulin, he receives a much larger dose of regular (rapid-acting) insulin than was ordered, 37 Units rather than 5 Units. The insulin metabolizes the patient's glucose too quickly; he becomes hypoglycemic and loses consciousness. Glucagon and 50% dextrose are administered and the patient recovers. This error can be avoided if you carefully check the order against the labels three times.

REVIEW and PRACTICE

INSULIN

In Exercises 1–14, refer to labels A–G. Select the label corresponding to each order. Then mark the desired amount of insulin on the syringe.

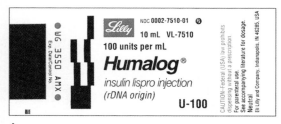

A

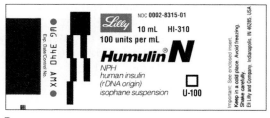

B

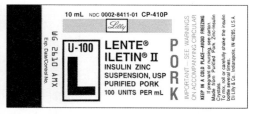

C

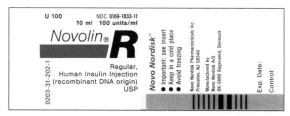

D

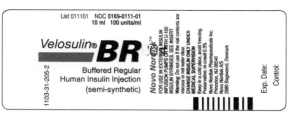

E

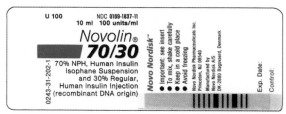

F

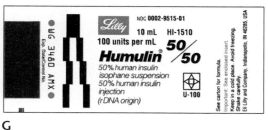

G

1. Ordered: *Novolin R 12 units sc ac breakfast*

   Select vial: _____

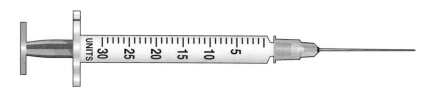

2. Ordered: *Humalog 5 units sc 15 minutes before lunch*

   Select vial: _____

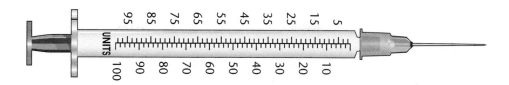

3. Ordered: *Lente Iletin II 35 units sc qd*

   Select vial: _____

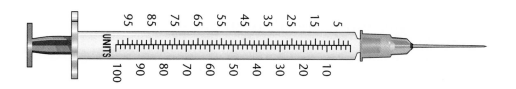

4. Ordered: *Humulin N 72 units sc qd*

   Select vial: _____

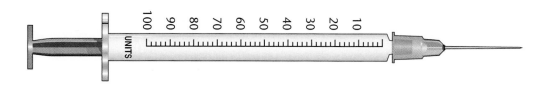

5. Ordered: *Humulin 50/50 42 units sc ac breakfast*

   Select vial: _____

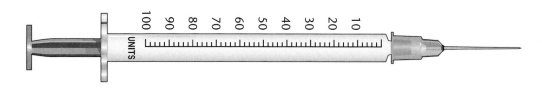

6. Ordered: *Velosulin BR 17 units ac breakfast*

   Select vial: _____

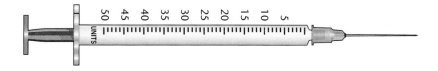

7. Ordered: *Novolin 70/30 53 units sc ac dinner*

   Select vial: _____

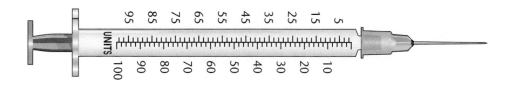

8. Ordered: *Novolin 70/30 R 26 units sc ac breakfast*

   Select vial: _____

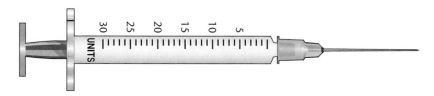

9. Ordered: *NPH insulin 44 units sc ac dinner*

   Select vial: _____

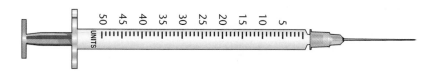

10. Ordered: *Humalog 15 units sc ac breakfast*

    Select vial: _____

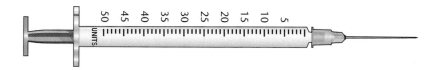

11. Ordered: *Lente Iletin II insulin 64 units sc qd*

    Select vial: _____

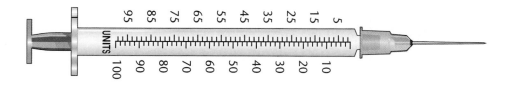

12. Ordered: *Humulin 50/50 injection 36 units sc ac dinner*

Select vial: _____

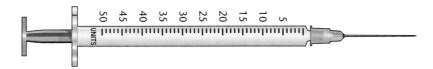

13. Ordered: *Velosulin BR 7 units sc stat*

Select vial: _____

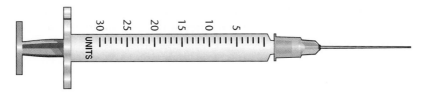

14. Ordered: *Novolin R 14 units sc ac breakfast*

Select vial: _____

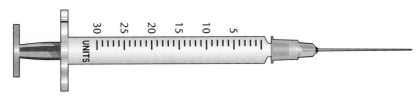

In exercises 15 and 16, first mark on the syringe the dose of rapid-acting insulin ordered. Then mark where the leading ring will be after you draw up the intermediate-acting insulin into the same syringe.

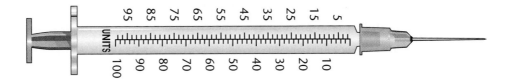

15. Novolin N 65 units and Novolin R 12 units

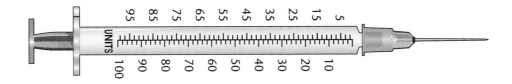

16. Humulin N 53 units and Humulin R 4 units

To check your answers, see page 357.

Other Medication Routes

Medications may be given by a variety of routes besides oral and common parenteral routes. These routes are used for intradermal injections, inhalants, and rectal and transdermal medications.

Intradermal Injections

Very small doses of medication can be injected under the first layer of the skin. This route is normally used for diagnostic testing, most often screening for tuberculosis or allergies. When an intradermal injection is required, the physician usually orders the intended diagnostic test, such as a Mantoux (PPD) test for tuberculosis. You determine the amount of solution to use by checking the vial label or the package insert. If a dose other than the standard diagnostic dose is to be administered, the physician will order the exact amount. No calculation is required. Intradermal injections are usually 0.1 mL or less. A tuberculin syringe is always used.

Inhalants

Inhaled medications are administered either by metered dose inhaler (MDI) or by nebulizer. Metered dose inhalers provide a measured dose of medication in each puff. The physician orders the number of puffs to be given. No calculation is necessary.

Medications given by nebulizer are supplied as liquids which are mixed with sterile saline solution. Single doses premixed with saline are available for most medications. A few are measured in the receptacle of the nebulizer, after which the correct amount of saline is added. Sterile saline is usually provided in 3 mL or 5 mL single-dose ampules.

Inhalant medications in multiple-dose containers are usually packaged with special droppers calibrated for the standard doses. If the dropper is not available or becomes contaminated, a sterile syringe may be used.

The physician usually specifies the solution strength and the amount of inhalant to administer. For example, the order *Mucomyst 20% 3 mL via nebulizer QID* is a complete order. When calculations are necessary, the same methods are used for inhalants as are used for parenteral medications.

> **EXAMPLE 1** Find the *amount to administer.*
>
> Ordered: *acetylcysteine 600 mg q4h inhalation*
>
> On hand: acetylcysteine 20% solution
>
> First convert the percent to g/mL:
>
> $$20\% \text{ solution} = \frac{20 \text{ g}}{100 \text{ mL}}$$
>
> Now use dimensional analysis to find the *amount to administer.* The *dosage ordered* is 600 mg, the *dose on hand* is 20 g, and the *dosage unit* is 100 mL.
>
> $$600 \text{ mg} \times \text{conversion factor} \times \frac{100 \text{ mL}}{20 \text{ g}} = A$$
>
> The conversion factor should relate g to mg so that it cancels these units. Using the factor $\dfrac{1 \text{ g}}{1000 \text{ mg}}$,
>
> $$600 \text{ mg} \times \frac{1 \text{ g}}{1000 \text{ mg}} \times \frac{100 \text{ mL}}{20 \text{ g}} = A$$
>
> $$^3\cancel{600} \text{ } \cancel{mg} \times \frac{1 \cancel{g}}{_1{}^5\cancel{1000} \text{ } \cancel{mg}} \times \frac{^1\cancel{20}{}^5 100 \text{ mL}}{\cancel{20} \text{ } \cancel{g}_1} = 3 \times 1 \text{ mL} = 3 \text{ mL}$$
>
> Administer 3 mL of acetylcysteine 20% solution.

Rectal Medications

Rectal medications are usually given in suppository form. Generally, suppositories cannot be accurately divided. Therefore, in most cases, only doses that are multiples of the available suppository strength may be administered.

EXAMPLE 1 Find the *amount to administer.*

Ordered: *Compazine 10 mg R BID*

On hand: Compazine 5-mg suppositories

$$10 \text{ mg} \times \frac{1 \text{ supp}}{5 \text{ mg}} = A$$

$$^{2}\cancel{10} \text{ } \cancel{mg} \times \frac{1 \text{ supp}}{\cancel{5} \text{ } \cancel{mg}_{1}} = 2 \times 1 \text{ supp} = 2 \text{ supp}$$

Administer 2 suppositories.

According to their manufacturers, some suppositories can be safely divided in half. However, they are not scored. Thus, the physician's order should specify that $\frac{1}{2}$ suppository is to be given. For example, if the order reads *Tigan 50 mg p.r. t.i.d.,* ask the physi-cian to clarify whether $\frac{1}{2}$ of a 100-mg suppository is acceptable. The order should then be rewritten: *Tigan 100 mg supp. Give $\frac{1}{2}$ supp.*

Transdermal Systems

Transdermal medications include patches, ointments, and creams. Patches usually consist of a special membrane which releases liquid medication at a constant rate. The patch has adhesive edges to hold it in place so that the membrane rests against the skin. The dosage strength of a transdermal patch is usually expressed in mg or mcg per hour. Patches cannot be divided. If a dose is larger than the amount provided by a single patch, you can use multiple patches. Before you administer a patch, be certain to remove any patches that are already in place and wipe off any residual medication.

EXAMPLE 1 Find the *amount to administer.*

Ordered: *Deponit 0.8 mg/hr topically*

On hand: Deponit 0.2 mg/hr and 0.4 mg/hr patches

$$0.8 \text{ mg/hr} \times \frac{1 \text{ patch}}{0.4 \text{ mg/hr}} = A$$

$$^{2}\cancel{0.8} \text{ } \cancel{mg} \text{ } \cancel{hr} \times \frac{1 \text{ patch}}{\cancel{0.4} \text{ } \cancel{mg} \text{ } \cancel{hr}_{1}} = 2 \times 1 \text{ patch} = 2 \text{ patches}$$

Administer 2 patches. While you could also administer four of the 0.2 mg/hr patches, you should use the least amount of medication possible to give the ordered dose.

Sometimes the ordered dose can be administered using a combination of patches. In these cases, use critical thinking skills to determine which combination will work.

EXAMPLE 2 Find the *amount to administer.*

Ordered: *Vivelle 0.125 mg/day*

On hand: Vivelle in four dosage strengths: 0.0375 mg/day, 0.05 mg/day, 0.075 mg/day, and 0.1 mg/day

Start with the patch that has the greatest dosage strength (0.1 mg/day). Because all the patches deliver more than 0.025 mg/day, none will work in combination with this patch. Next, try combinations with the 0.075 mg/day patch. Note that 0.075 + 0.05 = 0.125. Administer a combination of one 0.075 mg/day patch and one 0.05 mg/day patch.

REVIEW and PRACTICE

OTHER MEDICATION ROUTES

In Exercises 1–8, find the *amount to administer.*

1. Ordered: *acetylcysteine 1 g via nebulizer*
   On hand: acetylcysteine 20% solution

2. Ordered: *Albuterol 2.5 mg via nebulizer*
   On hand: Albuterol 5 mg/mL

3. Ordered: *Numorphan 10 mg p.r.*
   On hand: Numorphan 5 mg suppositories

4. Ordered: *RMS morphine supp 15 mg p.r.*
   On hand: RMS 5 mg, 10 mg, and 30 mg suppositories

5. Ordered: *Testoderm 0.8 mg/day top*
   On hand: Testoderm 0.4 mg/day patches

6. Ordered: *Catapres 0.5 mg/day top*
   On hand: Catapres TTS-1 (0.1 mg/day), TTS-2 (0.2 mg/day), TTS-3 (0.3 mg/day)

7. Ordered: *Alora 0.15 mg/day*
   On hand: Alora 0.05 mg/day, 0.075 mg/day, and 0.1 mg/day

8. Ordered: *Transderm Nitro 0.3 mg/hr top*
   On hand: Transderm Nitro 0.1 mg/hr, 0.2 mg/hr, and 0.6 mg/hr patches

To check your answers, see page 359.

CHAPTER *10* REVIEW

CHECK UP

In Exercises 1–20, find the *amount to administer*. Then select the proper syringe.

1. Ordered: *INFeD (iron dextran) 100 mg deep IM qd*
   On hand: INFeD 50 mg/mL

   Administer: _____ Syringe: _____

2. Ordered: *haloperidol decanoate 60 mg deep IM stat*
   On hand: haloperidol decanoate 50 mg/mL

   Administer: _____ Syringe: _____

3. Ordered: *Loxitane 30 mg IM bid*
   On hand: Loxitane 50 mg/mL

   Administer: _____ Syringe: _____

4. Ordered: *Epogen 1400 Units sc tiw*
   On hand: Epogen 2000 Units/mL

   Administer: _____ Syringe: _____

5. Ordered: *lidocaine 300 mg IM stat*
   On hand: lidocaine 20% solution

   Administer: _____ Syringe: _____

6. Ordered: *magnesium sulfate 250 mg IM qd*
   On hand: magnesium sulfate 10% solution

   Administer: _____ Syringe: _____

7. Ordered: *Levsin 0.4 mg IM bid*
   On hand: Levsin 0.5 mg/mL

   Administer: _____ Syringe: _____

8. Ordered: *Robinul 0.15 mg IM stat*
   On hand: Robinul 0.2 mg/mL

   Administer: _____ Syringe: _____

9. Order: *Prostigmin 0.75 mg IM q4h*
   On hand: Prostigmin 1:1000 solution

   Administer: _____ Syringe: _____

10. Ordered: *epinephrine 0.5 mg sc stat*
    On hand: epinephrine 1:200 solution

    Administer: _____ Syringe: _____

11. Ordered: *Adrenalin 0.2 mg sc stat*
    On hand: Adrenalin 1:2000 solution

    Administer: _____ Syringe: _____

12. Ordered: *Calciferol 24,000 IU IM qd*
    On hand: Calciferol 500,000 IU/5 mL

    Administer: _____ Syringe: _____

13. Ordered: *heparin sodium 7500 Units sc q8h*
    On hand: heparin 1:20,000 solution

    Administer: _____ Syringe: _____

14. Ordered: *heparin calcium 7500 Units sc q8h*
    On hand: heparin calcium 5000 Units/0.2 mL

    Administer: _____ Syringe: _____

15. Ordered: *Thorazine 10 mg deep IM qid*
    On hand: Refer to Label A.

    Administer: _____ Syringe: _____

16. Ordered: *Brethine 0.25 mg sc stat*
    On hand: Refer to Label B.

    Administer: _____ Syringe: _____

17. Ordered: *Imitrex 5 mg sc prn pain*
    On hand: Refer to Label C.

    Administer: _____ Syringe: _____

18. Ordered: *Dilaudid-HP 9 mg sc prn pain*
    On hand: Refer to Label D.

    Administer: _____ Syringe: _____

19. Ordered: *Epogen 2500 units sc tiw*
    On hand: Refer to Label E.

    Administer: _____ Syringe: _____

20. Ordered: *Engerix-B 10 mcg IM stat*
    On hand: Refer to Label F.

    Administer: _____ Syringe: _____

A

NSN 6505-01-156-1981
25mg/mL
NDC 0007-5062-01
THORAZINE®
CHLORPROMAZINE HCI INJECTION
10 mL Multi-Dose Vial
SB SmithKline Beecham

B

1 mL   1 mg/mL
Brethine®
terbutaline sulfate injection USP
For Subcutaneous Injection Only
Mfd. by:
Ciba-Geigy Ltd.
Basle, Switzerland
Geigy
643713

C

Imitrex® Injection
(sumatriptan succinate)
6 mg sumatriptan/0.5 mL
For subcutaneous injection only.
Glaxo Wellcome Inc.
Research Triangle Park, NC 27709
Made in England
NDC 0173-0449-02
Rev. 9/98

D

NDC 0044 - 1017 - 15
Dilaudid-HP®
hydromorphone HCI
Warning: May Be Habit Forming
50 mg/5 mL
FOR USE IN THE PREPARATION OF LARGE VOLUME PARENTERAL SOLUTIONS
Manufactured for:
Knoll Laboratories
A Division of Knoll Pharmaceutical Co.
Mount Olive, New Jersey 07828
By Abbott Laboratories, North Chicago, IL 60064, USA
6106005-2

E

NDC 55513-148-01   Store at 2° to 8°C
EPOGEN®
EPOETIN ALFA
S4
4,000 Units/mL   1 mL Single Use Vial
Caution: Federal law prohibits dispensing without prescription.
Amgen Inc. Thousand Oaks, CA 91320   U.S. License No. 1080
3107602

F

20mcg/mL
NDC 58160-860-16
HEPATITIS B VACCINE (RECOMBINANT)
ENGERIX-B®
25 Adult Doses
NSN 6505-01-311-5222
Store between 2°C and 8°C (35.6°F and 46.6°F).
Do not freeze. Discard if frozen.
20 mcg purified surface antigen (HBsAg) protein derived from *S. cerevisiae* eq. 1 dose; adsorbed onto 0.5 mg of aluminum as aluminum hydroxide; preserved with thimerosal 1:20,000 (mercury derivative).
Do not dilute; shake well before using.
For intramuscular administration only.
Adult Dosage: 20 mcg (1 mL) equals 1 dose. See complete prescribing information for vaccination schedule.
Caution: Federal law prohibits dispensing without prescription.
U.S. License 1090
Manufactured by SmithKline Beecham Biologicals
Rixensart, Belgium
Distributed by SmithKline Beecham Pharmaceuticals
Philadelphia, PA 19101
Engerix-B® is a SmithKline Beecham trademark.   525445
3 58160-860-16 4
LOT
EXP.

21. How much solution should be discarded from the prefilled syringe for the following order?
Ordered: *Lovenox 30 mg sc q12h*
Available: Refer to Label G.

G

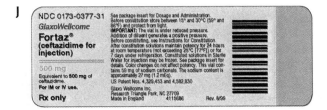

LOVENOX®
(enoxaparin sodium) Injection
40 mg/0.4 mL

Each 0.4 mL contains 40 mg of enoxaparin sodium derived from porcine intestinal mucosa in Water for Injection. See insert for directions for use.
FOR SUBCUTANEOUS INJECTION. Store at Controlled Room Temperature, 15 to 25°C (59 to 77°F) [see USP]. Rx only

NDC 0075-0620-40
1 Single Dose Prefilled Syringe — 0.4 mL
Made in France
RHÔNE-POULENC RORER
PHARMACEUTICALS INC.
COLLEGEVILLE, PA 19426   MP-5566B

LOVENOX®
(enoxaparin sodium) Injection
40 mg/0.4 mL

Each 0.4 mL contains 40 mg of enoxaparin sodium derived from porcine intestinal mucosa in Water for Injection. See insert for directions for use.
FOR SUBCUTANEOUS INJECTION. Store at Controlled Room Temperature, 15 to 25°C (59 to 77°F) [see USP]. Rx only

NDC 0075-0620-40
1 Single Dose Prefilled Syringe — 0.4 mL
Made in France
RHÔNE-POULENC RORER
PHARMACEUTICALS INC.
COLLEGEVILLE, PA 19426   MP-5566B

22. Explain which of the two medications represented by Labels H and I you would use for the following order.
Ordered: *Dilaudid 1.5 mg sc prn pain*

In Exercises 23–26, refer to label J and the package insert.

23. What diluents may be used to reconstitute Fortaz for IM use?

24. How much diluent should be added to the vial?

25. What is the strength of the solution?

26. How long will the solution retain its potency at room temperature?

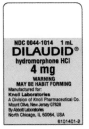

H

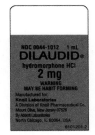

I

J

NDC 0173-0377-31
GlaxoWellcome
Fortaz®
(ceftazidime for injection)

500 mg
Equivalent to 500 mg of ceftazidime.
For IM or IV use.

Rx only

See package insert for Dosage and Administration. Before constitution store between 15° and 30°C (59° and 86°F) and protect from light.
IMPORTANT: The vial is under reduced pressure. Addition of diluent generates a positive pressure. Before constituting, see instructions for Constitution. After constitution solutions maintain potency for 24 hours at room temperature (not exceeding 25°C (77°F)) or for 7 days under refrigeration. Constituted solutions in Sterile Water for Injection may be frozen. See package insert for details. Color changes do not affect potency. This vial contains 59 mg of sodium carbonate. The sodium content is approximately 27 mg (1.2 mEq).
US Patent Nos. 4,329,453 and 4,582,830

Glaxo Wellcome Inc.
Research Triangle Park, NC 27709
Made in England   4115686   Rev. 8/99

Administration: FORTAZ may be given intravenously or by deep IM injection into a large muscle mass such as the upper outer quadrant of the gluteus maximus or lateral part of the thigh. Intra-arterial administration should be avoided (see PRECAUTIONS).
Intramuscular Administration: For IM administration, FORTAZ should be constituted with one of the following diluents: Sterile Water for Injection, Bacteriostatic Water for Injection, or 0.5% or 1% Lidocaine Hydrochloride Injection. Refer to Table 5.

Table 5: Preparation of Solutions of FORTAZ

Size	Amount of Diluent to be Added (mL)	Approximate Available Volume (mL)	Approximate Ceftazidime Concentration (mg/mL)
Intramuscular			
500-mg vial	1.5	1.8	280
1-gram vial	3.0	3.6	280
Intravenous			
500-mg vial	5.0	5.3	100
1-gram vial	10.0	10.6	100
2-gram vial	10.0	11.5	170
Infusion pack			
1-gram vial	100*	100	10
2-gram vial	100*	100	20
Pharmacy bulk package			
6-gram vial	26	30	200

COMPATIBILITY AND STABILITY:
Intramuscular: FORTAZ, when constituted as directed with Sterile Water for Injection, Bacteriostatic Water for Injection, or 0.5% or 1% Lidocaine Hydrochloride Injection, maintains satisfactory potency for 24 hours at room temperature or for 7 days under refrigeration. Solutions in Sterile Water for Injection that are frozen immediately after constitution in the original container are stable for 3 months when stored at -20°C. Once thawed, solutions should not be refrozen. Thawed solutions may be stored for up to 8 hours at room temperature or for 4 days in a refrigerator.

In Exercises 27–30, refer to label K and the package insert.

27. How much diluent should be used to reconstitute Ceptaz for IM use?

28. What solution strength should be written on the label of the vial?

29. If the Ceptaz is reconstituted at 0200 on 8/30/2002 and will be stored at room temperature, what expiration date and time should be written on the label?

30. For a 1-g dose, what is the *amount to administer*?

In Exercises 31–36, refer to labels L–Q. Select the label corresponding to each order. Then mark the desired amount of insulin on the syringe.

Administration: CEPTAZ may be given intravenously or by deep IM injection into a large muscle mass such as the upper outer quadrant of the gluteus maximus or lateral part of the thigh. Intra-arterial administration should be avoided (see PRECAUTIONS).

Table 5: Preparation of Solutions of CEPTAZ

Size	Amount of Diluent to Be Added (mL)	Volume to Be Withdrawn (mL)	Approximate Ceftazidime Concentration (mg/mL)
Intramuscular 1-gram vial	3.0	Total	250
Intravenous 1-gram vial	10.0	Total	90
2-gram vial	10.0	Total	170
Infusion pack 1-gram vial	100	—	10
2-gram vial	100	—	20
Pharmacy bulk package 10-gram vial	40	Amount needed	200

COMPATIBILITY AND STABILITY:
Intramuscular: CEPTAZ, when constituted as directed with Sterile Water for Injection, Bacteriostatic Water for Injection, or 0.5% or 1% Lidocaine Hydrochloride Injection, maintains satisfactory potency for 18 hours at room temperature or for 7 days under refrigeration. Solutions in Sterile Water for Injection that are frozen immediately after constitution in the original container are stable for 6 months when stored at -20°C. Components of the solution may precipitate in the frozen state and will dissolve on reaching room temperature with little or no agitation. Potency is not affected. Frozen solutions should only be thawed at room temperature. Do not force thaw by immersion in water baths or by microwave irradiation. Once thawed, solutions should not be refrozen. Thawed solutions may be stored for up to 12 hours at room temperature or for 7 days in a refrigerator.

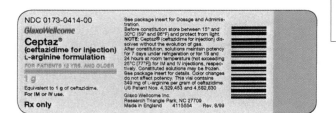

K

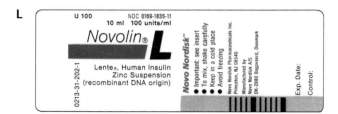

L

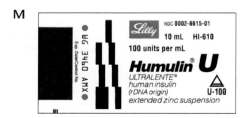

M

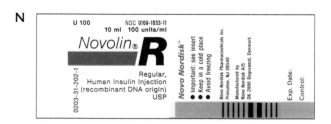

N

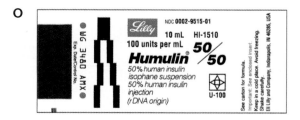

O

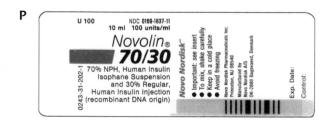

P

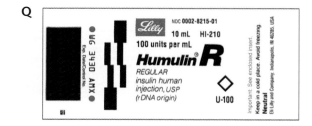

Q

31. Ordered: *Humulin R 11 units sc ac breakfast*

Select vial: _____

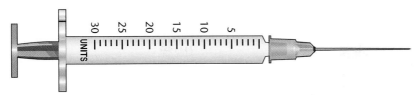

32. Ordered: *Humulin 50/50 48 units sc ac dinner*

Select vial: _____

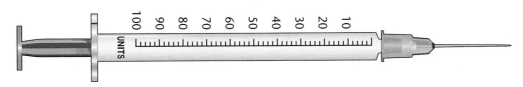

33. Ordered: *Novolin 70/30 57 units sc ac breakfast*

Select vial: _____

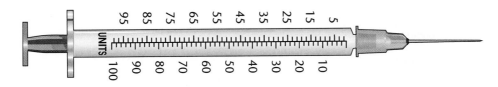

34. Ordered: *Humulin U 24 units sc qd*

Select vial: _____

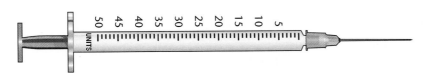

35. Ordered: *Novolin L 65 units sc ac dinner*

Select vial: _____

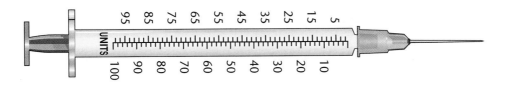

36. Ordered: *Novolin R insulin 21 units sc ac dinner*

Select vial: _____

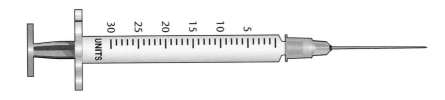

In exercises 37 and 38, first mark on the syringe the dose of rapid-acting insulin ordered. Then mark where the leading ring will be after you draw up the intermediate-acting insulin into the same syringe.

37. Humulin N 27 units and Humulin R 8 units

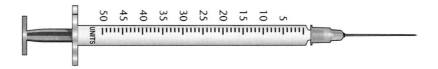

38. Novolin R 13 units and Novolin N 57 units

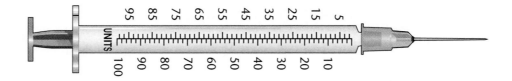

In Exercises 39–44, find the amount to administer.

39. Ordered: *acetylcysteine 800 mg via nebulizer*
On hand: acetylcysteine 10% solution

40. Ordered: *Albuterol 1.25 mg via nebulizer*
On hand: Albuterol 5 mg/mL

41. Ordered: *Thorazine 50 mg R*
On hand: Thorazine 25 mg and 100 mg suppositories

42. Ordered: *Dilaudid 6 mg R*
On hand: Dilaudid 3 mg suppositories

43. Ordered: *Androderm 5 mg/day top*
On hand: Androderm 2.5 mg/day patches

44. Ordered: *NitroDur 0.3 mg/hr top*
On hand: NitroDur 0.1 mg/hr and 0.2 mg/hr patches

CRITICAL THINKING

Ordered: *Humegon 75 IU IM tiw*
On hand: Refer to the label and package insert below.

1. How should you prepare this medication?

2. How much diluent should you use?

3. If you were not able to give the Humegon at the time it is mixed, and the patient will be returning tomorrow for the dose, what action should you take?

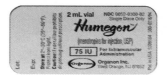

Dissolve the contents of one vial of Humegon® in one to two mL of sterile saline and **ADMINISTER INTRAMUSCULARLY** immediately. Any unused reconstituted material should be discarded. Parenteral drug products should be inspected visually for particulate matter and discoloration prior to administration, whenever solution and container permit.

CASE STUDY

A nurse receives the following order:

Primaxin 750 mg IM q12h

The patient is a 100-lb adult. The nurse has on hand Primaxin with the label below. Describe the actions she should take.

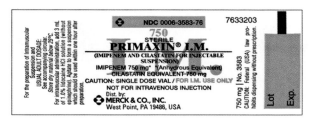

To check your answers, see page 359.

INTERNET ACTIVITY

Note: The Internet is a research tool from which to get basic information. Validate the accuracy of all Internet information.

You are working in a medical unit at a hospital where many patients newly-diagnosed with diabetes are treated. These patients need information about injecting their own insulin. You are looking for materials to teach them about the need to rotate insulin sites.

Assignment: Search the Internet for patient education materials about insulin site selection and rotation. Try the key words: insulin + site selection. Then try the key words: insulin + injection sites. Compare the information each of these combinations generates.

INTRAVENOUS DOSAGES 11

Objectives

When you have completed Chapter 11, you will be able to:

- Identify the components and concentrations of IV solutions.
- Distinguish basic types of IV equipment.
- Calculate IV flow rates for both electronically controlled and manually controlled IV devices.
- Adjust the flow rate for IV infusions.
- Calculate infusion time based on volume and flow rate.
- Calculate volume based on infusion time and flow rate.
- Measure heparin dosages and flow rates, verifying that they fall within the normal daily range.
- Calculate the hourly flow rate for IV infusions ordered in milligrams per minute.
- Calculate IV flow rates for medications ordered in mg/kg doses and for titrated medications.

Intravenous (IV) fluids are solutions, including medications, that are delivered directly into the bloodstream through a vein. Blood, a suspension, is also delivered intravenously. Fluids delivered directly into the bloodstream have a rapid effect, which is necessary during emergencies or other critical care situations when medications are needed. However, the results can be fatal if the wrong medication or dosage is given. Health care workers who administer or monitor solutions should know the principles discussed in this chapter.

Many IV drugs are available. Each has its own guidelines regarding its use, based on specifications developed by the manufacturers. The guidelines typically outline recommended dosages, infusion rates, compatibility, and patient monitoring. For example, some medications cannot be combined with others, or must be administered over a specific length of time. Furthermore, most states regulate who may administer IV medications and what training is required.

IV Solutions

IV solutions fall into four functional categories: replacement fluids, maintenance fluids, KVO fluids, and therapeutic fluids. *Replacement fluids* replace electrolytes and fluids lost or depleted due to hemorrhage, vomiting, or diarrhea. Examples include whole blood, nutrient solutions, or fluids administered to treat dehydration. *Maintenance fluids* help patients maintain normal electrolyte and fluid balance. They include IV fluids such as normal saline given during and after surgery. Some IVs provide access to the vascular system for emergency situations. Prescribed to keep the vein open (KVO or TKO), these *KVO fluids* include 5% dextrose in water. *Therapeutic fluids* deliver medication to the patient.

IV Labels

IV solutions are labeled with the name and exact amount of components in the solution. The label in Figure 11-1 is clearly marked as 5% Dextrose and Lactated Ringer's injection. Table 11-1 summarizes abbreviations often used for IV solutions.

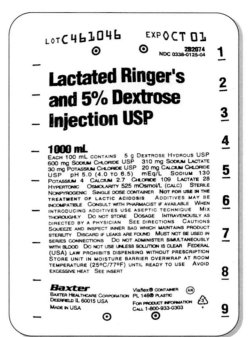

Figure 11-1

Table 11-1 Commonly Used Abbreviations

D	Dextrose
W, H$_2$O	Water
S	Saline
NS, NSS	Normal Saline (0.9% NaCl)
LR	Lactated Ringer's
RL	Ringer's Lactate
$\frac{1}{2}$ NS, $\frac{1}{2}$ NSS	half normal saline solution (0.45% NaCl)

Rule 11-1

In abbreviations for IV solutions, letters identify the component and numbers identify the concentration.

EXAMPLE 1 An order for 5% dextrose in lactated Ringer's solution might be abbreviated in any of the following ways:

D5LR   D$_5$LR   5%D/LR   D5%LR

IV Concentrations

Solutions may have different concentrations of dextrose (glucose) or saline (sodium chloride or NaCl). For example, 5% dextrose contains 5 g of dextrose per 100 mL (see Figure 11-2). Normal saline is 0.9% saline; it contains 900 mg, or 0.9 g, of sodium chloride per 100 mL (see Figure 11-3). In turn, 0.45% saline, or $\frac{1}{2}$ NS, has 450 mg of sodium chloride per 100 mL—half the amount of normal saline. Other saline concentrations include 0.33% saline (or $\frac{1}{3}$ NS) and 0.225% saline (or $\frac{1}{4}$ NS).

Figure 11-2

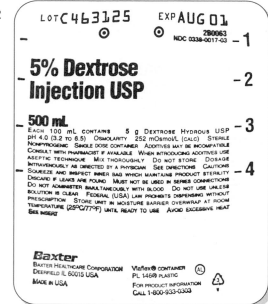

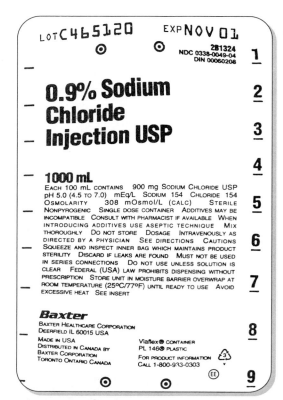

Figure 11-3

EXAMPLE 1 How much dextrose is contained in *500 mL D5W*?

D5W represents 5% dextrose in water; it has 5 g of dextrose per 100 mL of water. Using a ratio proportion,

500 mL:? g::100 mL:5 g

? g × 100 mL = 500 mL × 5 g

? = 25

25 g of dextrose is contained in 500 mL D5W.

A patient's fluid and electrolyte balance helps determine the solution's concentration. Calcium, potassium, chloride, phosphorus, and magnesium are electrolytes that can be added to an IV solution to help correct a fluid or chemical imbalance.

IV solutions are classified as *isotonic, hypotonic,* or *hypertonic,* depending on their effect on the fluid content of cells. Isotonic IV solutions, such as D5W, NS, and lactated Ringer's, do not affect the fluid balance of the surrounding cells or tissues. The fluid in hypotonic IV solutions such as 0.45% NS and 0.33% sodium chloride moves across the cell membrane into surrounding cells and tissues. This movement restores the proper fluid level in cells and tissues of patients who are dehydrated. By contrast, hypertonic IV solutions such as 3% saline draw fluids from cells and tissues across the cell membrane into the bloodstream. They are helpful for patients with severe fluid shifts, such as those caused by burns.

Rule 11-2

Patients with normal electrolyte levels are likely to receive isotonic solutions. Those with high electrolyte levels will receive hypotonic solutions. Those with low electrolyte levels will receive hypertonic solutions.

Compatibility

Medications, electrolytes, and nutrients are additives that can be combined with IV solutions. Potassium chloride, vitamins B and C, and antibiotics are common additives. While additives are often prepackaged in the solution, you may need to mix the additive and IV solution yourself. The physician's order will tell you how much additive to administer, the amount and type of basic IV solution to use, and the length of time over which the additive/IV mixture should infuse. For example, an order may call for 20 mEq of potassium chloride in 1000 mL 5% dextrose and normal saline over 8 hours, or

1000 mL D5NS c̄ 20 mEq KCl over 8 h

Rule 11-3

Before combining any medications, electrolytes, or nutrients with an IV solution, be sure the components are compatible.

If you mix an IV base solution with an additive that is incompatible, you place the patient's health at serious risk. Verify compatibility by checking with a compatibility chart, a drug reference book, or the pharmacy.

Table 11-2 Verifying Compatibility

The following are a few examples of incompatible combinations:

Ampicillin	5% dextrose in water
Cefotaxime sodium	Sodium bicarbonate
Diazepam	Potassium chloride
Dopamine HCl	Sodium bicarbonate
Penicillin	Heparin
Penicillin	Vitamin B complex
Sodium bicarbonate	Lactated Ringer's
Tetracycline HCl	Calcium chloride

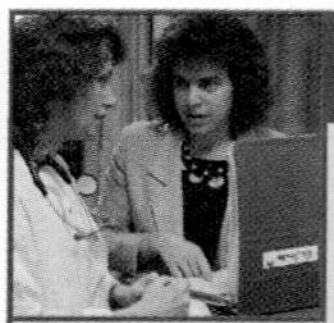

Checking Compatibility

A patient in respiratory distress with congestive heart failure is started on D5/0.45% NaCl. The next day she is diagnosed with an upper respiratory infection. The physician orders:
500 mg ampicillin IVPB q6h

The nurse begins to administer the ampicillin. She notices that the solution in the tubing has become cloudy.

Think Before You Act

The nurse suspects that the additive is not compatible with the IV solution. She uses a compatibility chart to verify her suspicions, then calls the physician to obtain a new order. In this case, the nurse was fortunate that a change in the fluid's appearance alerted her to the problem. However, in many cases, failing to verify compatibility **before** introducing an additive can have severe consequences for the patient, including death.

IV Equipment

IV equipment is available in several forms. Some are completely manual, while others include electronic components.

The Primary Line

The typical IV setup consists of a bag or bottle of IV solution and tubing. IV bags come in different sizes, often containing 500 or 1000 cc (mL) of solution. You should mark them at regular time intervals to record the amount of solution that is being infused. Your facility will have specific guidelines for you to follow.

The tubing, which is the primary line, usually includes a drip chamber, clamp, and injection ports (see Figure 11-4). The drip chamber attaches to the IV bag. To measure the flow rate, squeeze and release the drip chamber until it is half filled with IV solution. Fluid in the chamber makes it easy to count the drops that fall into it from the bag. Use roller and screw clamps to set or adjust the flow rate of the IV solution. A slide clamp shuts off the IV solution flow completely without disturbing the flow rate setting at the roller or screw clamp (see Figure 11-5). Injection ports allow you

Figure 11-4
A typical IV setup.

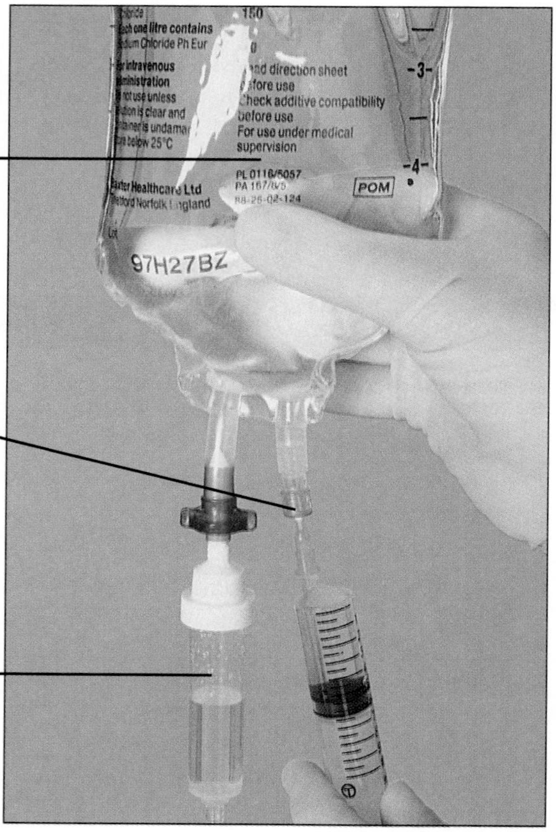

IV Solution Bag

Injection Port

Drip Chamber

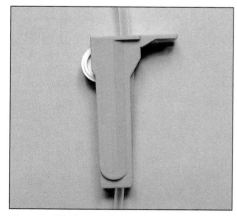

Figure 11-5a   *Roller clamp.*

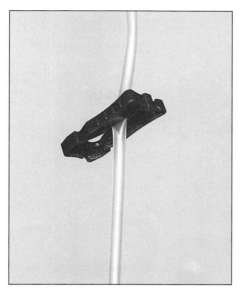

Figure 11-5b *Slide clamp.*

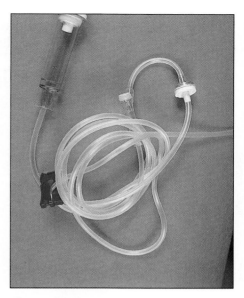

Figure 11-6 *IV tubing.*

to inject medications or compatible fluids into the primary line or to attach a second IV line. IV bags may have ports for additives injected directly into the solution.

Tubing is available in two sizes: macrodrip or microdrip (see Figure 11-6). Macrodrip tubing allows larger drops to form before falling into the drip chamber. It is used for infusions of 80 mL/hour or more and is always used for operating room infusions. Microdrip tubing allows smaller drops to enter the drip chamber. It is used for volumes of less than 80 mL/hour and is often used for KVO infusions. Microdrip tubing is especially useful for pediatric and critical care IVs, when very small volumes are used and accuracy is extremely important. Accidental increases in volume can be fatal in these situations.

Monitoring IV Equipment

In many cases, IVs are monitored manually. The bag is hung 36 inches above the patient's heart to allow gravity to draw the fluid through the tubing and into the vascular system. Whoever administers and monitors the IV adjusts the flow rate using roller or screw clamps.

Electronic devices—rate controllers, infusion pumps, syringe pumps, and patient-controlled analgesia (PCA) devices—can be used to regulate the flow of IV infusions. These devices often use tubing specific to the equipment. Some types of tubing may be used only with specific pumps (see Figures 11-7, 11-8, 11-9, and 11-10).

Rate controllers rely on gravity to infuse the solution, but no clamp is used to adjust the flow rate. Tubing is threaded through the controller, where a pincher maintains a pre-set flow rate. The controller is attached to a sensor that measures the drops or volume of solution that is delivered. An alarm sounds when the preset flow rate cannot be maintained.

Infusion pumps apply pressure sufficient to deliver a set volume of liquid every minute into the vein. They can introduce liquid into a central vein, where pressure is much higher than in peripheral veins. The desired flow rate is set on an infusion pump, either in mL/hr or by dosage. The unit does not rely on gravity, but forces the IV solution through the tubing. A sensor detects when the IV bag is empty or the flow is too rapid. An alarm sounds if the flow rate cannot be maintained or if the bag is empty. A rate that is too slow may indicate too much resistance in the vein, suggesting blockage, a kink in the tubing, or that the IV catheter has come out of the vein. In some cases, the equipment

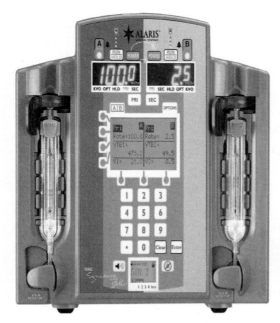

Figure 11-7   *Rate controller.*

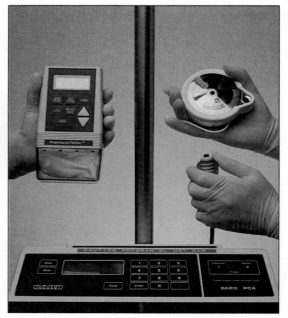

Figure 11-8   *Infusion pump.*

will continue to pump the IV fluid, even though the catheter is out of the vein. Thus, when you use an infusion pump, you must monitor the patient regularly for signs of infiltration (such as swelling, coolness, or discomfort).

Syringe pumps allow you to insert a syringe in the pump unit (see Figure 11-9). The syringe can deliver medication or fluids that cannot be combined with other medications or solutions. Syringe pumps are useful for pediatric medications as well as for medications that must be administered at a precisely controlled rate. Syringe pumps are often used in cases when a medication must be administered over half an hour or less; they are also used for longer time periods as well.

Patient Controlled Analgesia (PCA) devices are used by patients in pain, including pain from cancer or surgery (see Figure 11-10). PCA pumps allow patients to control their own medication within limits preset according to the physician's order. By pressing a button on a handheld device, a patient administers medication. The PCA helps monitor the effectiveness of the pain relief prescription, recording the number of times the patient uses the device.

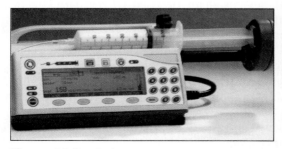

Figure 11-9   *Syringe pump.*

Figure 11-10   *PCA pump.*

Volume-control sets such as Buretrol, Soluset, and Volutrol are used with manual IV setups and electronic rate controllers to improve accuracy, especially for small volumes of medication or fluid (see Figure 11-11). They are calibrated in 1-mL increments, with a total volume capacity ranging from 100–150 mL. Medication is injected through an injection port into a burette—a chamber that holds a smaller controlled amount of fluid. An exact amount of IV fluid is added as a diluent to the burette chamber, where it is mixed. The fluid is delivered to the patient in microdrips. Burettes are often used in critical care or pediatric IVs because of their accuracy.

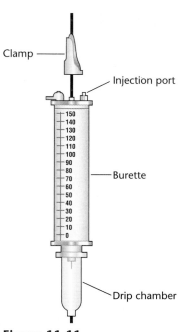

Figure 11-11

Volume control set.

Secondary Lines ("Piggybacks")

A secondary line, also known as a piggyback or IVPB, is an IV setup that attaches to a primary line (see Figure 11-12). It can be used to infuse medications or other compatible fluids on an intermittent basis, such as q6h. Although shorter than primary tubing, secondary tubing has the same basic components. IVPB bags are smaller, often holding 50, 100, or 150 cc of fluid. The ADD-Vantage® system from Abbott Laboratories is a secondary system. It uses a specially designed IV bag into which you add medication directly from the vial, often in powdered form. Any mixing takes place in the bag. The solution is then infused, with the medication vial remaining in place.

Peripheral and Central IV Therapy

Peripheral IV therapy accesses the circulatory system through a peripheral vein. Sites are usually located in the hand, forearm, foot, and leg. Because peripheral veins can be difficult to locate in small or premature infants, a peripheral IV line may be set up using a vein in the scalp.

Central IV therapy provides direct access to major veins. A central line is used when the patient needs large amounts of fluids, a rapid infusion of medication, infusion of highly concentrated solutions, or long-term IV therapy. Central lines can be inserted using a catheter through the chest wall or by threading a catheter through a peripheral vein. In newborn infants, a central line can be inserted into the umbilical vein or artery. These procedures are usually performed by a physician. Peripherally inserted central catheters (PICC) are inserted in arm veins and threaded into a central vein, often by specially trained nurses.

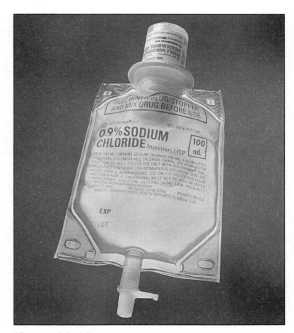

Figure 11-12 *ADD-Vantage® system.*

If you flush (or irrigate) an IV needle or catheter that is clogged, you may push a clot into the circulatory system, causing an embolism—an obstruction of a blood vessel that can be fatal. You also increase the risk of infection.

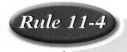

Rule 11-4

Never flush a sluggish IV with a syringe.

Pain or swelling near an IV site may indicate an infiltration or phlebitis. An infiltration occurs when the needle or catheter is dislodged from the vein or penetrates the vein. Fluid is then infused into the surrounding tissue. Signs of infiltration include swelling, discomfort, and coolness at the infiltration site, as well as a sizable decrease in flow rate. Phlebitis is an inflammation of the vein. It can develop when the vein is irritated by IV additives, by movement of the needle or catheter, or during long-term IV therapy. In most cases of phlebitis, patients will complain of pain at or near the site. Other signs include heat, redness, and swelling of the injection site. In the case of either infiltration or phlebitis, stop the IV infusion and restart it in another limb. In the case of phlebitis, also notify the patient's physician.

REVIEW and PRACTICE

IV EQUIPMENT

In Exercises 1–8, identify the IV equipment that you would use in each instance.

1. Add a dose of medication to an existing line.

2. Adjust the flow rate of an IV solution.

3. Stop the IV flow without disturbing the flow rate.

4. Introduce IV fluid into a central vein.

5. Set up tubing to infuse D5W at the rate of 40 mL/h.

6. Allow patient to self-administer medication for pain.

7. Administer a small amount of fluid over 15 minutes.

8. Dilute a powdered medication in an IV bag.

Provide a brief response to each of the following questions.

9. When would central IV therapy be used?

10. Describe what you look for when you monitor an IV.

11. How might you recognize infiltration?

12. What are three possible causes of phlebitis?

To check your answers, see page 362.

Calculating Flow Rates

An order for IV fluids indicates the flow rate—the amount of fluid that is to be infused over a certain time period. The amount of time listed in the physician's order may be expressed in hours or minutes. By controlling the flow rate, you control the speed with which medication is administered.

Rule 11-5

The flow rate can be expressed as $F = \dfrac{V}{T}$, where

F = flow rate

V = volume of fluid to infuse

T = time period of the infusion

EXAMPLE 1 Find the flow rate in mL/h.

Ordered: *1000 mL D5W to infuse over 8 h*

The volume to infuse (V) is 1000 mL. The time period of the infusion (T) is 8 hours.

$$F = \frac{V}{T} = \frac{1000 \text{ mL}}{8 \text{ h}} = \frac{\overset{125}{\cancel{1000}} \text{ mL}}{\underset{1}{\cancel{8}} \text{ h}} = \frac{125 \text{ mL}}{1 \text{ h}}$$

The flow rate is 125 mL/h.

Flow Rates for Electronic Regulation

Most electronic devices that regulate the flow of IV infusions measure the flow in milliliters per hour, or mL/h. Sometimes an order will call for an infusion to last less than an hour. However, you still calculate an hourly flow rate.

Rule 11-6

To find the flow rate F for electronic devices that measure an infusion in milliliters per hour, find $\dfrac{V}{T}$

$$\frac{\text{volume to infuse}}{\text{time period of infusion}} = \frac{V}{T}$$

where T = 1 hour and V is rounded to the nearest mL.

EXAMPLE 1 Find the flow rate.

Ordered: *500 mL 5%D 0.45%S over 3 hours by infusion pump*

The volume to infuse is 500 mL and the time period of infusion is 3 h.

$$\frac{\text{volume to infuse}}{\text{time period of infusion}} = \frac{500 \text{ mL}}{3 \text{ h}} = \frac{166.7 \text{ mL}}{1 \text{ h}}$$

Rounding to the nearest mL, the flow rate is 167 mL/h. You could also solve this problem using a fraction proportion.

$$\frac{500 \text{ mL}}{3 \text{ h}} = \frac{V}{1 \text{ h}}$$

$$500 \text{ mL} \times 1 \text{ h} = 3 \text{ h} \times V$$

$$\frac{500 \text{ mL}}{3} = V$$

$$166.67 \text{ mL} = V$$

EXAMPLE 2 Find the flow rate.

Ordered: *500 mg ampicillin in 100 mL NS to infuse over 30 min*

The volume to infuse is 100 mL. The time period of the infusion is 30 minutes. First convert 30 min to 0.5 h.

$$\frac{\text{volume to infuse}}{\text{time period of infusion}} = \frac{100 \text{ mL}}{0.5 \text{ h}} = \frac{200 \text{ mL}}{1 \text{ h}}$$

The flow rate is 200 mL/h.

Instead of converting minutes to hours and then calculating the flow rate, you can combine these steps by using dimensional analysis. You would multiply $\frac{\text{volume to infuse}}{\text{time period of infusion}}$ by a conversion factor. Thus,

$$\frac{100 \text{ mL}}{30 \text{ min}} \times \frac{60 \text{ min}}{1 \text{ h}} = \frac{100 \text{ mL}}{{}_{1}\cancel{30 \text{ min}}} \times \frac{\overset{2}{\cancel{60 \text{ min}}}}{1 \text{ h}} = \frac{200 \text{ mL}}{1 \text{ h}}$$

Once you calculate the flow rate, you set the infusion device to regulate the IV flow. For electronic regulators, enter the calculated flow rate according to the manufacturer's instructions. Most pumps or controllers also require you to enter the total volume of solution to be infused.

Flow Rates for Manual Regulation

For a manually regulated IV, the flow rate is expressed as the quantity of drops per minute, or gtt/min. Once you know the desired flow rate, you adjust the roller or screw clamp so that the desired number of drops fall per minute. The calibration of the tubing is an important factor. IV tubing packages are labeled with the drop factor: the number of drops per milliliter, or gtt/mL of IV solution (Figures 11-13 and 11-14). Macrodrip tubing has larger drops and one of three drop factors: 10 gtt/mL, 15 gtt/mL, or 20 gtt/mL. Microdrip tubing has smaller drops; its drop factor is always 60 gtt/mL. When microdrip tubing is used, the drops per minute equals milliliters per hour, or mL/h (Figure 11-15).

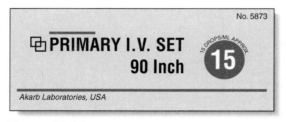

Figure 11-13

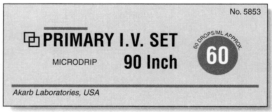

Figure 11-14

Figure 11-15

Macrodrop and microdrop calibration.

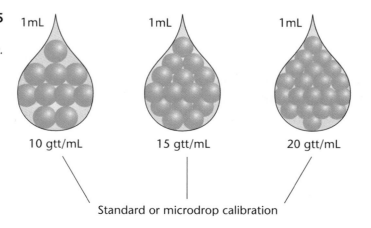

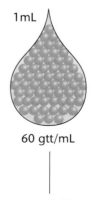

Rule 11-7

To find the flow rate F for manually regulated IVs, when the time duration of infusion is listed in minutes, calculate

$$C \times \frac{\text{volume to infuse}}{\text{time period of infusion}} = F$$

where C = calibration of the tubing in gtt/mL. The volume (V) of the flow rate is rounded to the nearest drop; the time (T) is 1 minute.

EXAMPLE 1 Calculate the flow rate if you are using macrodrip tubing calibrated to 10 gtt/mL.

Ordered: *500 mg ampicillin in 100 mL NS to infuse over 30 min*

The tubing calibration C is $\frac{10 \text{ gtt}}{1 \text{ mL}}$. The volume to infuse is 100 mL. The time period of the infusion is 30 minutes.

$$\frac{10 \text{ gtt}}{1 \text{ mL}} \times \frac{100 \text{ mL}}{30 \text{ min}} = F$$

$$\frac{^1\cancel{10} \text{ gtt}}{1 \cancel{\text{mL}}} \times \frac{100 \cancel{\text{mL}}}{_3\cancel{30} \text{ min}} = 1 \text{ gtt} \times \frac{100}{3 \text{ min}} = \frac{100 \text{ gtt}}{3 \text{ min}} = \frac{33.3 \text{ gtt}}{1 \text{ min}}$$

Rounding to the nearest drop, the flow rate F is 33 gtt/min.

When the infusion time is listed in hours, include the conversion factor $\frac{1 \text{ h}}{60 \text{ min}}$ in your calculation to cancel the necessary units of measurement. Another approach would be to convert the infusion time from hours to minutes, then calculate according to Rule 11-7.

Rule 11-8

To find the flow rate F for manually regulated IVs, when the time duration of infusion is listed in hours, calculate

$$C \times \frac{\text{volume to infuse}}{\text{time period of infusion}} \times \frac{1 \text{ h}}{60 \text{ min}} = F$$

where C = calibration of the tubing in gtt/mL. The volume (V) of the flow rate is rounded to the nearest drop; the time (T) is 1 minute.

EXAMPLE 1 Calculate the flow rate if you are using macrodrip tubing calibrated to 15 gtt/mL.

Ordered: *250 mL NS to infuse over 3 h*

The tubing calibration C is $\frac{15 \text{ gtt}}{1 \text{ mL}}$. The volume to infuse is 250 mL. The time period of the infusion is 3 hours.

$$\frac{15 \text{ gtt}}{1 \text{ mL}} \times \frac{250 \text{ mL}}{3 \text{ h}} \times \frac{1 \text{ h}}{60 \text{ min}} = F$$

$$\frac{^5\cancel{15} \text{ gtt}}{1 \cancel{\text{mL}}} \times \frac{^{25}\cancel{250} \cancel{\text{mL}}}{3 \cancel{\text{h}}} \times \frac{1 \cancel{\text{h}}}{_6\cancel{60} \text{ min}} =$$

$$5 \text{ gtt} \times 25 \times \frac{1}{6 \text{ min}} = \frac{125 \text{ gtt}}{6 \text{ min}} = \frac{20.8 \text{ gtt}}{1 \text{ min}}$$

Rounding to the nearest drop, the flow rate is 21 gtt/min.

$\overline{\text{EXAMPLE 2}}$ Calculate the flow rate for the previous order if the tubing has a drop factor of 20 gtt/mL.

Substituting $C = \dfrac{20 \text{ gtt}}{1 \text{ mL}}$,

$$\frac{20 \text{ gtt}}{1 \text{ mL}} \times \frac{250 \text{ mL}}{3 \text{ h}} \times \frac{1 \text{ h}}{60 \text{ min}} = F$$

$$\frac{{}^{1}\!\!\cancel{20} \text{ gtt}}{1 \cancel{mL}} \times \frac{250 \cancel{mL}}{3 \cancel{h}} \times \frac{1 \cancel{h}}{{}_{3}\!\cancel{60} \text{ min}} =$$

$$1 \text{ gtt} \times \frac{250}{3} \times \frac{1}{3 \text{ min}} = \frac{250 \text{ gtt}}{9 \text{ min}} = \frac{27.8 \text{ gtt}}{1 \text{ min}}$$

Rounding to the nearest drop, the flow rate is 28 gtt/min.

For manually regulated IVs, count the number of drops that fall into the drip chamber. Then adjust the clamp for the desired flow rate. Rather than count drops for a full minute, you may divide the volume to infuse by 4 and count drops for 15 seconds. For example, if the desired flow rate is 24 gtt/min, you may set the clamp for 6 gtt per 15 seconds.

Adjusting the Flow Rate

Because any device can malfunction, you should check at least once every hour that the IV is infusing at the desired flow rate. If you find that the infusion is behind or ahead of schedule, you may need to adjust the rate. Hospital policy will dictate whether you may adjust the IV flow rate or whether you should notify the patient's physician.

Rule 11-9

To adjust the flow rate, recalculate the infusion using the remaining volume and the remaining time.

$\overline{\text{EXAMPLE 1}}$ The original order reads: *1500 mL NS over 12 hours.* Using 20 gtt/mL tubing, you manually set the IV to deliver 42 gtt/min. After three hours, you observe that 1200 mL of fluid remains in the IV bag. According to hospital policy, you can reset the flow rate, provided that the change does not exceed 25%. What adjustment should you make?

Calculate how much fluid should have been administered to the patient. You expect the IV to deliver 42 gtt/min. Therefore after three hours, the patient should have received

$$3 \text{ h} \times \frac{60 \text{ min}}{1 \text{ h}} \times \frac{42 \text{ gtt}}{1 \text{ min}} \times \frac{1 \text{ mL}}{20 \text{ gtt}} = \text{number of mL infused}$$

$$3 \cancel{h} \times \frac{{}^{3}\!\cancel{60} \text{ min}}{1 \cancel{h}} \times \frac{42 \cancel{gtt}}{1 \cancel{min}} \times \frac{1 \text{ mL}}{{}_{1}\!\cancel{20} \text{ gtt}} =$$

$$3 \times 3 \times 42 \times 1 \text{ mL} = 378 \text{ mL}$$

(Notice that $\dfrac{1 \text{ mL}}{20 \text{ gtt}}$ was used rather than $\dfrac{20 \text{ gtt}}{1 \text{ mL}}$ so that units would cancel.) The patient should have received 378 mL of fluid. Therefore, 1122 mL should remain in the IV bag, not 1200 mL. The patient received less fluid than was ordered.

To adjust the flow rate, recalculate using the remaining volume (1200 mL), the remaining time (9 hours), and the existing drop factor (20 gtt/mL). From Rule 11-8,

$$\frac{20 \text{ gtt}}{1 \text{ mL}} \times \frac{1200 \text{ mL}}{9 \text{h}} \times \frac{1 \text{ h}}{60 \text{ min}} = \text{new flow rate}$$

$$\frac{^{1}\cancel{20} \text{ gtt}}{1 \text{ m\cancel{L}}} \times \frac{^{400}\cancel{1200} \text{ m\cancel{L}}}{_{3}\cancel{9} \text{ h}} \times \frac{1 \cancel{\text{h}}}{_{3}\cancel{60} \text{ min}} =$$

$$1 \text{ gtt} \times \frac{400}{3} \times \frac{1}{3 \text{ min}} = \frac{400 \text{ gtt}}{9 \text{ min}} = \frac{44.4 \text{ gtt}}{1 \text{ min}}$$

The adjusted flow rate is 44 gtt/min. However, before you reset the flow rate, determine if it is within 25% of the original flow rate of 42 gtt/min. Because 25% × 42 = 10.5, any flow rate that differs from 42 gtt/min by less than 10.5 gtt/min is within 25% of the original flow rate.

Because 44 − 42 = 2, the flow rate of 44 gtt/min is acceptable.

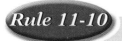

Rule 11-10

When adjusting the flow rate,

1. Do not increase or decrease the flow rate by more than 25% of the original rate.
2. Always check the guidelines at your facility before adjusting the flow rate.
3. Spread the adjustment over the entire remaining time.

CRITICAL THINKING ON THE JOB

Adjusting the Flow Rate

Earlier in the day, Pat set up an IV based on the following physician's order: *750 mL D5N5 to infuse over 8 hours.* Pat calculated that the patient should receive 94 mL of fluid per hour, with a flow rate of 16 gtt/min.

After four hours (half the time ordered for the infusion), Pat observed that 450 mL remained in the IV bag. Only half the fluid, or 375 mL should have remained in the bag. The patient had received 75 mL less fluid than expected. Pat decided to reset the flow rate for the next hour so that the patient would receive the original 94 mL per hour plus the 75 mL that should have already been administered, a total of 169 mL. After the next hour, Pat planned to reset the IV to the original flow rate of 16 gtt/min. Pat calculated the new flow rate,

$$\frac{10 \text{ gtt}}{1 \text{ mL}} \times \frac{169 \text{ mL}}{1 \text{ h}} \times \frac{1 \text{ h}}{60 \text{ min}} =$$

$$\frac{28.17 \text{ gtt}}{1 \text{ min}} =$$

28 gtt/min

Thus, Pat adjusted the flow rate to 28 gtt/min.

Think Before You Act

Pat's error could have serious consequences for the patient by providing far too much solution in a limited time period. The new flow rate of 28 gtt/min is a 75% increase over the original flow rate of 16 gtt/min, well beyond safety guidelines. Instead of making up the entire schedule in one hour, Pat should have adjusted the remainder of the entire schedule. The IV bag still had 450 mL of fluid with 4 hours of infusion time remaining. The calculation should be

$$\frac{10 \text{ gtt}}{1 \text{ mL}} \times \frac{450 \text{ mL}}{4 \text{ h}} \times \frac{1 \text{ h}}{60 \text{ min}} =$$

$$\frac{18.75 \text{ gtt}}{1 \text{ min}} =$$

19 gtt/min

The increase from 16 gtt/min to 19 gtt/min is a 19% increase, within the acceptable amount of change.

CALCULATING FLOW RATES

In Exercises 1–4, find the flow rate in mL/h.

1. Ordered: *1000 mL LR over 6 h*

2. Ordered: *300 mL NS over 2 h*

3. Ordered: *3000 mL 0.45% NS q24h*

4. Ordered: *40 mEq KCl in 100 mL NS over 45 min*

In Exercises 5–10, calculate the flow rate for IVs using electronic devices.

5. Ordered: *1500 mL RL over 12 h, using an infusion pump*

6. Ordered: *1000 mL NS over 12 h, using an infusion pump*

7. Ordered: *750 mL NS over 8 h, using an electronic controller set in mL/h*

8. Ordered: *20 mEq KCl in 50 mL NS over 30 min, using an electronic rate controller set in mL/h*

9. Ordered: *1800 mL 0.45% S per day by infusion pump*

10. Ordered: *250 mL D5W over 3 h by infusion pump*

In Exercises 11–20, calculate the flow rate for manually regulated IVs.

11. Ordered: *1000 mL NS over 24 h, tubing is 20 gtt/mL*

12. Ordered: *400 mL RL over 8 h, tubing is 10 gtt/mL*

13. Ordered: *1500 mL 0.45% S over 12 h, tubing is 15 gtt/mL*

14. Ordered: *250 mL D5W over 3 h, tubing is 10 gtt/mL*

15. Ordered: *40 mEq KCl in 100 mL NS over 40 min, tubing is 20 gtt/mL*

16. Ordered: *500 mL NS over 8 h, tubing is 15 gtt/mL*

17. Ordered: *3000 mL NS over 24 h,* Refer to Label A.

18. Ordered: *50 mL penicillin IV over 1 h,* Refer to Label B.

19. Ordered: *750 mL 5%D NS over 5 h,* Refer to Label C.

20. Ordered: *100 mL gentamicin over 30 min,* Refer to Label D.

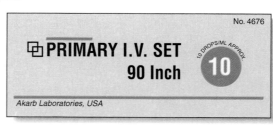

A

B

C

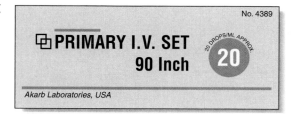

No. 4389

⊞ **PRIMARY I.V. SET**
90 Inch **20** 20 DROPS/ML APPROX.

Akarb Laboratories, USA

D

No. 5873

⊞ **PRIMARY I.V. SET**
90 Inch **15** 15 DROPS/ML APPROX.

Akarb Laboratories, USA

In Exercises 21–22, calculate the flow rate in gtt/min.

21. Ordered: *1000 mL D5W over 9 h, using an electronic controller set in gtt/min, tubing calibration is 15 gtt/mL*

22. Ordered: *750 mL RL over 8 h by electronic rate controller set in gtt/min, tubing calibration is 15 gtt/mL*

In Exercises 23–24, calculate the original flow rate. Then determine if an adjustment is necessary and calculate the adjusted flow rate.

23. Ordered: *375 mL RL over 3 h* (10 gtt/mL tubing)
After one hour, 175 mL has infused.

24. Ordered: *1000 mL NS over 10 h* (20 gtt/mL tubing)
With five hours remaining, 550 mL of NS remains in the IV bag.

To check your answers, see page 362.

Infusion Time and Volume

An order may call for a certain amount of fluid to infuse at a specific rate, without specifying the duration. You will need to calculate the duration so that you can monitor the IV properly. For example, the order may be a standing order that will continue until further notice. When you set up the IV, you will need to mark the bag so that others will know when it needs replacing. In other cases, you may know the duration and the flow rate, and will need to calculate the volume.

Infusion Time

If you know the desired flow rate and the total amount of fluid to be administered, then you can use a fraction proportion, a ratio proportion, or dimensional analysis to find the total infusion time. All methods lead to the same result.

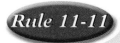

Rule 11-11

Ways to calculate the total infusion time for an IV, where $\frac{V}{T}$ is the flow rate, include

1. the fraction proportion method

$$\frac{V}{T} = \frac{\text{total volume to infuse}}{\text{total time to infuse}}$$

2. the ratio proportion method

V:T::total volume:total time

3. dimensional analysis

$$\text{total volume} \times \frac{T}{V} = \text{total time}$$

$\boxed{\text{EXAMPLE 1}}$ Find the total time to infuse.

Ordered: *1000 mL NS to infuse at a rate of 75 mL/h*

The total volume is 1000 mL. The flow rate is 75 mL/h, so that V = 75 mL and T = 1 h. Using a fraction proportion,

$$\frac{75 \text{ mL}}{1 \text{ h}} = \frac{1000 \text{ mL}}{\text{total time to infuse}}$$

75 mL × total time to infuse = 1 h × 1000 mL

total time to infuse = 13.33 h

Note that 0.33 hours does not represent 33 minutes. Instead,

0.33 h = 0.33 × 60 min = 20 min

The total time to infuse is 13 hours and 20 minutes.

$\boxed{\text{EXAMPLE 2}}$ Find the total time to infuse.

Ordered: *750 mL LR to infuse at a rate of 25 gtt/min, the tubing is 15 gtt/mL*

The total volume is 750 mL. The flow rate is 25 gtt/min, so that V = 25 gtt and T = 1 min. Using dimensional analysis,

$$750 \text{ mL} \times \frac{1 \text{ min}}{25 \text{ gtt}} = \text{total time (minutes)}$$

The tubing calibration, $\frac{15 \text{ gtt}}{1 \text{ mL}}$, provides a conversion factor that cancels *gtt* and *mL*, leaving the answer in *min*.

$$750 \text{ mL} \times \frac{15 \text{ gtt}}{1 \text{ mL}} \times \frac{1 \text{ min}}{25 \text{ gtt}} =$$

$$^{30}\cancel{750} \text{ } \cancel{mL} \times \frac{15 \text{ } \cancel{gtt}}{1 \text{ } \cancel{mL}} \times \frac{1 \text{ min}}{_1\cancel{25} \text{ } \cancel{gtt}} = 30 \times 15 \times 1 \text{ min} = 450 \text{ min}$$

In turn, 450 min = 7 h 30 min. Using dimensional analysis reduces rounding, leading to a more accurate calculation.

Infusion Volume

If you know the desired flow rate and the total time during which a fluid is to be administered, then you can calculate the total volume of fluid to administer.

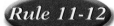
Rule 11-12

To calculate the total volume of fluid to administer, where $\frac{V}{T}$ is the flow rate, multiply

$$\frac{V}{T} \times \text{total time to infuse} = \text{total volume to infuse}$$

$\boxed{\text{EXAMPLE 1}}$ An infusion pump is set at 35 mL/h. How much 0.9% S will infuse over 5 h?

$$\frac{V}{T} = \frac{35 \text{ mL}}{1 \text{ h}} \text{ and total time to infuse is 5 h. Thus,}$$

$$\frac{35 \text{ mL}}{1 \text{ h}} \times 5 \text{ h} = \frac{35 \text{ mL}}{1 \text{ } \cancel{h}} \times 5 \text{ } \cancel{h} = 35 \text{ mL} \times 5 = 175 \text{ mL}$$

175 mL of 0.9% S will infuse over 5 h.

EXAMPLE 2 An IV is set up to infuse RL over 12 h at a rate of 25 gtt/min. The calibration of the tubing is 10 gtt/mL. How much RL will infuse?

Here, $\dfrac{V}{T} = \dfrac{25 \text{ gtt}}{1 \text{ min}}$ and total time to infuse is 12 h. Thus,

$$\frac{25 \text{ gtt}}{1 \text{ min}} \times 12 \text{ h} = \text{total volume to infuse}$$

You need a conversion factor that introduces *mL* and cancels *gtt*. Use the reciprocal of the tubing's calibration, $\dfrac{1 \text{ mL}}{10 \text{ gtt}}$. The conversion factor $\dfrac{60 \text{ min}}{1 \text{ h}}$ will cancel *min* and *h*. Thus,

$$\frac{1 \text{ mL}}{10 \text{ gtt}} \times \frac{25 \text{ gtt}}{1 \text{ min}} \times \frac{60 \text{ min}}{1 \text{ h}} \times 12 \text{ h} = \text{total volume to infuse}$$

$$\frac{1 \text{ mL}}{_1\cancel{10} \text{ gtt}} \times \frac{25 \cancel{\text{gtt}}}{1 \cancel{\text{min}}} \times \frac{^6\cancel{60} \cancel{\text{min}}}{1 \cancel{\text{h}}} \times 12 \cancel{\text{h}} =$$

$$1 \text{ mL} \times 25 \times 6 \times 12 = 1800 \text{ mL}$$

1800 mL of RL will infuse over 12 hours.

REVIEW and PRACTICE

INFUSION TIME AND VOLUME

In Exercises 1–4, find the total time to infuse.

1. Ordered: *1000 mL NS at 83 mL/h using an infusion pump*

2. Ordered: *500 mL LR at 125 gtt/min using microdrip tubing*

3. Ordered: *750 mL .45% NS at 31 gtt/min.* Refer to Label A.

4. Ordered: *1000 mL at 22 gtt/min.* Refer to Label B.

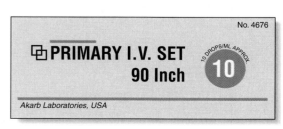

A

B

In Exercises 5–8, find when the infusion will be completed.

5. Ordered: *1500 mL D5W with 30 mEq KCl/ liter at a rate of 36 gtt/min.* You start the infusion at noon, with 15 gtt/mL tubing.

6. Ordered: *2000 mL NS via infusion pump at 98 mL/h.* You start the infusion at 1530.

7. Ordered: *750 mL RL at 31 gtt/min.* You start the IV at 1000, with 10 gtt/mL tubing.

8. Ordered: *250 mL via a microdrip set at 40 gtt/min.* You start the infusion at 2140.

In Exercises 9–12, find the total volume to administer.

9. 75 mL/h 0.45% NS for 2 h 30 min using a rate controller

10. D5RL set at 15 gtt/min for 8 h using 20 gtt/mL

11. D5W at 125 mL/h for 12 hours using an infusion pump

12. An antibiotic solution infused over 2 h at 15 gtt/min using a microdrip set

To check your answers, see page 363.

Saline and Heparin Locks

You can administer medication to a patient on a regular, though not continuous, schedule by using a saline or heparin lock. To create a lock, attach an infusion port to an already-inserted IV needle or catheter. This port allows you to inject medications directly into the vein using a syringe or to infuse IV medications intermittently. Physicians' orders will list *IV push* or *bolus* for medications that are injected into an IV line or through a saline or heparin lock.

Fluids do not flow continuously through the IV needle or catheter when a lock is used. To prevent blockage of the line, the device must be flushed two or three times a day or after administering medication. A saline lock uses saline as the irrigant. A heparin lock uses heparin, an anticoagulant that retards clot formation. Hospital policy and the device will dictate the amount and concentration of irrigant to use. Saline or heparin fills the the infusion port and IV catheter, preventing blood from entering and becoming trapped. If blood were trapped, a clot would form, blocking the catheter.

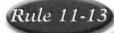

Rule 11-13

If you meet resistance when flushing a saline or heparin lock, stop the procedure immediately so that you do not force a clot into the bloodstream.

PATIENT EDUCATION

Instruct patients who are sent home with a saline or heparin lock to care for the device and administer their medications. Teach them about infiltration and phlebitis, and to contact their physician immediately should signs of either problem arise.

1. Avoid getting the injection site wet when bathing or washing hands.

2. Collect all necessary supplies before irrigating the lock or administering medication.

3. Irrigate the device at least twice a day to prevent clotting around the needle or catheter. Develop a schedule.

4. Clean the injection port with an antiseptic swab before injecting the irrigant or prescribed medication.

5. Before administering medication, flush a heparin lock with 1 to 10 mL NS to clear any residual heparin.

6. Hold the injection port steady while gently inserting the needle into the center of the port. If there is resistance, withdraw the needle and reinsert it in a different spot.

7. Once a syringe needle is inserted, pull the plunger back. Watch for blood in the chamber to confirm access to the vein. This step must be followed for every injection with the device.

8. After injecting the saline, withdraw the syringe. Inject the medication according to the physician's instructions.

9. After withdrawing the syringe, flush any residual medication from the device.

10. If heparin is used as an irrigant, inject it according to the physician's instructions. Then withdraw the syringe.

11. After completing the injections, swab the port with an antiseptic wipe. Replace the sterile cap.

Heparin Calculations

Heparin is measured in USP units (U). When intended as an irrigant, it is often packaged in vials of 10 to 100 units (see Figure 11-16). It may be administered intermittently as an IV medication to slow clot formation in a heparin lock (see Figure 11-17). When used for anticoagulant therapy, heparin may be administered safely to adults at a dosage of 20,000–40,000 U per 24 hours. Before administering heparin, verify that the dosage ordered falls within this range.

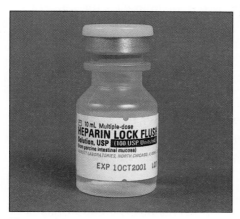

Figure 11-16

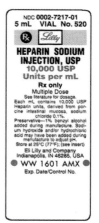

Figure 11-17

In Chapters 7 and 8, you used the formula method and dimensional analysis to calculate how many mL of solution were needed to administer a dose of heparin. Calculating the flow rate is very similar. Before, the desired dose D represented only a quantity of units. Here, the desired dose D represents a flow rate, a quantity of units per time period.

Rule 11-14

To calculate the rate at which to administer a solution containing IV heparin when an electronic device that measures an infusion in mL per hour is used, find A,

$$D \times \frac{Q}{H} = A$$

where D is the rate of the *desired dose,* Q is the *dosage unit,* H is the *dose on hand,* and A is the rate of the *amount to administer.*

EXAMPLE 1 Find the hourly rate to administer IV heparin.

Ordered: *1000 U/h IV heparin using an infusion pump*

On hand: 50,000 U heparin in 1000 mL D5W

The rate of the desired dose D is $\dfrac{1000\ U}{1\ h}$. The dosage unit Q is 1000 mL. The dose on hand H is 50,000 Units of heparin.

$$D \times \frac{Q}{H} = A$$

$$\frac{1000\ U}{1\ h} \times \frac{1000\ mL}{50,000\ U} = \frac{^1\cancel{1000}\ \cancel{U}}{1\ h} \times \frac{^{20}\cancel{1000}\ mL}{_{1}{}_{50}\cancel{50,000}\ \cancel{U}} = \frac{20\ mL}{1\ h}$$

In this example, to administer 1000 Units of IV heparin per hour, you would administer the solution at the rate of 20 mL/h.

When you manually regulate the IV, you use a similar calculation. However, you need to include conversion factors so that the flow rate will be expressed in gtt/min.

Rule 11-15

To calculate the rate to administer a solution containing IV heparin for manually regulated IVs,

1. if the duration of infusion is listed in hours, find A,

$$C \times D \times \frac{Q}{H} \times \frac{1\ h}{60\ min} = A$$

where C is the calibration of the tubing in gtt/min, D is the rate of the *desired dose*, Q is the *dosage unit*, H is the *dose on hand*, and A is the rate of the *amount to administer*.

2. if the duration of infusion is listed in minutes, find A,

$$C \times D \times \frac{Q}{H} = A$$

EXAMPLE 1   Find the rate to administer IV heparin.

Ordered: *1000 U/h IV heparin using 15 gtt/mL macrodrip tubing*

On hand: 50,000 U heparin in 1000 mL D5W

The tubing calibration C is 15 gtt/mL; the rate of the *desired dose* D is $\frac{1000\ U}{1\ h}$; the *dosage unit* Q is 1000 mL; and the *dose on hand* H is 50,000 Units of heparin.

$$C \times D \times \frac{Q}{H} \times \frac{1\ h}{60\ min} = A$$

$$\frac{15\ gtt}{1\ mL} \times \frac{1000\ U}{1\ h} \times \frac{1000\ mL}{50,000\ U} \times \frac{1\ h}{60\ min} =$$

$$\frac{^1\cancel{15}\ gtt}{\cancel{mL}} \times \frac{^{5}\cancel{20}\cancel{1000}\ \cancel{U}}{1\ \cancel{h}} \times \frac{^1\cancel{1000}\ \cancel{mL}}{_{150}\cancel{50,000}\ \cancel{U}} \times \frac{1\ \cancel{h}}{_{1}\cancel{460}\ min} =$$

$$1\ gtt \times 5 \times 1 \times \frac{1}{1\ min} = \frac{5\ gtt}{1\ min}$$

This example is the same as the previous one except you are using macrodrip tubing rather than an infusion pump. In this case, you would administer the solution at the rate of 5 gtt/min in order to administer 1000 U of heparin per hour.

Rule 11-16

To calculate the hourly dose, multiply the total dosage by the hourly flow rate, so that

$$\frac{H}{Q} \times \frac{V}{T} = D$$

where H is the *dose on hand* (the total *amount to administer*), Q is the *dosage unit* for the total amount, V is the volume of the dose, T is the (time) duration of the dose, and D is the rate of the *desired dose*.

EXAMPLE 1   What is the hourly dose?

Ordered: *30,000 U of IV heparin in 500 mL D5W to infuse at 25 mL/h*

The total *amount to administer* H is 30,000 U, the *dosage unit* Q is 500 mL, the volume of the dose V is 25 mL, the duration of the dose T is 1 h.

$$\frac{30,000\ U}{500\ mL} \times \frac{25\ mL}{1\ h} = D$$

$$\frac{^{60}30{,}000 \text{ U}}{_{1}\cancel{500} \text{ mL}} \times \frac{25 \cancel{\text{ mL}}}{1 \text{ h}} = 60 \text{ U} \times \frac{25}{1 \text{ h}} = \frac{1500 \text{ U}}{1 \text{ h}}$$

Before you administer heparin at a rate of 1500 U/h, confirm if this is a safe rate. Multiplying by 24 h/day,

$$\frac{1500 \text{ U}}{1 \text{ h}} \times \frac{24 \text{ h}}{1 \text{ day}} = \frac{36{,}000 \text{ U}}{1 \text{ day}}$$

36,000 U/day falls within the safe daily range for IV heparin.

EXAMPLE 2   What is the hourly dose?

Ordered: *15,000 U of IV heparin in 1500 mL D5W to infuse at 30 gtt/min*

On hand: macrodrip tubing calibrated to 15 gtt/mL

The total *amount to administer* H is 15,000 U, the *dosage unit* Q is 1500 mL, the volume of the dose V is 30 gtt, the duration of the dose T is 1 min.

$$\frac{15{,}000 \text{ U}}{1500 \text{ mL}} \times \frac{30 \text{ gtt}}{1 \text{ min}} = D$$

Use the tubing calibration $\frac{1 \text{ mL}}{15 \text{ gtt}}$ to cancel *gtt* and *mL*. Also use $\frac{60 \text{ min}}{1 \text{ h}}$ so that your answer will measure U/h.

$$\frac{15{,}000 \text{ U}}{1500 \text{ mL}} \times \frac{30 \text{ gtt}}{1 \text{ min}} \times \frac{1 \text{ mL}}{15 \text{ gtt}} \times \frac{60 \text{ min}}{1 \text{ hr}} =$$

$$\frac{^{10}15{,}000 \text{ U}}{_{1}\cancel{1500} \cancel{\text{ mL}}} \times \frac{^{2}30 \cancel{\text{ gtt}}}{1 \cancel{\text{ min}}} \times \frac{1 \cancel{\text{ mL}}}{_{1}\cancel{15} \cancel{\text{ gtt}}} \times \frac{60 \cancel{\text{ min}}}{1 \text{ h}} =$$

$$10 \text{ U} \times 2 \times 1 \times \frac{60}{1 \text{ h}} = \frac{1200 \text{ U}}{1 \text{ h}}$$

As before, confirm if the rate of 1200 U/h is a safe rate.

$$\frac{1200 \text{ U}}{1 \text{ h}} \times \frac{24 \text{ h}}{1 \text{ day}} = \frac{28{,}800 \text{ U}}{1 \text{ day}}$$

28,800 U/day falls within the safe daily range for IV heparin.

REVIEW and PRACTICE

HEPARIN CALCULATIONS

In Exercises 1–4, find the flow rate.

1. Ordered: *Heparin 1000 U/h IV using an infusion pump*
   On hand: 20,000 U in 1500 mL 5% DW

2. Ordered: *Heparin 1000 U/h IV*
   On hand: 20,000 U in 500 mL D5W, microdrip tubing

3. Ordered: *Heparin 850 U/h IV*
   On hand: 40,000 U in 1500 mL 5% DW, 15 gtt/mL tubing

4. Ordered: *Heparin 1500 U/h IV*
   On hand: 30,000 U in 500 mL 5% D 0.45%NS, 10 gtt/mL tubing

In Exercises 5–8, find the hourly dosage for the heparin orders. Then determine whether the dosage is safe.

5. An IV with 60,000 U in 1500 mL 5% DW infusing at 25 mL/h

6. An IV set up delivering 45 gtt/min from 25,000 U in 2500 mL D5NS using microdrip tubing

7. 40,000 U in 1800 mL 5% DW delivered at 25 gtt/min using 10 gtt/mL tubing

8. 30,000 U in 1500 mL 5% D 0.45%NS delivered at 20 gtt/min using 10 gtt/mL tubing

To check your answers, see page 363.

Critical Care IV

By necessity, IV medications used in critical care settings are fast-acting and potent. Because they enter the bloodstream directly, only a small amount is required to have an effect. IV medications are given to alter or maintain life-sustaining functions such as heart rate, cardiac output, blood pressure, or respiration. Because of their narrow margin of safety, you must have the right medication for the right patient in the correct concentration. Be equally certain that you are administering the proper dosage at the proper rate.

Critical care drugs are administered by IV push or bolus. However, they can be delivered via continuous IV. Using a volume-controlled burette, electronic infusion device, or microdrip tubing will improve the precision of the dosage.

Per Minute Orders

Earlier you learned to calculate flow rates for heparin, using Units to measure the volume to administer. Use the same steps to calculate critical care medications. In most cases, measure the *amount to administer* in either *mg* or *mcg*. Many IV medication orders express an amount of medication to be delivered per minute. You need to convert this rate to mL/h. For manually regulated IVs, you will convert mL/h to gtt/min.

Rule 11-17

To convert a per minute order to an hourly flow rate, convert the order to mL/min, then to mL/h. To combine these steps, find

$$D \times \frac{Q}{H} \times \frac{60 \text{ min}}{1 \text{ h}} = A$$

where D is the rate of the *desired dose*, Q is the *dosage unit*, H is the *dose on hand*, and A is the flow rate of the *amount to administer.*

EXAMPLE 1 Find the hourly flow rate.

Ordered: *5000 mg Esmolol in 500 mL D5W at 8 mg/min via infusion pump*

The rate of the *desired dose* is 8 mg/min; the *dosage unit* Q is 500 mL, and the *dose on hand* H is 5000 mg.

$$\frac{8 \text{ mg}}{\text{min}} \times \frac{500 \text{ mL}}{5000 \text{ mg}} \times \frac{60 \text{ min}}{1 \text{ h}} = A$$

$$\frac{8 \cancel{\text{ mg}}}{\cancel{\text{min}}} \times \frac{\overset{1}{\cancel{500}} \text{ mL}}{\underset{1}{\cancel{10}} \cancel{5000} \cancel{\text{ mg}}} \times \frac{\overset{6}{\cancel{60}} \cancel{\text{ min}}}{1 \text{ h}}$$

$$8 \times 1 \text{ mL} \times \frac{6}{1 \text{ h}} = \frac{48 \text{ mL}}{1 \text{ h}}$$

The hourly flow rate is 48 mL/h.

EXAMPLE 2 Find the flow rate in gtt/min for the order from Example 1 if the equipment to be used is macrodrip tubing at 20 gtt/mL.

Here, flow rate will be expressed in gtt/min. Thus, you do not need to use $\frac{60 \text{ min}}{1 \text{ h}}$ to convert the rate to hours. However, use the conversion factor $\frac{20 \text{ gtt}}{1 \text{ mL}}$ to convert the rate to drops.

$$\frac{8 \text{ mg}}{\text{min}} \times \frac{500 \text{ mL}}{5000 \text{ mg}} \times \frac{20 \text{ gtt}}{1 \text{ mL}} = A$$

$$\frac{8 \text{ mg}}{\text{min}} \times \frac{^{1}500 \text{ mL}}{_{1}{^{10}}5000 \text{ mg}} \times \frac{^{2}20 \text{ gtt}}{1 \text{ mL}} =$$

$$\frac{8}{\text{min}} \times 1 \times 2 \text{ gtt} = \frac{16 \text{ gtt}}{\text{min}}$$

Orders Based on Body Weight

Many medication orders, especially pediatric and geriatric orders, are based on body weight. Body weight calculations are relevant to IV medications and many other parenteral and oral medications. Chapter 12 discusses these calculations further.

An order based on body weight will often state an amount of medication per weight of the patient per unit of time. For example, a recommended daily dosage of a medication may be 5 mg/kg/day. If the patient weighs 50 kg, then you can use a proportion to calculate the daily dosage.

$$\frac{5 \text{ mg}}{1 \text{ kg}} = \frac{? \text{ mg}}{50 \text{ kg}}$$
$$5 \text{ mg} \times 50 \text{ kg} = 1 \text{ kg} \times ? \text{ mg}$$
$$250 = ?$$

The daily dose in this case is 250 mg of medication.

If you know the patient's weight in pounds, then convert the weight to *kg*. (Recall from Chapter 3 that 1 kg = 2.2 lb.) The recommended dosage may use a different time period. For example, you may need an hourly flow rate, but the order refers to a daily dosage. You would convert from days to hours. If the order lists an hourly flow rate, the recommended dosage is a daily amount, and you are using microdrip tubing at 60 gtt/mL, first convert the dosage to hours and then to minutes.

Most drug orders already factor in the patient's body weight; therefore, in most cases you will not have to perform this calculation. However, you have already learned the techniques needed to factor in a patient's weight when calculating the amount to administer.

EXAMPLE 1 Find the flow rate for an adult who weighs 187 lb.

Ordered: *Zofran 0.15 mg/kg IV over 15 min, started 30 min prior to chemo; repeat x 2 at 4h & 8h*

On hand: Refer to the label below. Use macrodrip tubing calibrated for 20 gtt/mL. The injection should be diluted with 50 mL of 5% DW.

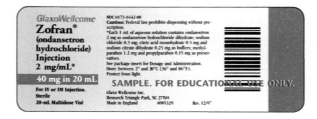

First convert the patient's weight to kg.

$$\frac{2.2 \text{ lb}}{1 \text{ kg}} = \frac{187 \text{ lb}}{? \text{ kg}}$$

2.2 lb × ? kg = 1 kg × 187 lb

? = 85

The patient weighs 85 kg. Next, determine how many mg of Zofran have been ordered.

$$\frac{0.15 \text{ mg}}{1 \text{ kg}} = \frac{? \text{ mg}}{85 \text{ kg}}$$

0.15 mg × 85 kg = 1 kg × ? mg

12.75 = ?

You want to administer 12.8 mg of Zofran over 15 minutes. Now calculate the amount of mL to administer. The vial contains 40 mg/20 mL and has been diluted in 50 mL of 5% DW. Thus, the solution now has a dosage strength of 40 mg/70 mL.

$$\frac{12.8 \text{ mg}}{? \text{ mL}} = \frac{40 \text{ mg}}{70 \text{ mL}}$$

12.8 mg × 70 ml = ? mL × 40 mg

22.4 = ?

You want to administer 22.4 mL of Zofran over 15 minutes. The tubing is calibrated for 20 gtt/mL. Therefore,

$$C \times \frac{\text{volume to infuse}}{\text{time to infuse}} = \frac{V}{T}$$

$$\frac{20 \text{ gtt}}{1 \text{ mL}} \times \frac{22.4 \text{ mL}}{15 \text{ min}} =$$

$$\frac{\overset{4}{\cancel{20}} \text{ gtt}}{1 \cancel{mL}} \times \frac{22.4 \cancel{mL}}{\underset{3}{\cancel{15}} \text{ min}} = 29.9 \text{ gtt/min}$$

Here, the flow rate for administering the Zofran is 30 gtt/min.

Titrated Medications

Some critical care medications are administered at varying rates, depending on their effect on bodily functions such as heart rate and blood pressure. For example, one effect of a medication may be to raise the patient's heart rate. If the heart rate rises past a certain range, then the amount of the medication must be lowered. The rates of such titrated (or regulated) medications have an upper and lower range. You must carefully monitor and adjust the rate of these medications.

When administering titrated medications, calculate flow rates for the lowest and highest dosages. Frequently you start administering at the lower end and increase incrementally over time until the desired effect, such as a particular heart rate, is achieved. When medications are titrated for a certain effect, you must calculate the total amount the patient has received. Start by measuring the total mL of infused solution. Infusion pumps have indicators that can measure the total mL of solution.

Rule 11-18

If you know the total amount of medication in the total volume of solution as well as the volume of solution that the patient has received, then you can use a proportion to calculate the amount of medication the patient has received (the dose).

$$\frac{\text{total amount of medication}}{\text{total volume of solution}} = \frac{\text{amount of medication received}}{\text{volume of solution received}}$$

EXAMPLE 1 ▷ A pregnant patient has been given increasing rates of Pitocin to induce labor. Since her arrival at the hospital, she has received 50 mL of a solution of Pitocin that contains 20 units in 1000 mL LR. How much Pitocin has she received?

The total amount of medication is 20 units, the total volume of solution is 1000 mL, and the volume of solution received is 50 mL.

$$\frac{20 \text{ U}}{1000 \text{ mL}} = \frac{? \text{ U}}{50 \text{ mL}}$$

20 U × 50 mL = 1000 mL × ?

1000 = 1000 × ?

1 = ?

The patient has received 1 unit of Pitocin.

REVIEW and PRACTICE

CRITICAL CARE IV

In Exercises 1–4, find the flow rates appropriate to the IV equipment used. Round per minute rates to the nearest drop.

1. Ordered: *1.5 g Unasyn in 50 mL 5%DW infusing at 0.05 g/min*
   a. infusion pump   **b.** macrodrip tubing at 20 gtt/mL

2. Ordered: *250 mg dobutamine HCl in 50 mL LR infusing at 1.5 mg/min*
   a. syringe pump   **b.** microdrip tubing

3. Ordered: *2000 mg lidocaine in 500 mL NS infusing at 2 mg/min*
   a. infusion pump   **b.** macrodrip tubing at 10 gtt/mL

4. Ordered: *3000 mg lidocaine in 750 mL D5W infusing at 3 mg/min*
   a. infusion pump   **b.** macrodrip tubing at 15 gtt/mL

In Exercises 5–8, find the appropriate flow rate.

5. Ordered: *Garamycin 3 mg/kg/day IVPB q8h in 30 mL D5W over 30 min*
   On hand: Garamycin Injectable 2-mL vial with 40 mg/mL. The patient weighs 44 lb. Use microdrip tubing. The injection should be diluted with 28 mL of 5% DW.

6. Ordered: *Cytoxan 5 mg/kg IV b.i.w. in 100 mL LR over 1 hour*
   On hand: Cytoxan 500-mg vial which should be dissolved in 25 mL of sterile water. The patient weighs 126 lb. Use macrodrip tubing, 15 gtt/mL. Dilute the dissolved Cytoxan in 100 mL of LR.

7. Ordered: *Retrovir 5 mg/kg/day IV q4h in 120 mL D5W over 1 hour*
   On hand: Retrovir IV, 20-mL vial with 10 mg/mL. The patient weighs 135 lb. Use macrodrip tubing, 10 gtt/mL. Dilute the desired dose in 120 mL of D5W.

8. Ordered: *Mezlin 250 mg/kg/day IV q6h in 80 mL NS over 1 hour*
   On hand: Mezlin 20 g vial which should be reconstituted with 10 mL of sterile water for each g. The patient weighs 152 lb. Use macrodrip tubing, 15 gtt/mL. Dilute the desired dose in 80 mL NS.

In Exercises 9–12, find the amount of medication that has already been administered to the patient.

9. Ordered: *Lidocaine 2 g in 1000 mL D5W*
   The patient has received 400 mL.

10. Ordered: *Remicade 300 mg in 250 mL NaCl*
    The patient has received 150 mL.

11. Ordered: *Dobutrex 500 mg in 500 mL D5W*
    The patient has received 120 mL.

12. Ordered: *Gentamicin 80 mg in 150 mL D5W*
    The patient has received 105 mL.

To check your answers, see page 363.

CHAPTER *11* REVIEW

CHECK UP

In Exercises 1–6, calculate the flow rate for orders to be administered by an infusion pump.

1. *3000 mL D5W q24h*

2. *500 mL LR q8h*

3. *1200 mL 0.45% NS q12h*

4. *250 mL NS q4h*

5. *1 g Claforan in 100 mL D5W over 90 min*

6. *500 mg ampicillin in 50 mL D5W over 30 min*

In Exercises 7–12, find the flow rate for the orders, rounded to the nearest drop.

7. *2200 mL RL q24h* (15 gtt/mL tubing)

8. *300 mL NS q8h* (10 gtt/mL tubing)

9. *1000 mL D5W q6h* (15 gtt/mL tubing)

10. *1800 mL D5/$\frac{1}{2}$ NS q12h* (20 gtt/mL tubing)

11. *1500 mL $\frac{1}{3}$ NS q8h* (10 gtt/mL tubing)

12. *300 mL D5/Ringer's q6h* (microdrip tubing)

In Exercises 13–14, calculate the original flow rate. Then determine if an adjustment is necessary and calculate the adjusted flow rate. Determine if the rate can be adjusted safely.

13. Ordered: *1000 mL RL over 8 h* (15 gtt/mL tubing)
    After 2 hours, 125 mL has infused.

14. Ordered: *2500 mL NS over 24 h* (10 gtt/mL tubing)
    After 3 hours, 200 mL has infused.

In Exercises 15–18, find the total time to infuse.

15. Ordered: *1000 mL D5/0.45% NS at 125 mL/h via infusion pump*

16. Ordered: *800 mL $\frac{1}{4}$ NS at 50 gtt/min* (15 gtt/mL tubing)

17. Ordered: *600 mL LR at 7 gtt/min* (10 gtt/mL tubing)

18. Ordered: *1200 mL D5/NS at 70 gtt/min* (microdrip tubing)

In Exercises 19–22, find when the infusion will be completed.

19. 800 mL via infusion pump at 90 mL/h, starting at 0820

20. 1000 mL at 25 gtt/min (20 gtt/mL tubing), starting at 1300

21. 500 mL at 17 gtt/min (15 gtt/mL tubing), starting at 2230

22. 750 mL at 35 gtt/min (microdrip tubing), starting at 1600

In Exercises 23–26, find the total volume to administer.

23. $\frac{1}{4}$NS at 125 mL/h over 5 h 30 min via infusion pump

24. RL at 17 gtt/min over 12 h via 15 gtt/mL tubing

25. NS at 24 gtt/min over 7 h 30 min via 20 gtt/mL tubing

26. D5W at 8 gtt/min over 8 h 20 min via 10 gtt/mL tubing

In Exercises 27–30, find the flow rate.

27. Ordered: *Heparin 1500 U/h IV*
    On hand: 50,000 U in 1000 mL D5W, 15 gtt/mL tubing

28. Ordered: *Heparin 1500 U/h IV*
    On hand: 100,000 U in 1000 mL NS, 20 gtt/mL tubing

29. Ordered: *Heparin 1200 U/h IV*
    On hand: 40,000 U in 500 mL D5W via infusion pump

30. Ordered: *Heparin 800 U/h IV*
    On hand: 20,000 units in 1000 mL NS using microdrip tubing

In Exercises 31–34, find the hourly dosage for the heparin orders. Determine whether the dosage is within the safe daily range for adults.

31. 20,000 U in 1000 mL D5W infusing at 30 gtt/min using 20 gtt/mL tubing

32. 30,000 U in 1000 mL NS infusing at 7 gtt/min using 10 gtt/mL tubing

33. 40,000 U in 1000 mL NS infusing at 40 gtt/min via microdrip tubing

34. 50,000 U in 500 mL D5W infusing at 10 mL/h via infusion pump

In Exercises 35–38, find the flow rates appropriate to the IV equipment used.

35. Ordered: *nitroprusside sodium 50 mg in 500 mL D5W at 0.35 mg/min*
    a. infusion pump　　　　　　　　　　　b. macrodrip tubing at 15 gtt/mL

36. Ordered: *dopamine 800 mg in 500 mL NS at 0.9 mg/min*
    a. infusion pump　　　　　　　　　　　b. microdrip tubing

37. Ordered: *Isuprel 1 mg in 250 mL D5W at 3 mcg/min*
    a. infusion pump　　　　　　　　　　　b. macrodrip tubing at 10 gtt/mL

38. Ordered: *4 g lidocaine in 1000 mL NS at 3 mg/min*
    a. infusion pump　　　　　　　　　　　b. macrodrip tubing at 20 gtt/mL

In Exercises 39–40, find the appropriate flow rate.

39. Ordered: *Ticar 200 mg/kg/day IV q4h in 60 mL LR over 90 min*
    On hand: Ticar 3 g vial. Each g is reconstituted with 4 mL of diluent. The patient weighs 182 lb.
    Use macrodrip tubing, 20 gtt/mL. Dilute the reconstituted Ticar in 48 mL of LR.

40. Ordered: *Septra 15 mg/kg/day IV q8h in D5W over 1 hr*
    On hand: Septra 5-mL vial, with 80 mg/mL. The patient weighs 108 lb. Use macrodrip tubing, 15 gtt/mL. Each 5 mL should be added to 75 mL of D5W.

In Exercises 41–42, find the amount of medication that has already been administered to the patient.

41. Ordered: *magnesium sulfate 20 g in 500 mL LR*
    The patient has received 200 mL.

42. Ordered: *nitroprusside 50 mg in 500 mL D5W*
    The patient has received 30 mL.

CRITICAL THINKING

A patient with malignant hypertension is being treated in the critical care unit. The physician writes the following order: *Nipride 50 mg in 500 mL D5W to start at 1 mcg/kg/min, and titrate to maintain the systolic BP under 140.* (When you measure a patient's blood pressure, the first number represents the systolic blood pressure.) The patient weighs 176 pounds. According to the product insert, the maximum safe dose of Nipride is 10 mcg/kg/min.

1. At what rate should you initially set the infusion?

2. What is the maximum safe rate for the infusion?

3. At 1600, the patient's BP is 210/105. The Nipride infusion is running at 360 mL/h. What should you do?

4. At 2000, the patient's BP is 170/90. The Nipride infusion is running at 480 mL/h. What should you do?

CASE STUDY

A patient has a PCA pump with morphine sulfate 50 mg in 500 mL W. Hospital policy requires you to document the dose of morphine administered during your shift. When you came on duty, the pump showed that 227 mL had infused. At the end of your shift the pump shows that 272 mL have infused. How much morphine did the patient receive during your shift?

To check you answers, see page 364.

INTERNET ACTIVITY

Note: The Internet is a research tool from which to get basic information. Validate the accuracy of all Internet information.

You are working in an intensive care unit that uses many IV critical care drugs. Checking the safe ranges of these drugs during emergency situations is both inconvenient and time consuming. You and your coworkers decide to search the Internet for guides to dosages of commonly used drugs. Try finding answers to the following questions on-line:

1. What is the usual adult loading dose of amiodarone IV?
2. If you are administering nitroglycerine IV and titrating the dose,
   a. By how many mcg can you increase the dose at a time?
   b. How often can you increase the dose?
3. What treatment must be in place before tubocurarine is given?

PEDIATRIC CONCERNS

12

Objectives

When you have completed Chapter 12, you will be able to:

- Explain why pediatric dosages must be calculated based on the individual patient.
- Determine a safe dose for pediatric patients.
- Calculate pediatric dosages based on body weight.
- Find a patient's body surface area (BSA).
- Calculate pediatric dosages based on a patient's BSA.
- Describe volume limitations for parenteral injections.
- Calculate infusion rates for children.

General Concerns in Calculating Pediatric Dosages

Administering incorrect amounts of medication to adults can be harmful. However, the risk of harm to pediatric patients is far greater due to their size and the way they metabolize (break down and absorb) medications. If you prepare or administer medication, you have full responsibility for providing a safe amount. You must clarify all confusing drug orders, calculate with absolute accuracy, compare the dosage ordered with safe dosages listed in drug literature, and seek assistance from your supervisor or the ordering physician if you have any concerns about the order or its administration. No matter how rushed you may feel, you may not take short cuts with any pediatric medications.

When you calculate drug dosages, do not consider a child to be a small adult. The average child does not metabolize drugs the way an adult does. For example, many organ systems in infants and toddlers are immature. Children show significant differences in their responses to medications. A newborn does not metabolize drugs the way a ten-year-old child does. Infants born prematurely metabolize drugs differently than full-term infants of the same age. Variations for children are so great that no foolproof formula exists to determine the amount of medication a child should receive.

Absorption is the process by which a drug moves from the site where it is given into the bloodstream. Oral medications are absorbed through the gastrointestinal (GI) system, while topical medications are absorbed through the skin. Intravenous (IV) medications bypass the absorption process because they enter the bloodstream directly through the veins.

Stomach pH (acidity), which is greater immediately after birth, can deactivate certain medications. Infants and children are more likely to experience diarrhea. As a result, medications pass through the GI tract more quickly, reducing the time during which they can be absorbed. Topical medications may be absorbed more completely in infants because of their thin skin. The absorption rate for IM medications depends on blood flow and muscle mass, both of which are reduced in infants. An IV is the most reliable route for administering medications to newborns and infants because the medication goes directly to the blood stream. However, because of their size, an infant's veins are more fragile than an adult's and can be hard to use.

PATIENT EDUCATION

Family members or others who care for children at home must understand and follow directions when they administer drugs. Talk to parents or caretakers about the following:

1. Explain how much medication to administer at one time, how often during the day, and for how many days. Give parents or caretakers this information in writing. Have them repeat this information, especially if their English or literacy skills are limited.

2. Discuss expected side effects. Provide a telephone number or resource for them to call in case of unexpected or serious side effects. Explain how to reach a Poison Control Center.

3. Children should never be given someone else's medication. They react differently to medications than adults.

4. Over-the-counter, herbal, and alternative remedies should never be given to a child under age two without first speaking to a health care provider.

5. Parents must check dosage information on over-the-counter medications. The amount to administer changes with age and weight. Some medications may *not* be administered to children below a certain age (often two) without first checking with a physician.

6. Demonstrate how to measure doses accurately. Calibrated equipment should be used. Droppers are not automatically interchangeable between medications.

7. The full course of prescription medications such as antibiotics must be administered, even if the child appears to be well or resists taking the medication. Do not refer to medication as candy.

8. Replace childproof caps properly.

Dosages Based on Body Weight

Many pediatric dosages are based on a child's body weight. Others are based on a child's body surface area, or BSA.

Body Weight Calculations

In Chapter 11, you learned to calculate orders for IV medications based on body weight. The same methods apply to many pediatric orders, including oral and parenteral dosages.

Rule 12-1

To calculate the *amount to administer*, based on body weight,

1. Convert the patient's body weight to kg.

2. Calculate the *desired dose*, D, multiplying
$$\frac{mg}{kg} \times kg = desired\ dose \quad or \quad \frac{mcg}{kg} \times kg = desired\ dose$$

3. Confirm whether or not the *desired dose* is safe. If unsafe, consult the physician who wrote the order.

4. Calculate the *amount to administer,* using fraction proportions, ratio proportions, or the formula method.

EXAMPLE 1 Calculate the *amount to administer* to a three-year-old child who weighs 34 lb.

Ordered: *Hyoscyamine sulfate 77 mcg sc 1 h pre-anesthesia*

On hand: Levsin Injection 0.5 mg/mL

You need to confirm if this order is a safe amount. Check the package insert or a drug reference. For pediatric patients over 2 years of age, the recommended dose when Levsin is used as a pre-anesthetic medication, is 5 mcg/kg. Convert the patient's weight to kg.

$$1 \text{ kg:2.2 lb::? kg:34 lb}$$

$$2.2 \text{ lb} \times ? \text{ kg} = 1 \text{ kg} \times 34 \text{ lb}$$

$$? = 15.45$$

Next, calculate the *desired dose.*

$$\frac{5 \text{ mcg}}{1 \text{ kg}} \times 15.45 \text{ kg} = \frac{5 \text{ mcg}}{1 \text{ kg}} \times 15.45 \text{ kg} = 77.25 \text{ mcg}$$

This recommended dose rounds to 77 mcg. The order, which is also for 77 mcg, is a safe order. Next, you need to convert 77 mcg to mg, the unit of the dose on hand.

$$77 \text{ mcg} \div 1000 = 0.077 \text{ mg}$$

Now calculate the *amount to administer.*

$$\frac{0.5 \text{ mg}}{1 \text{ mL}} = \frac{0.077 \text{ mg}}{? \text{ mL}}$$

$$0.5 \text{ mg} \times ? \text{ mL} = 1 \text{ mL} \times 0.077 \text{ mg}$$

$$? = 0.154$$

You would administer 0.154 mL of injection. This amount rounds to 0.15 mL, which you can administer subcutaneously.

EXAMPLE 2 Suppose the original order read:

Hyoscyamine sulfate 5 mcg/kg/day sc 1 h pre-anesthesia

This ordered dose matches the dose in the package insert and the PDR. You can combine all your calculations using dimensional analysis. Start with the formula method, $D \times \frac{Q}{H} = A$. Write D as $\frac{5 \text{ mcg}}{1 \text{ kg}}$ times the patient's weight, or $\frac{5 \text{ mcg}}{1 \text{ kg}} \times \frac{1 \text{ kg}}{2.2 \text{ lb}} \times \frac{34 \text{ lb}}{1}$. Thus,

$$\frac{5 \text{ mcg}}{1 \text{ kg}} \times \frac{1 \text{ kg}}{2.2 \text{ lb}} \times \frac{34 \text{ lb}}{1} \times \frac{1 \text{ mL}}{0.5 \text{ mg}} = A$$

The last factor, $\frac{Q}{H}$, is the reciprocal of the dosage strength. The amount you will administer is measured in mL. You need a conversion factor relating mg to mcg, leaving mL for your answer.

$$\frac{5 \text{ mcg}}{1 \text{ kg}} \times \frac{1 \text{ kg}}{2.2 \text{ lb}} \times \frac{34 \text{ lb}}{1} \times \frac{1 \text{ mg}}{1000 \text{ mcg}} \times \frac{1 \text{ mL}}{0.5 \text{ mg}} = A$$

$$\frac{\overset{1}{5 \text{ mcg}}}{1 \text{ kg}} \times \frac{1 \text{ kg}}{2.2 \text{ lb}} \times \frac{34 \text{ lb}}{1} \times \frac{1 \text{ mg}}{\underset{200}{1000} \text{ mcg}} \times \frac{1 \text{ mL}}{0.5 \text{ mg}} =$$

$$1 \times \frac{1}{2.2} \times 34 \times \frac{1}{200} \times \frac{1 \text{ mL}}{0.5} = \frac{34 \text{ mL}}{220} = 0.154 \text{ mL}$$

As before, the amount to administer is 0.15 mL.

The physician's order in this example and the next are written with quantity per kg per day. In practice, orders are seldom written in this format, but rather in the format you see in Example 1. Knowing how to perform the calculations in Examples 2 and 3, however, help you determine if the total quantity ordered is safe.

EXAMPLE 3   Find the *amount to administer.* The patient is a 55-lb child.

Ordered: *Cefaclor susp 20 mg/kg/day po q8h*

On hand: Refer to label below.

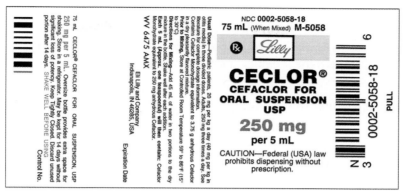

First convert the child's weight to kg.

1 kg:2.2 lb::? kg:55 lb

2.2 lb × ? kg = 1 kg × 55 lb

? = 25

The patient weighs 25 kg. Now find the daily dosage.

$$\frac{20 \text{ mg}}{1 \text{ kg}} \times 25 \text{ kg} = \frac{20 \text{ mg}}{1 \text{ kg}} \times 25 \text{ kg} = 500 \text{ mg}$$

Next, find the daily amount to administer in mL.

$$D \times \frac{Q}{H} = 500 \text{ mg} \times \frac{5 \text{ mL}}{250 \text{ mg}} = {}^{2}500 \text{ mg} \times \frac{5 \text{ mL}}{{}_{1}250 \text{ mg}} = 10 \text{ mL}$$

This daily amount, 10 mL, is divided into three doses of 3.3 mL.

ERROR ALERT!

Convert ounces carefully.

The weight of babies is often measured in pounds and ounces. Because 16 oz = 1 lb, an ounce is not a tenth of a pound. A baby whose weight is 8 lb 6 oz *does not* weigh 8.6 lb. Convert 6 ounces to pounds using $\frac{1 \text{ lb}}{16 \text{ oz}}$ as the conversion factor. Here,

$6 \text{ oz} \times \frac{1 \text{ lb}}{16 \text{ oz}} = 0.375 \text{ lb}$. Thus, 8 lb 6 oz = 8.375 lb.

Premature infants are often weighed in grams.

EXAMPLE 1   Convert the weight of a 3 lb 10 oz premature baby to g. Round to the nearest tenth.

First convert the baby's weight to a decimal.

$$10 \text{ oz} = \frac{10}{16} \text{ lb} = 0.625 \text{ lb}$$

Thus, 3 lb 10 oz = 3.625 lb. Now convert 3.625 lb to kg.

1 kg:2.2 lb::? kg:3.625 lb

2.2 lb × ? kg = 1 kg × 3.625 lb

? = 1.647 kg

Multiply by 1000 to convert from kg to g,

1.647 kg × 1000 = 1647 g

Safe Dosages

Pediatric drug orders may be written in several ways. If you measure or administer the medication, you have the responsibility to check whether the dose is the standard safe dose.

Rule 12-2

Before administering a pediatric dose, check the drug label, package insert, or drug literature to determine whether the dose is safe.

EXAMPLE 1 Determine whether the following order is safe for an 8-week-old baby who weighs 11 lb 7 oz. If the order is safe, find the *amount to administer.*

Ordered: *Amoxil 75 mg po q12h*

On hand: Refer to label below.

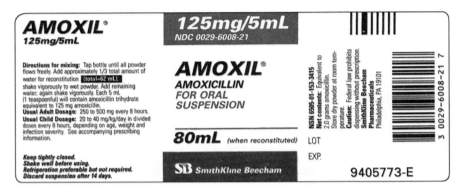

Convert the baby's weight, noting that

$$7 \text{ oz} = \frac{7}{16} \text{ lb} = 0.4375 \text{ lb}$$

Thus,

1 kg:2.2 lb::? kg:11.4375 lb

2.2 lb × ? kg = 1 kg × 11.4375 lb

? = 5.2

The baby weighs 5.2 kg. The drug label lists a range of child dosages. Because the patient is a young infant, however, check the package insert for more information. It indicates that the upper dosage of Amoxil is 30 mg/kg/day divided into two doses q12h. Therefore, the maximum daily dosage for the patient is

$$\frac{30 \text{ mg}}{1 \text{ kg}} \times 5.2 \text{ kg} = 156 \text{ mg}$$

Dividing 156 mg by 2 (the number of doses), the maximum safe dose is 78 mg, when administered twice a day. Thus, 75 mg administered twice per day, is below the upper limit.

Now find the *amount to administer.*

$$75 \text{ mg} \times \frac{5 \text{ ml}}{125 \text{ mg}} = 3 \text{ mL}$$

Administer 3 mL of the reconstituted Amoxil every 12 hours. If the order had been written q8h instead of q12h, it would have been unsafe. An individual dose of 75 mg is safe, but three doses leads to 225 mg per day, above the maximum safe dosage of 156 mg per day.

EXAMPLE 2 Determine whether the following order is safe for a 2-year-old child who weighs 27 lb and has a mild, upper respiratory tract infection. If the order is safe, find the *amount to administer.*

Ordered: *EryPed drops 120 mg po q6h*

On hand: Refer to the label below.

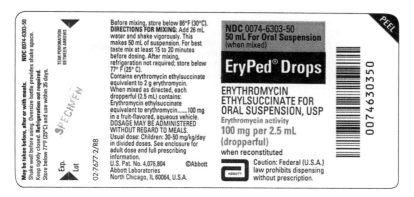

First convert the child's weight to kg.

1 kg:2.2 lb::? kg:27 lb

2.2 lb × ? kg = 1 kg × 27 lb

? = 12.27

The child weighs approximately 12.27 kg. The drug label indicates that the dosage range for this patient is 30 to 50 mg/kg/day. *When the recommended daily dosage is a range, you must calculate whether the ordered dosage is within that range.* The lower recommended dosage is 30 mg/kg/day.

$$\frac{30 \text{ mg}}{1 \text{ kg}} \times 12.27 \text{ kg} = 368.1 \text{ mg}$$

The upper recommended dosage is 50 mg/kg/day.

$$\frac{50 \text{ mg}}{1 \text{ kg}} \times 12.27 \text{ kg} = 613.5 \text{ mg}$$

The recommended dosage for the patient ranges from 368.1 mg to 613.5 mg per day. The order calls for four doses/day of 120 mg, a total of 480 mg/day. This amount is in the recommended range. (If the dosage is outside the recommended range, consult the physician.) Now find the *amount to administer.*

$$120 \text{ mg} \times \frac{2.5 \text{ mL}}{100 \text{ mg}} = 3 \text{ mL}$$

Administer 3 mL of reconstituted solution every six hours. The dropper packaged with the EryPed holds up to 2.5 mL. The calibrations on the dropper will help you determine the best way to measure the 3 mL of solution.

Rule 12-3

Before administering a combination drug, check the maximum safe dose or safe range for each drug component. Only administer the drug if all the components can be given safely.

EXAMPLE 1 Determine whether the following order is safe for a child weighing 38 lb. If it is, find the *amount to administer.*

Ordered: *Pediazole susp 5 mL po qid*

On hand: Refer to the label and package insert on the following page.

Before mixing, store below 86°F (30°C).
Directions for mixing: **Total amount of water to be added is 110 mL.** Add approximately half of the total amount of water for reconstitution and shake well. Add the remainder of the water and again shake well. This makes 200 mL of suspension.

Contains erythromycin ethylsuccinate equivalent to 8 g erythromycin, and sulfisoxazole acetyl equivalent to 24 g sulfisoxazole.

When mixed as directed, each teaspoonful (5 mL) of Pediazole Suspension contains erythromycin ethylsuccinate equivalent to 200 mg erythromycin, and sulfisoxazole acetyl equivalent to 600 mg sulfisoxazole.

Usual dose: **See package enclosure for dosage and full prescribing information.**

TO PATIENT: **Shake before using.** Oversize bottle provides shake space. Keep tightly closed. Store in the refrigerator. Use within 14 days. Unused portion should be discarded after 14 days.

6505-01-144-5318

© 1998 Abbott
02-8171-2

ROSS PRODUCTS DIVISION
ABBOTT LABORATORIES
COLUMBUS, OHIO 43215-1724 USA

200 mL when mixed   NDC 0074-8030-53

Pediazole®

suspension

erythromycin ethylsuccinate
and sulfisoxazole acetyl
for oral suspension

200 mg erythromycin activity
and the equivalent of
600 mg sulfisoxazole per

5 mL reconstituted

ROSS
PEDIATRICS

℞ only

DOSAGE AND ADMINISTRATION

PEDIAZOLE SHOULD NOT BE ADMINISTERED TO INFANTS UNDER 2 MONTHS OF AGE BECAUSE OF CONTRAINDICATIONS OF SYSTEMIC SULFONAMIDES IN THIS AGE GROUP.

For Acute Otitis Media in Children: The dose of Pediazole can be calculated based on the erythromycin component (50 mg/kg/day) or the sulfisoxazole component (150 mg/kg/day to a maximum of 6 g/day). The total daily dose of Pediazole should be administered in equally divided doses three or four times a day for 10 days. Pediazole may be administered without regard to meals.

First convert the child's weight to kg.

1 kg:2.2 lb::? kg:38 lb

2.2 lb × ? kg = 1 kg × 38 lb

? = 17.27

The child weighs 17.27 kg. Pediazole is a combination drug. According to the package insert, the recommended doses of the components are 50 mg/kg/day of erythromycin ethylsuccinate and 150 mg/kg/day of sulfisoxalzole acetyl.

$$\frac{50 \text{ mg}}{1 \text{ kg}} \times 17.27 \text{ kg} = 863.5 \text{ mg}$$

$$\frac{150 \text{ mg}}{1 \text{ kg}} \times 17.27 \text{ kg} = 2590.5 \text{ mg}$$

The maximum daily dosages are 863.5 mg/day of erythromycin ethylsuccinate and 2590.5 mg of sulfisoxalzole acetyl.

The order calls for 5 mL of Pediazole four times per day. According to the label, each 5 mL of reconstituted Pediazole contains 200 mg of erythromycin and 600 mg of sulfisoxazole. The daily dosages ordered, then, are 800 mg of erythromycin and 2400 mg of sulfisoxazole. The dosage of erythromycin is below the maximum safe dose of 863.5 mg/day. The dosage of sulfisoxazole is below the maximum safe dose of 2590.5 mg/day. The dosage of each component is within the recommended range. You may administer the medication.

The physician's order is already written as a volume of Pediazole. No further calculation is needed. Administer 5 mL, or 1 tsp, of Pediazole orally four times per day.

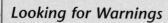

CRITICAL THINKING ON THE JOB

Looking for Warnings

Elena received an order to administer 1.5 mL of Pediazole to a 7-week-old infant who weighs 12 lb. The schedule on the package insert (see previous example) has an instruction to adjust the dosage by body weight. She notices that for a 13-lb infant, the recommended dosage is 2.5 mL every six or eight hours. Her first instinct tells her that 1.5 mL seems like a safe amount to administer.

Think Before You Act

Fortunately, Elena acts on more than instinct. Reading the dosage and administration section of the package insert, she finds a warning that Pediazole should not be administered to patients less than 2 months of age. This patient, 7 weeks old, should not receive Pediazole. Elena contacts the physician to discuss the order further.

REVIEW and PRACTICE

DOSAGES BASED ON BODY WEIGHT

In Exercises 1–8, convert the following weights to kg.

1. 66 lb

2. 77 lb

3. 54 lb

4. 37 lb

5. 16 lb 4 oz

6. 11 lb 10 oz

7. 9 lb 14 oz

8. 14 lb 5 oz

In Exercises 9–18, determine if the order is safe. If it is, then determine the *amount to administer.*

9. The patient is a 3-day-old newborn who weighs 6 lb 5 oz.
   Ordered: *Nebcin 5 mg IM q12h*
   On hand: Nebcin multidose vial, 20 mg/2 mL. According to the package insert, a premature or full-term neonate up to 1 week of age may be administered up to 4 mg/kg/day in 2 equal doses every 12 hours.

10. The patient is a 4-year-old child who weighs 32 lb.
    Ordered: *Proventil 1 tsp syrup po tid*
    On hand: Proventil Syrup, 2 mg/5 mL. According to the package insert, for children 2 to 6 years of age, dosing should be initiated at 0.1 mg/kg of body weight three times a day. This starting dose should not exceed 2 mg three times per day.

11. The patient is a 5-year-old child who weighs 34 lb and has a severe infection.
    Ordered: *Augmentin 225 mg po q8h*
    On hand: Refer to Label A. According to the package insert, the dosing regimen for pediatric patients aged 12 weeks and older, but less than 40 kg, is 40 mg/kg/day q8h.

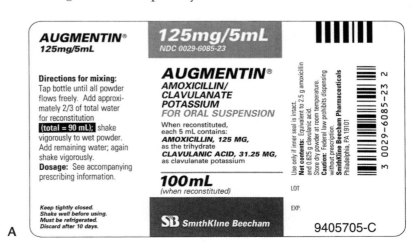

A

12. The patient is a 7-year-old child who weighs 52 lb.
    Ordered: *Kantrex 175 mg IV bid over 60 minutes bid*
    Available: Refer to Labels B and C. The contents are mixed with diluent to produce 100 mL of solution.

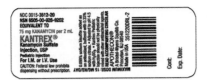

B

Intravenous Administration: The dose should not exceed 15 mg/kg per day and must be administered slowly. The solution for intravenous use is prepared by adding the contents of a 500-mg vial to 100 to 200 mL of sterile diluent such as Normal Saline or 5% Dextrose in Water, or the contents of a 1.0-g vial to 200 to 400 mL of sterile diluent. The appropriate dose is administered over a 30- to 60-minute period. The total daily dose should be divided into 2 or 3 equally divided doses.

In pediatric patients the amount of diluent used should be sufficient to infuse the kanamycin sulfate over a 30- to 60-minute period.

Kanamycin sulfate Injection, USP should not be physically mixed with other antibacterial agents but each should be administered separately in accordance with its recommended route of administration and dosage schedule.

C

13. The patient is an 8-year-old child who weighs 55 lb who is being treated to prevent tuberculosis.
    Ordered: *Nydrazid 250 mg IM stat*
    On hand: Refer to Labels D and E.

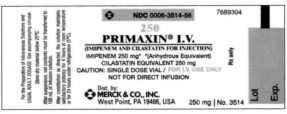

D

14. The patient is a 44-lb child who is $5\frac{1}{2}$ years old.
    Ordered: *Tolectin 100 mg po qid*
    On hand: Tolectin 200-mg scored tablets. The package insert indicates that for children two years and older, the usual dose ranges from 15 to 30 mg/kg/day.

For Preventative Therapy of Tuberculosis

Before isoniazid preventive therapy is initiated, bacteriologically positive or radiographically progressive tuberculosis must be excluded. Appropriate evaluations should be performed if Extra pulmonary tuberculosis is suspected.

Adults over 30 Kg: 300 mg per day in a single dose.

Infants and Children: 10 mg/kg (up to 300 mg daily) in a single dose.

In situations where adherence with daily preventative therapy cannot be assured, 20-30 mg/kg (not to exceed 900 mg) twice weekly under the direct observation of a health care worker at the time of administration[8].

Continuous administration of isoniazid for a sufficient period of time is an essential part of the regimen because relapse rates are higher if chemotherapy is stopped prematurely. In the treatment of tuberculosis, resistant organisms may multiply and the emergence during the treatment may necessitate a change in the regimen.

For following patient compliance: the Potts-Cozart test[9], a simple colorimetric[6] method of checking for isoniazid in the urine, is a useful tool for assuring patient compliance, which is essential for effective tuberculosis control. Additionally, isoniazid test strips are also available to check patient compliance.

Concomitant administration of pyridoxine (B[6]) is recommended in the malnourished and in those predisposed to neuropathy (e.g., alcoholics and diabetics).

E

15. The patient is a 5-month-old baby who weighs 14 lb.
    Ordered: *Primaxin IV 15 mg/kg over 30 min q6h*
    On hand: Refer to Label F. The package insert indicates that for children 3 months of age and older, the recommended dose is 15-25 mg/kg/dose administered every six hours. The contents of the vial are restored with 100 mL of diluent.

F

16. The same patient from Exercise 15 is given the following order: *Primaxin 200 mg IV q6h*

17. The patient is a one-year-old child who weighs 18 lb. The patient has a mild ear infection.

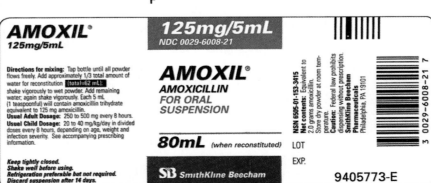

G

Ordered: *Amoxil susp 150 mg po q12h*
On hand: Refer to label G. According to the package insert, the following are usual dosages for children over 3 months of age: For mild to moderate ear/nose/throat infections, either 25 mg/kg/day in divided doses every 12 hours, or 20 mg/kg/day in divided doses every 8 hours. For lower respiratory tract infections, 45 mg/kg/day in divided doses every 12 hours.

18. The same patient from Exercise 17 is given the following order for a moderate ear infection: *Amoxil susp 50 mg po q8h*

To check you answers, see page 365.

Dosages Based on Body Surface Area (BSA)

Some medications are prescribed based on a patient's body weight. Others factor in both weight and height to determine a patient's body surface area, or BSA. Many pediatric medications use a patient's BSA to determine the daily dosage. BSA is also important for burn victims and for patients undergoing chemotherapy, radiation treatments, and open heart surgery.

Calculating a Patient's BSA

A patient's BSA is stated in square meters, or m². You can calculate the BSA using one of the two formulas listed in Rule 12-4. Your calculator should have a program or button that will help you find a square root ($\sqrt{}$). You can also use a special chart called a nomogram.

Rule 12-4

To determine a patient's BSA (body surface area),

1. if you know the height in cm and weight in kg, calculate

$$\text{BSA} = \sqrt{\frac{\text{height (cm)} \times \text{weight (kg)}}{3600}} \ \text{m}^2$$

2. if you know the height in inches and weight in pounds, calculate

$$\text{BSA} = \sqrt{\frac{\text{height (in)} \times \text{weight (lb)}}{3131}} \ \text{m}^2$$

EXAMPLE 1 Find the body surface area for a child who is 85 cm tall and weighs 13.9 kg.

Use the first of the formulas from Rule 12-4.

$$\text{BSA} = \sqrt{\frac{85 \times 13.9}{3600}} \ \text{m}^2 = \sqrt{\frac{1181.5}{3600}} \ \text{m}^2 = 0.572 \ \text{m}^2 = 0.57 \ \text{m}^2$$

EXAMPLE 2 Find the body surface area for a baby who is 24 inches tall and who weighs 12.2 lb.

Use the second of the formulas from Rule 12-4.

$$\text{BSA} = \sqrt{\frac{24 \times 12.2}{3131}} \ \text{m}^2 = \sqrt{\frac{292.8}{3131}} \ \text{m}^2 = 0.305 \ \text{m}^2 = 0.31 \ \text{m}^2$$

Finding the Amount to Administer

Rule 12-5

To calculate the *amount to administer,*

1. Calculate the patient's BSA.

2. Calculate the desired dose:

   dosage ordered × BSA = desired dose

3. Confirm whether or not the desired dose is safe. If unsafe, consult the physician who wrote the order.

4. Calculate the *amount to administer,* using fraction proportions, ratio proportions, or the formula method.

EXAMPLE 1   Find the recommended first dose in mg of CeeNU for a child whose height is 38 in and whose weight is 47 lb. CeeNu is available in 100-mg, 40-mg, and 10-mg capsules. According to the package insert, the first recommended dose of CeeNU is a single oral dose providing 130 mg/m^2.

Because the recommended dose is per m^2, you need to find the patient's BSA. You know the patient's height and weight in inches and pounds. Use the second formula in Rule 12-4.

$$BSA = \sqrt{\frac{\text{height (in)} \times \text{weight (lb)}}{3131}} \ m^2$$

$$BSA = \sqrt{\frac{38 \times 47}{3131}} \ m^2 = \sqrt{\frac{1786}{3131}} \ m^2 = 0.755 \ m^2$$

Next, calculate the desired dose.

$$\frac{130 \ mg}{m^2} \times 0.755 \ m^2 = 98.15 \ mg$$

REVIEW and PRACTICE

DOSAGES BASED ON BODY SURFACE AREA (BSA)

In Exercises 1–8, use the appropriate formula to calculate the BSA for patients with the following height and weight.

1. 88 cm and 13.2 kg

2. 115 cm and 21 kg

3. 38 cm and 6 kg

4. 48 cm and 10 kg

5. 52 in and 64 lb

6. 43 in and 35 lb

7. 22 in and 18 lb

8. 26 in and 21 lb

In Exercises 9–12, calculate the *amount to administer.*

9. The child's BSA is 0.82 m^2. The recommended dosage is 175 mcg/m^2.

10. The child's BSA is 0.65 m^2. The recommended dosage is 0.4 mg/m^2.

11. The child's height is 62 cm and weight is 5 kg. The recommended dosage is 50 mcg/m^2.

12. The child's height is 41 inches and weight is 63 lb. The recommended dosage is 0.2 mg/m^2.

IM and IV Medications

You must always consider the age and size of the patient when you determine the amount to administer. To increase the precision of any injections, *always round your pediatric dosage calculations to the nearest hundredth.*

IM Medications

When you calculate dosages for pediatric injections, use the same methods that you use for adults.

Rule 12-6

The total volume of a pediatric injection is limited based on the size and age of the child. The length and gauge of the needle also vary with the age and size of the child as well as the location of the injection.

Table 12-1 summarizes the maximum volume that is appropriate for a pediatric injection. For premature infants, weight is an important factor.

Table 12-1 Pediatric Injections

Stage of Development	Maximum Volume of IM Injection
Infant	0.5–1 mL
Toddler, walking more than 1 year	1 mL
Preschooler and elementary school age	1–1.5 mL

EXAMPLE 1 Find the *amount to administer.* The patient is a 5-year-old child who weighs 44 lb.

Ordered: *Zinacef 50 mg/kg/day IM q6h*

Available: Refer to the label below. According to the package insert, Zinacef may be given to pediatric patients above 3 months of age at the rate of 50-100 mg/kg/ day in divided doses every 6 to 8 hours.
Notice that the dosage ordered corresponds to the low end of this range and is a safe order.

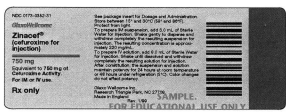

First convert the child's weight from lb to kg.

1 kg:2.2 lb::? kg:44 lb

2.2 lb × ? kg = 1 kg × 44 lb

? = 20 kg

Now, find the daily dosage.

$$\frac{50 \text{ mg}}{1 \text{ kg}} \times 20 \text{ kg} = \frac{50 \text{ mg}}{1 \text{ kg}} \times 20 \text{ kg} = 1000 \text{ mg}$$

Next, find the desired dose. There are 4 doses each day (q6h). Because 1000 ÷ 4 = 250, each dose is 250 mg. After reconstitution, the Zinacef has a dosage strength of 220 mg/mL. Finding the *amount to administer* for each dose,

$$250 \text{ mg} \times \frac{1 \text{ mL}}{220 \text{ mg}} = {}^{25}\cancel{250} \cancel{\text{mg}} \times \frac{1 \text{ mL}}{22\cancel{220} \cancel{\text{mg}}} = 1.14 \text{ mL}$$

By Table 12-1, this amount is an appropriate volume to administer to a 5-year-old child.

IV Medications

The amount to administer of pediatric IVs is smaller than the amounts for adults. Your calculations must be even more accurate because there is less room for error. Volume-control sets (see Chapter 11) used with microdrip tubing that measures 60 gtt/mL, increase the accuracy and safety of IV medications for children. They help to prevent accidental fluid overload.

Many pediatric IV orders are based on the child's body weight. You convert weight from lb to kg, use the converted weight to find the daily dosage, find the individual dose and the volume to infuse, and calculate the gtt/min rate.

EXAMPLE 1 | A medication is ordered at the rate of 25 mg/kg/day for a 33-lb patient. Find the gtt/min flow rate for microdrip tubing if the dosage strength is 50 mg/1 mL, and the dosage is given in 3 doses over 10 minutes per dose.

First convert the patient's weight:

$$33 \text{ lb} \times \frac{1 \text{ kg}}{2.2 \text{ lb}} = 15 \text{ kg}$$

Then find the daily dosage.

$$\frac{25 \text{ mg}}{1 \text{ kg}} \times 15 \text{ kg} = \frac{25 \text{ mg}}{1 \cancel{\text{kg}}} \times 15 \cancel{\text{kg}} = 375 \text{ mg}$$

The daily dosage is 375 mg. The individual dose is 375 mg ÷ 3 = 125 mg. Next, find the volume to infuse.

$$\frac{125 \text{ mg}}{1 \text{ dose}} \times \frac{1 \text{ mL}}{50 \text{ mg}} = \frac{{}^{5}\cancel{125} \cancel{\text{mg}}}{1 \text{ dose}} \times \frac{1 \text{ mL}}{{}_{2}\cancel{50} \cancel{\text{mg}}} = \frac{5 \text{ mL}}{2 \text{ dose}} = 2.5 \text{ mL/dose}$$

The volume to infuse is 2.5 mL. Finally, find the flow rate F by using the formula from Rule 11-7 where the calibration C is 60 gtt/mL, the volume to infuse is 2.5 mL, and the time to infuse is 10 minutes.

$$C \times \frac{\text{volume to infuse}}{\text{time period of infusion}} = F$$

$$\frac{60 \text{ gtt}}{1 \text{ mL}} \times \frac{2.5 \text{ mL}}{10 \text{ min}} = \frac{{}^{6}\cancel{60} \text{ gtt}}{1 \cancel{\text{mL}}} \times \frac{2.5 \cancel{\text{mL}}}{{}_{1}\cancel{10} \text{ min}} = \frac{15 \text{ gtt}}{1 \text{ min}}$$

The flow rate is 15 gtt/min.

For orders that are based on body surface area, the steps are similar. You calculate the patient's BSA before finding the daily dosage. All other steps are the same.

Daily Maintenance Fluid Needs (DMFN)

Children's bodies contain a higher percentage of water than adults' bodies. They are more at risk for fluid overload, dehydration, or electrolyte imbalances. Therefore, you must monitor not only the amount of medication but also the amount of fluid the child receives. Fluids may be calculated based on body weight, body surface area (BSA), metabolism, or age.

Daily maintenance fluid needs (DMFN) represent the fluid a patient needs over 24 hours. It combines maintenance fluids, medications, diluent for medications, and fluids used to flush the injection port. The amount of maintenance fluid required varies according to weight, with the smallest children requiring 100 mL/kg/day. DMFN does not include fluids needed to replace those lost to vomiting, diarrhea, or fever. These are called replacement fluids and are based on each patient's condition.

Rule 12-7

To calculate daily maintenance fluid needs (DMFN) based on weight,

1. if the child weighs up to 10 kg, find

$$\frac{100 \text{ mL}}{1 \text{ kg}} \times \text{kg} = \text{DMFN in mL}$$

2. if the child weighs 10 to 20 kg, find

$$1000 \text{ mL} + [\frac{50 \text{ mL}}{1 \text{ kg}} \times (\text{kg} - 10)] = \text{DMFN in mL}$$

3. if the child weighs over 20 kg, find

$$1500 + [\frac{20 \text{ mL}}{1 \text{ kg}} \times (\text{kg} - 20)] = \text{DMFN in mL}$$

EXAMPLE 1 Find the DMFN for a child who weighs

    a. 7 kg   **b.** 16 kg   **c.** 24 kg

a. The child weighs less than 10 kg.

$$\frac{100 \text{ mL}}{1 \text{ kg}} \times 7 \text{ kg} = 700 \text{ mL}$$

b. The child weighs between 10 and 20 kg.

$$1000 \text{ mL} + [\frac{50 \text{ mL}}{1 \text{ kg}} \times (16 - 10)] =$$

$$1000 \text{ mL} + [\frac{50 \text{ mL}}{1 \text{ kg}} \times 6] = 1000 \text{ mL} + 300 \text{ mL} = 1300 \text{ mL}$$

c. The child weighs over 20 kg.

$$1500 \text{ mL} + [\frac{20 \text{ mL}}{1 \text{ kg}} \times (24 - 20)] =$$

$$1500 \text{ mL} + [\frac{20 \text{ mL}}{1 \text{ kg}} \times 4] = 1500 \text{ mL} + 80 \text{ mL} = 1580 \text{ mL}$$

EXAMPLE 2 What is the microdrip tubing flow rate for DMFN for a child who weighs 14 kg?

Find the DMFN. The child weighs between 10 and 20 kg.

$$1000 \text{ mL} + [\frac{50 \text{ mL}}{1 \text{ kg}} \times (14 - 10)] =$$

$$1000 \text{ mL} + [\frac{50 \text{ mL}}{1 \text{ kg}} \times 4] = 1000 \text{ mL} + 200 \text{ mL} = 1200 \text{ mL}$$

Next, find the microdrip tubing flow rate for 1200 mL/day

$$\frac{1200 \text{ mL}}{1 \text{ day}} \times \frac{1 \text{ day}}{24 \text{ h}} \times \frac{1 \text{ h}}{60 \text{ min}} \times \frac{60 \text{ gtt}}{1 \text{ mL}} =$$

$$\frac{1200 \times 60 \text{ gtt}}{24 \times 60 \text{ min}} = \frac{50 \text{ gtt}}{1 \text{ min}}$$

The flow rate is 50 gtt/min. Recall from Chapter 11 that for microdrip tubing, $\frac{mL}{h} = \frac{gtt}{min}$. In this example, the patient should receive

$$\frac{1200 \text{ mL}}{24 \text{ h}} = \frac{50 \text{ mL}}{1 \text{ h}} = \frac{50 \text{ gtt}}{1 \text{ min}}$$

Rule 12-8

For pediatric patients, the amount of solution in the IV tubing must be considered when determining infusion times and volumes.

Five feet of standard IV tubing contains about 10 mL of solution. If this tubing is used along with a volume-control chamber, a child will not begin receiving medication until the 10 mL of solution already in the tubing has infused. Low-volume (small-diameter) tubing, contains only 0.3 mL of solution per 5 feet, and effectively eliminates this problem.

REVIEW and PRACTICE

IM AND IV MEDICATIONS

In Exercises 1–4, find the *amount to administer*. Assume the amount of medication is safe.

1. The patient weighs 47 lb.
   Ordered: *antibiotic 3 mcg/kg/day IM divided in two equal doses*
   On hand: antibiotic in 50 mcg/mL vials

2. The patient weighs 27 kg.
   Ordered: *muscle relaxant 10 mg/kg/day IV stat*
   On hand: muscle relaxant in 50 mg/mL suspension.

3. The patient is 42 inches tall and weighs 71 lb.
   Ordered: *chemotherapy medication 6 mg/m²/day IV q12h*
   On hand: chemotherapy medication 200 mcg/mL for IV use.

4. The patient is 86 cm tall and weighs 12 kg.
   Ordered: *antibiotic 25 mg/m²/day IV q6h*
   On hand: antibiotic 2 mg/mL for IV use.

In Exercises 5–12, determine if the order is safe. If it is, then determine the *amount to administer*.

5. The patient weighs 14 kg.
   Ordered: *Nebcin 2 mg/kg IM q8h*
   On hand: Nebcin 80 mg/2 mL multi-dose vial. The package insert indicates that the usual dosage for pediatric patients is 6 to 7.5 mg/kg/day in 3 or 4 equally divided doses.

6. The patient weighs 61 lb.
   Ordered: *Mefoxin 1 g IV 30 min pre-op*
   On hand: Mefoxin 2 g/50 mL for injection. The package insert indicates that the usual dosage for pediatric patients (3 months and older) is 30 to 40 mg/kg doses.

7. The patient weighs 26 kg and has a severe infection.
   Ordered: *Mandol 700 mg IV q6h*
   On hand: Refer to Label A. The package insert indicates that for severe infections, a child may be administered up to 150 mg/kg/day.

8. The patient weighs 73 lb.
   Ordered: *Zofran 3.3 mg IV post-op over 4 min*
   On hand: Refer to Label B. Package insert indicates that for post-operative treatment of nausea and vomiting, the recommended IV dosage for pediatric patients is a single 0.1-mg/kg dose for patients who weigh 40 kg or less, and a single 4-mg dose for patients who weigh more than 40 kg. The rate of administration should not be less than 30 seconds, preferably over 2 to 5 minutes.

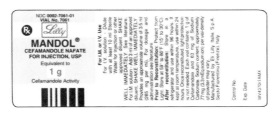

A

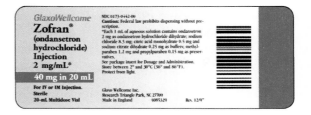

B

9. The patient is 34 cm tall and weighs 5 kg.
   Ordered: *Cerubidine 25 mg/m² IV qw*
   On hand: Cerubidine for injection. When reconstituted, each mL contains 5 mg of drug. The recommended pediatric dosage is 25 mg/m² IV the first day every week.

10. The patient, who is over one-year-old, is 42 inches tall and weighs 45 lb.
    Ordered: *Oncaspar 2500 IU/m² IM every 14 days*
    On hand: Oncaspar 5 mL/vial, 750 IU/mL. The recommended pediatric dosage is 2500 IU/m² for children whose BSA is greater than or equal to 0.6 m² and 82.5 IU/kg for children whose BSA is less than 0.6 m².

11. The patient is 78 cm tall and weighs 15 kg.
    Ordered: *Oncovin 1 mg IV qw*
    On hand: Refer to Label C. The usual dose is 1.5–2 mg/m² for patients weighing more than 10 kg.

12. The patient is 51 inches tall and weighs 86 lb.
    Ordered: *Adriamycin 80 mg IV once every 21 days*
    On hand: Refer to Label D. The usual dose is 60–75 mg/m².

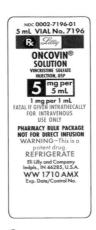

C

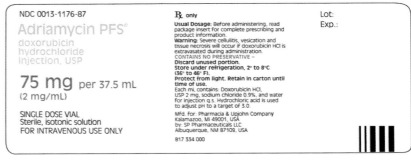

D

In Exercises 13–14, find the gtt/min flow rate.

13. The patient weighs 42 lb. The medication is ordered at the rate of 30 mg/kg/day, with microdrip tubing. The dosage strength is 2 mg/mL.

14. The patient weighs 31 kg. The medication is ordered at the rate of 22 mg/kg/day, with microdrip tubing. The dosage strength is 5 mg/2 mL.

In Exercises 15–18, calculate the child's daily maintenance fluid needs, based on the following weights.

15. 8 kg   16. 33 kg   17. 37 lb   18. 58 lb

In Exercises 19–22, find the microdrip tubing flow rate for DMFN for pediatric patients, based on the following weights.

19. 21 kg   20. 15 kg   21. 17 lb   22. 41 lb

To check you answers, see page 366.

CHAPTER *12* REVIEW

CHECK UP

In Exercises 1–4, convert the following weights to kg.

1. 49 lb
2. 61 lb
3. 6 lb 9 oz
4. 12 lb 13 oz

In Exercises 5–8, calculate the BSA for patients with the following height and weight.

5. 105 cm and 19 kg
6. 74 cm and 12.1 kg
7. 41 in and 33 lb
8. 30 in and 23 lb

In Exercises 9–10, calculate the child's daily maintenance fluid needs, based on the following weights. Then find the microdrip tubing flow rate for DMFN.

9. 24 kg
10. 39 lb

In Exercises 11–20, determine if the order is safe. If it is, then determine the *amount to administer*.

11. The child weighs 30 lb.
Ordered: *Depakene syrup 100 mg po q12h*
On hand: Depakene syrup 250 mg/5 mL. According to the package insert, the initial daily dose for pediatric patients is 15 mg/kg/day.

12. The patient is a four-year-old child who weighs 16 kg.
Ordered: *Ventolin syrup 1.6 mg po tid*
On hand: Ventolin syrup 2 mg/5 mL. According to the package insert, for children from 2 to 6 years of age, dosing should be initiated at 0.1 mg/kg of body weight three times a day. This starting dosage should not exceed 2 mg three times a day.

13. The patient is a six-day-old newborn who weighs 7 lb 12 oz.
Ordered: *Nebcin 7.5 mg IM q12h*
On hand: Nebcin multidose vial, 20 mg/2 mL. According to the package insert, a premature or full-term neonate up to 1 week of age may be administered up to 4 mg/kg/day in 2 equal doses every 12 hours.

14. The patient is 72 cm tall and weighs 16 kg.
Ordered: *Oncaspar 1300 IU IM every 14 days*
On hand: Oncaspar 5 mL/vial, 750 IU/mL. The recommended pediatric dosage is 2500 IU/m^2 for children whose BSA is greater than or equal to 0.6 m^2 and 82.5 IU/kg for children whose BSA is less than 0.6 m^2.

15. The child weighs 31 kg.
Ordered: *Biaxin susp 225 mg po q12h x10*
On hand: Refer to Label A. According to the package insert, the usual recommended daily dosage for children is 15 mg/kg/day for 10 days.

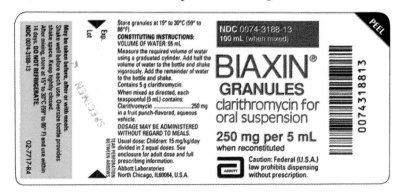

A

16. The child weighs 66 lb.
    Ordered: *Cedax susp 270 mg po qd 1h p̄ breakfast*
    On hand: Refer to Label B. According to the package insert, the usual recommended daily dosage for children who weigh 45 kg or less is 9 mg/kg QD.

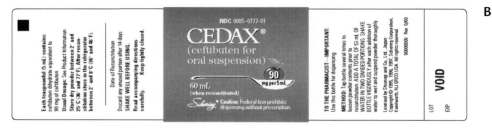

B

17. The patient is a 58-lb child undergoing hemodialysis.
    Ordered: *Mefoxin 1 g IV q4d*
    On hand: Refer to Label C. The Mefoxin is reconstituted to a strength of 180 mg/mL. According to the package insert, the recommended dosage for pediatric patients three months and older who are undergoing hemodialysis is 80 to 160 mg/kg of body weight per day divided into four to six equal doses. The total daily dosage should not exceed 12 grams.

18. The patient is a 25-kg child receiving myelosuppressive chemotherapy.
    Ordered: *Neupogen 125 mcg IVPB over 30 minutes*
    On hand: Refer to Label D. According to the package insert, for patients receiving myelosuppressive chemotherapy, the recommended daily starting dose is 5 mcg/kg/day, administered as a single daily injection by SC bolus injection, by short IV infusion (15 to 30 minutes), or by continuous SC or continuous IV infusion.

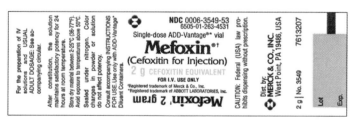

C

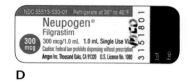

D

CRITICAL THINKING

You are preparing doses for two pediatric patients who are each undergoing treatment for a brain tumor. According to the PDR, the recommended dose for CeeNu is 130 mg/m² po once every six weeks.

The first patient is six years old, 37 inches tall, and weighs 42 lbs. Her order is for 90 mg. The second patient is thirteen years old, 150 cm, and weighs 45 kg. His order is for 180 mg. CeeNU is available in three dosage strengths: 100 mg capsules, 40 mg capsules, and 10 mg capsules (see labels E, F, and G).

1. Determine if the two orders are correct and safe.

2. How would you fill the order for the first patient?

3. How would you fill the order for the second patient?

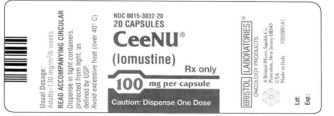

E

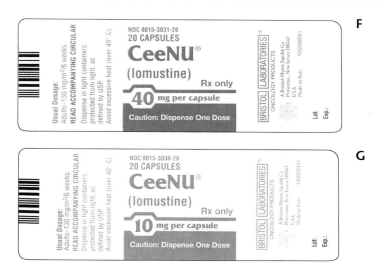

F

G

CASE STUDY

You are working on a pediatric ICU where your patient is a 3-year-old boy who has a staphylococcal skin infection in the area surrounding his incision. His attending physician has prescribed the following treatment. You know from his chart that he weighs 40 lbs.

Ordered: *Rocephin 1200 mg IV over 30 minutes bid*

On hand: Refer to Label H. According to the package insert, for pediatric patients with skin infections, the recommended total daily dose is 50 to 75 mg/kg/day given once a day (or in equally divided doses twice a day). The total daily dose should not exceed 2 grams. The Rocephin is reconstituted to a dosage strength of 40 mg/mL.

1. What is the recommended range of doses for this patient?

2. Calculate the flow rate for the infusion pump used to deliver this order.

3. Is this order a safe dose for your patient? If it is not a safe dose, what steps should you take?

To check your answers, see page 367.

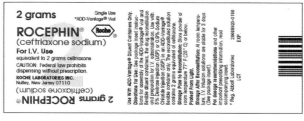

H

INTERNET ACTIVITY

Note: The Internet is a research tool from which to get basic information. Validate the accuracy of all Internet information.

You have just been assigned to work in a clinic that specializes in the treatment of children with leukemia. You know that in the past thirty years, great progress has been made in treating childhood leukemia, but you want to know more about the disease, including symptoms, treatments, and the reactions children might have to medications. Locate on the Internet sites that can help you learn more about childhood leukemia.

Hint: try key words such as *leukemia* and *pediatric*.

GERIATRIC CONCERNS

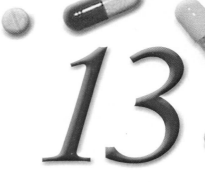

13

Objectives

When you have completed Chapter 13, you will be able to:

- Evaluate whether prescribed doses are safe for geriatric patients, including those with renal impairment.
- Identify factors that affect the absorption, metabolism, and excretion of drugs in geriatric patients.
- Compare actual and ideal body weight.
- Identify health factors that could affect a geriatric patient's ability to self-administer medications.
- Take appropriate actions to reduce polypharmacy in geriatric patients.

The geriatric population—people over the age of 65—is among the fastest-growing segments of our society. In recent years, they represented a little more than 10 percent of our population. In coming years, however, the geriatric population will be over 20 percent of our total population. Currently, geriatric patients account for an even higher percentage of medications—more than 30 percent of prescription medications in the United States.

Geriatric patients are more susceptible to side effects. In fact, many hospitalizations are due to adverse reactions that geriatric patients have to medications. Body changes, the onset of disease, and the ability to participate actively with their own care will vary widely among geriatric patients. You must exercise extra caution when calculating dosages for geriatric patients and when you teach them about their medications.

Age-Related Changes

A person's body changes with age. For example, the elderly have thinner, more fragile skin. The loss of subcutaneous fat contributes to wrinkles; it also makes damaging the skin easier. Topical medications are more likely to be distributed throughout a geriatric patient's entire body, especially if large amounts are applied or if they are applied too often. Fragile skin is more susceptible to irritation by medications or by the adhesives used in transdermal patches. Thus, site rotation is more important in the elderly.

When intravenous medications are given, the IV catheter and tubing must be well supported, often by more tape or an arm board, in order to prevent pulling the tape from the fragile skin. With less subcutaneous tissue to support the IV catheter, medication is more likely to escape into surrounding tissues.

You may need to modify injection techniques. For thin patients with little subcutaneous fat, the angle of a subcutaneous injection may need to be smaller to prevent inadvertently injecting medication into a muscle. When you select a site for an intramuscular injection, consider each patient's decreased muscle mass. For example, gluteal muscles may be a poor injection site for patients who are wheelchair bound. You must also consider the appropriate needle length for each individual patient.

Oral medications can present problems for geriatric patients. Some patients have difficulty swallowing due to weaker contractions of the esophagus caused by stroke or other diseases. Other patients have a fear of swallowing and may resist taking pills.

Creatinine Clearance

Liver and kidney functions are often reduced in elderly patients. Decreased liver function results in slower metabolism of certain drugs, delaying or prolonging the desired effect of the medication. It can also lead to a higher level of drug in the blood system, producing more intense results. In some cases, the absorption of the medication may be decreased.

Decreased kidney function, along with decreased cardiac output, slows the excretion of medications from the body. Slower excretion (resulting from decreased kidney function) and a reduced metabolism (resulting from decreased liver function) combine their effects. Medication accumulates in the body, causing increased side effects or even toxicity.

When a medication is prescribed, subsequent doses are given to maintain a certain blood level of medications. They are timed to be administered as the first dose is "wearing off" from being metabolized and excreted. You learned this concept in Chapter 10, in the discussion of combination insulins. If the first or previous dose has not been completely metabolized or excreted, as is often the case with geriatric patients, then the second or subsequent dose may raise medication levels to an unsafe level.

Many chronic diseases common in the elderly can damage the kidneys. These diseases include hypertension, diabetes, and congestive heart failure. Also, some commonly used drugs, such as Lasix and aminoglycoside antibiotics, can further impair kidney function. Geriatric patients who have these diseases or are prescribed these medications must be monitored especially closely for their kidney function.

Many package inserts discuss safe dosage levels based on creatinine clearance. Creatinine is a byproduct found in the blood as a result of muscle metabolism. Creatinine clearance (CL_{CR}) is an indicator of the rate at which the kidneys filter the blood. Creatinine clearance often decreases with age because the elderly tend to have lower

CRITICAL THINKING ON THE JOB

Consulting the Physician

While transcribing orders for Mrs. Bekins, who is 83 years old and weighs 118 lbs., Karen notes that one of Mrs. Bekins' diagnoses is chronic renal failure. Mrs. Bekins has been given the following drug order: *Tazidime 1 g IV q8h* for pneumonia.

Karen knows that safe doses of antibiotics are often lower for patients with kidney disease than usual prescribed doses. From the package insert, she knows the recommended maintenance dose for Tazidime should be adjusted based on CL_{CR}. According to a table in the insert, for creatine clearance levels of 31 to 50 mL/min, the recommended dosage is 1 g q12h; for levels of 16 to 30 mL/min, the dosage is 1 g q24h; for levels 6 to 15 mL/min, the dosage is 500 mg q24h; and for levels < 5 mL/min, the dosage is 500 mg q48h.

Karen is able to determine that the patient's creatinine clearance level is 9.5 mL/min. This value is between 6 and 15 mL/min. Therefore, the safe dose of Tazidime for the patient is 500 mg q24h. This amount is considerably less than the one indicated by the drug order.

Think Before You Act

Karen immediately contacts the physician to discuss the order. As it turns out, the physician did not consider the chronic renal failure when prescribing the medication for the pneumonia. A new order is written: *Tazidime 500 mg q24h*

If Karen had administered the original amount of Tazidime, Mrs. Bekins would probably have developed an accumulation of the drug, producing symptoms of toxicity such as seizures. By using her critical thinking skills, Karen helped the patient to receive the correct dosage.

muscle mass, thus producing less creatinine. In addition the filtration rate of their kidneys is often slower. For many, this decrease is a normal part of the aging process. The creatinine clearance level of an elderly patient with normal renal function is often lower than the level of an average younger adult.

If a patient has decreased kidney function, then the amount of creatinine excreted through the urine will decrease. At the same time, the amount of creatinine in the blood (or serum creatinine level) will be higher.

The creatinine clearance level is calculated using information that comes from an analysis of blood and urine samples. You may not know this information for every patient. The physician will usually factor in a patient's creatinine clearance when preparing a drug order. If you have any questions about administering a medication when creatinine clearance is a factor, speak with your supervisor or the physician who wrote the order.

Ideal and Actual Body Weight

A geriatric patient's body generally has a decreased proportion of lean body mass and water, along with an increased proportion of body fat. These proportions alter the distribution of drugs.

Some water-soluble drugs, such as aminoglycosides (antibiotics) and digitalis preparations (cardiac medications), are strongly bound to lean tissues. Because the elderly have less lean tissue, more of these water-soluble drugs remain in the circulating blood. Higher levels can lead to toxicity. Thus, you must monitor serum drug levels (the level of drug dissolved in the blood).

Fat-soluble drugs are distributed to body fat. Because the elderly have a larger proportion of body fat, these drugs are distributed to more tissues. The drugs do not remain in the body fat, but are slowly released back into circulation. Thus, fat-soluble drugs have a longer duration of action, resulting in residual effects such as drowsiness.

For medications strongly bound to lean tissues (water soluble), the dose for an overweight patient should be based on the *ideal body weight*. For patients whose weight is below ideal, the *actual* weight should be used. For medications strongly bound to body fat (fat soluble), the dose is based on the *actual* weight.

Table 13–1 provides samples of ideal body weights. Many height-weight tables are available. Some distinguish between men and women, others among people with small, medium, and large body frames. Tables also cover different age ranges. Check with your facility to determine which height-weight table you should use.

Table 13-1 Suggested Weights for Adults (35 Years and Over)

Height (without shoes)	Weight in Pounds (without clothes)	Height	Weight	Height	Weight
		5'5"	126-162	6'0"	155-199
		5'6"	130-167	6'1"	159-205
5'0"	108-138	5'7"	134-172	6'2"	164-210
5'1"	111-143	5'8"	138-178	6'3"	168-216
5'2"	115-148	5'9"	142-183	6'4"	173-222
5'3"	119-152	5'10"	146-188	6'5"	177-228
5'4"	122-157	5'11"	151-194	6'6"	182-234

Note: The higher weights in the ranges generally apply to men, who tend to have more muscle and bone; the lower weights more often apply to women, who have less muscle and bone.

Source: *Nutrition and Your Health: Dietary Guidelines for America,* 3rd Edition, 1990, U.S. Department of Agriculture; U.S. Department of Health and Human Services; Home and Garden Bulletin, No. 232.

EXAMPLE 1 A 78-year-old male, 5'4" tall, and weighing 180 lb, is given the following order. He has normal renal function and is being treated for a serious, but not life-threatening, infection.

Ordered: *Garamycin 70 mg IM q8h*

On hand: Garamycin Injectable, 40 mg/mL. According to the package insert, for patients with normal renal function, the usual dosage for serious infections is 1 mg/kg q8h. The dosage for obese patients should be based on lean body mass. For a 5'4" patient, the ideal weight range is 122 to 157 lb.

Because 122 lb = 55 kg and 157 lb = 71 kg, after rounding, the safe dose for this patient is from 55 to 71 mg q8h. The dosage ordered, 70 mg, falls within that range and is safe. The *amount to administer* per dose is

$$70 \text{ mg} \times \frac{1 \text{ mL}}{40 \text{ mg}} = 1.75 \text{ mL}$$

ERROR ALERT!

For medications that are strongly bound to lean body tissue, calculate an overweight patient's dose on ideal body weight, not actual weight.

Suppose your patient is a 75-year-old female, 5'1" tall, and weighing 190 lb. Her CL_{CR} is 30 mL/min. She is prescribed an initial daily dose of 0.25 mg of Lanoxin injection.

According to the package insert, the level of Lanoxin is based on the patient's creatinine clearance and lean body weight, not actual body weight. The patient's safe dose is 125 mcg/day (0.125 mg/day), half the amount prescribed. By getting too much medication, the patient suffers digoxin toxicity. The physician who initially ordered the Lanoxin made the first error. Still, the person who administered the Lanoxin should have checked the safety of the amount.

REVIEW and PRACTICE

AGE-RELATED CHANGES

In Exercises 1–4, determine if the *dosage ordered* is safe. Use the height-weight chart from Table 13–1, as needed.

1. The patient: 92-year-old female, 5'6" tall, 130 lb, and CL_{CR} of 61 mL/min.
   Ordered: *Amikacin 375 mg IM q12h*
   According to the package insert, patients with normal renal function may be administered 7.5 mg/kg q12h or 5 mg/kg q8h. This patient has normal renal function.

2. The patient: 76-year-old female, 5'2" tall, 126 lb, and CL_{CR} of 50 mL/min.
   Ordered: *Tazidime 1 g IV q12h*
   According to the package insert, for creatinine clearance levels of 31 to 50 mL/min, the recommended dosage is 1 g q12h; for levels of 16 to 30 mL/min, the dosage is 1 g q24h; for levels 6 to 15 mL/min, the dosage is 500 mg q24h; and for levels < 5 mL/min, the dosage is 500 mg q48h.

3. The patient: 68-year-old male, 5'7" tall, 188 lb, CL_{CR} of 60 mL/min, and impaired renal function.
   Ordered: *Vancocin HCl 150 mg IV q6h*

According to the package insert, the daily dosage for patients with normal renal function is 2 g divided into doses q6h or q12h. The daily dosage for patients with impaired renal function is 1545 mg/24h for creatinine clearance of 100 mL/min; 1390 mg/24h for 90 mL/min; 1235 mg/24h for 80 mL/min; 1080 mg/24h for 70 mL/min; 925 mg/24h for 60 mL/min; 770 mg/24h for 50 mL/min; 620 mg/24h for 40 mL/min; 425 mg/24h for 30 mL/min; 310 mg/24h for 20 mL/min; and 155 mg/24h for 10 mL/min.

4. The patient: 79-year-old female, 5′ tall, 110 lb, CL_{CR} of 90 mL/min, and normal renal function.
   Ordered: *Vancocin HCI 0.5 g IV q6h*
   See Exercise 3 above for information about the recommended daily dosage.

In Exercises 5–6, determine if the *dosage ordered* is safe. Then find the *amount to administer*.

5. The patient: 75-year-old female, 5′3″ tall, 198 lb, CL_{CR} of 56 mL/min, diagnosed with hypertension and renal impairment.
   Ordered: *Vasotec 2.5 mg po qd*
   On hand: Vasotec 5 mg scored tablets
   According to the package insert, the usual dose for patients with normal renal function (over 80 mL/min creatinine clearance) is 5 mg/day; for mild impairment (over 30 and up to 80 mL/min), 5 mg/day; for moderate to severe impairment (30 or less mL/min), 2.5 mg/day.

6. The patient: 81-year-old male, 5′ tall, 138 lb, CL_{CR} of 63 mL/min, and renal impairment.
   Ordered: *Ticarcillin 2 g IV q4h*
   On hand: Ticar 1 gram vial, 200 mg/mL when reconstituted
   According to the package insert, the usual dose, after the initial loading dose, for patients with infections complicated by renal insufficiency, is 3 g q4h with creatinine clearance over 60 mL/min; 2 g q4h for 30 to 60 mL/min; 2 g q8h for 10 to 30 mL/min; 2 g q12h for less than 10 mL/min; other amounts for patients with complications.

Working with Geriatric Patients

You may be called upon to educate geriatric patients and their families about their medications (see Table 13–2). You may also find yourself responsible for monitoring how effectively patients and their families follow directions for administering medications.

Table 13-2 Teaching Patients About Medications

Name of the medication

Purpose of taking the medication

How to store the medication

How long the patient will need to take the medication

How and when to take the medication

How to know if the medication is effective

Required follow-up (lab tests, doctor appointments)

Possible side effects and what to do about them

Interactions with other drugs and foods

Symptoms to report to the doctor

What to do if a dose is missed

Keeping a list of all medications

When you work with geriatric patients, show them respect. Encourage them, if they are able, to participate in planning their schedule. Listen to their concerns. Recommend that they use the same pharmacy to fill all prescriptions. Encourage them to have one doctor as their primary physician to monitor and approve all medications. Remind them to keep a list of all their medications and to take the list when they see their primary physician and all their specialists.

Be aware of factors that can interfere with their ability to learn about their medications or to administer their own medications. If patients are unable to administer a medication, or if memory or sensory problems make self-medication impossible, then family members will need to be included in the planning and training.

In some cases, geriatric patients may have decreased manual dexterity that can interfere with their ability to inject medications, administer eye drops, or even open bottles. Patients may need to specifically ask their pharmacist for bottle caps that are not child-proof. Patients with difficulty swallowing will need information about which medications may be crushed and mixed with applesauce or pudding. In addition, they need information about which medications may not be broken or crushed.

Many patients cannot read small print. Medications may need to be labeled so that they can easily be read and will clearly describe the purpose of each medication. Do not assume patients can distinguish between colors of tablets; white and yellow may be confused, as may blue and green, or orange and pink.

Geriatric patients often have some form of hearing loss. They may even try to hide their hearing loss from you. Have patients repeat to you the information that you give them. They may also have short-term memory loss. Determine if they need written directions and explanations. Help them work with memory tools, like medication calendars that tell them which medications to take each day. Pharmacies often sell weekly dispensers that have a container for each day of the week; patients or family members can prepare in advance the medications for the week (see Figure 13-1).

Figure 13.1

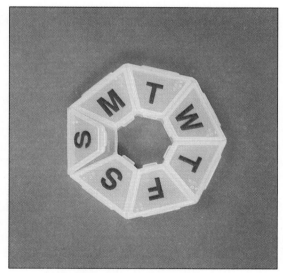

Instruct patients who regularly take prescription medications not to take over-the-counter or herbal medications without first checking with their physician. They should not take more of any medication than is indicated by the label. They should avoid any medications that have expired (show them how to read the expiration date). They should never borrow medications, especially prescription ones, from anyone else.

Polypharmacy

Many geriatric patients take several medications. They often have more than one physician: an internist who is their primary physician and one or more specialists who treat very specific diseases and ailments. Polypharmacy refers to the practice of taking many medications at a time.

Many patients take over a dozen prescription medications each year and numerous over-the-counter medications or natural supplements. They may use medications that were initially prescribed years earlier and are past their expiration date. They may borrow medications. Because of financial pressures, they may also look for ways to limit physician costs by using older medications instead of visiting the physician. They may also order medications by mail or through the Internet, without having direct contact with the pharmacist. In addition, some medications may be prescribed without consideration of their interaction with other medications the patient is already taking.

Drug Interactions

Each additional medication a patient takes increases the likelihood of a drug interaction. These interactions can interfere with the effectiveness of one or more medications. They can also cause serious or even fatal side effects.

Rule 13-1

To identify cases of polypharmacy and reduce the risk of drug interactions, ask elderly patients about

1. all medications they take which are prescribed by either their primary physician or specialists.

2. any over-the-counter medications they take, including vitamins, laxatives, and allergy medications.

3. any social drugs which they use, including alcohol, tobacco, and marijuana.

4. medications that they borrow from family and friends.

5. herbal and home remedies that they use, including natural supplements such as ginseng, gingko biloba, and St. John's Wort.

Adverse drug reactions can be caused by a variety of factors. These include advanced age, small body size, multiple illnesses (including chronic problems), multiple medications, living alone (patients with failing memories or mental capacities), and malnutrition. Elderly patients often take more than one medication to treat the same problem. Sometimes they have neglected to inform a new physician about medications prescribed by other physicians.

Sometimes multiple medications are needed to bring a problem under control. The patient may then continue to take all the medications, even though only one or two are still needed. This overuse is especially common with patients being treated for high blood pressure, constipation, or behavioral problems that occur with dementia.

Health care providers should periodically review with their elderly patients the list of medications the patients are taking. They should look especially for medications that are no longer needed as well as for multiple medications being used to treat the same condition.

Drugs for Elderly Patients to Avoid

Treatment for elderly patients in long term care facilities is regulated by the Omnibus Budget Reconciliation Act (OBRA). The Health Care Financing Administration (HCFA) interprets these regulations and produces guidelines for state health departments. These guidelines include a list of medications that should be avoided for elderly patients (see Table 13–3) as well as a list of medications that should be avoided in certain diseases (see Table 13–4).

Table 13-3 Drugs That Should Be Avoided for Elderly Patients

Due to high risk for adverse effects that may cause significant harm to the elderly, it is recommended that these drugs be avoided. Safer alternatives are available for all of them.

amitriptyline (Elavil)

antihistamines (Benadryl, Vistaril, Atarax, Periactin, Phenergan, Polaramine, Chlor-Trimeton)

barbiturates (Nembutal, Seconal) except phenobarbital

carisoprodol (Soma)

chlordiazepoxide (Librium)

chlorpropamide (Diabinese)

chlorzoxazone (Paraflex)

cyclobenzaprine (Flexeril)

diazepam (Valium)

diphenhydramine (Benadryl) used as a hypnotic

disopyramide (Norpace)

doxepin (Sinequan)

ergot mesyloids (Cyclospasmol, Hydergine)

gastrointestinal antispasmodics (Bentyl, Donnatal, Levsin, Levsinex, Librax, Pro-Banthine)

indomethacin (Indocin)

meperidine (Demerol)

meprobamate (Equanil, Miltown)

metaxalone (Skelaxin)

methocarbamol (Robaxin)

methyldopa (Aldomet)

oxybutynin (Ditropan)

pentazocine (Talwin)

phenylbutazone (Butazolidin)

propoxyphene (Darvocet)

reserpine (Serpasil, Hydropres)

ticlopidine (Ticlid)

trimethobenzamide (Tigan)

Table 13-4 Drugs To Be Avoided in Specific Diseases

These drugs are likely to cause significant adverse effects in elderly patients with the diseases noted.

Severe Risk		Less Severe Risk	
benign prostatic hypertrophy	antihistamines, anti-Parkinson's drugs, GI antispasmodics, antidepressants	benign prostatic hypertrophy	narcotics
cardiac dysrhythmia	tricyclic antidepressants	constipation	antihistamines, anti-Parkinson's drugs, GI antispasmodics, antidepressants
clotting disorders	antiplatelet drugs	diabetes mellitus	steroids, beta blockers
COPD	hypnotics, sedatives, beta blockers	GI diseases	aspirin, potassium supplements
GI diseases	NSAIDs	insomnia	decongestants, bronchodilators, some antidepressants
seizures	metoclopramide (Reglan)	seizures	antipsychotics

CHAPTER *13* REVIEW

CHECK UP

In Exercises 1–6, determine if the *dosage ordered* is safe. If the order is safe, then find the *amount to administer*. Assume that the patients have impaired renal functions.

1. The patient: 85-year-old male, 6'1" tall, 210 lb, CL_{CR} of 64 mL/min.
   Ordered: *Cartrol 2.5 mg PO Q24H*
   On hand: Cartrol 2.5 mg/tablet
   According to the package insert, the usual dosage interval for 2.5 mg is as follows: for patients with creatinine clearance above 60 mL/min is 24 hours; for 20 to 60 mL/min, 48 hours; and for less than 20 mL/min, 72 hours.

2. The patient: 68-year-old female, 5'5" tall, 166 lb, CL_{CR} of 60 mL/min.
   Ordered: *Capastat 500 mg IM qd*
   On hand: Capastat sulfate, diluted to 300 mg/mL
   According to the package insert, the estimated daily dosage required to maintain a steady level of drug is 1.29 mg/kg for creatinine clearance of 0 mL/min; 2.43 mg/kg for 10 mL/min; 3.58 mg/kg for 20 mL/min; 4.72 mg/kg for 30 mL/min; 5.87 mg/kg for 40 mL/min; 7.01 mg/kg for 50 mL/min; and 8.16 mg/kg for 60 mL/min.

3. The patient: 82-year-old female, 4'10" tall, 102 lb, CL_{CR} of 26 mL/min.
   Ordered: *Acyclovir sodium (Zovirax) 450 mg IV q12h infused over 1 hr*
   On hand: Zovirax for Injection, 50 mg/mL when reconstituted
   According to the package insert, the recommended dose for this diagnosis for patients with normal renal function is 10 mg/kg q8h. The dose is adjusted as follows for patients with impaired renal function: For creatinine clearance over 50 mL/min, 100% of the recommended dose every 8 hours; from 25-50 mL/min, 100% of the recommended dose every 12 hours; from 10-25 mL/min, 100% of the recommended dose every 24 hours; for 0-10 mL/min, 50% of the recommended dose every 24 hours.

4. The patient: 73-year-old male, 5'8" tall, 154 lb, CL_{CR} of 49 mL/min, diagnosed with a complicated urinary tract infection.
   Ordered: *Fortaz 1 g IV qd*
   On hand: Fortaz for injection, reconstituted at 10 mg/mL
   According to the package insert, the usual recommended dosage for patients with complicated urinary tract infections is 500 mg-1g given q8-12h. For patients with renal insufficiency, the following maintenance dosages are recommended (however, if the usual dosage is less, administer the lower amount): for creatinine clearance of 31-50 mL/min, 1 g q12h; for 16-30 mL/min, 1 g q24h; for 6-15 mL/min, 500 mg q24h; for less than 5 mL/min, 500 mg q48h.

5. The patient: 79-year-old male, 5'9" tall, 149 lb, CL_{CR} of 55 mL/min. The patient does not have a life-threatening infection.
   Ordered: *Mandol 2 g IV q6h*
   On hand: Mandol reconstituted to 1 g/10 mL
   According to the package insert, for patients with renal impairment and less severe infections, the following maintenance dosages are recommended: for creatinine clearance of over 80 mL/min, 1-2 g q6h; for 50-80 mL/min, 0.75-1.5 g q6h; for 25-50 mL/min, 0.75-1.5 g q8h; for 10-25 mL/min, 0.5-1 g q8h; for 2-10 mL/min, 0.5-0.75 g q12h, for less than 2 mL/min, 0.25-0.5 g q12h.

6. The patient: 92-year-old female, 5'1" tall, 112 lb, CL_{CR} of 32 mL/min.
   Ordered: *Timentin 2 g IV q4h*
   On hand: Timentin reconstituted to 20 mg/mL
   According to the package insert, for patients with renal impairment, the following maintenance dosages are recommended: for creatinine clearance over 60 mL/min, 3.1 g q4h; for 30 to 60 mL/min, 2 g q4h; for 10 to 30 mL/min, 2 g q8h; for less than 10 mL/min, 2 g q12h. For patients with more advanced impairments, lower dosages are recommended.

CRITICAL THINKING

Mr. Peron, who is 68 years old, has a serious infection. He also has impaired renal function. Mr. Peron is 6'1" tall; he weighs 220 lbs. His CL_{CR} is 82 mL/min.
Ordered: *Garamycin 100 mg IV q8h*

According to the package insert, the usual dose for a patient with a serious infection and normal renal function is 1 mg/kg q8h. For patients with renal impairment, the following adjustments are recommended: for creatinine clearance over 100 mL/min, 100% of the usual dose; for 70-100 mL/min, 80%; for 55-70 mL/min, 65%; for 45-55 mL/min, 55%; for 40-45 mL/min, 50%; for 35-40 mL/min, 40%; for 30-35 mL/min, 35%; for 25-30 mL/min, 30%; for 20-25 mL/min, 25%; for 15-20 mL/min, 20%; for 10-15 mL/min, 15%; for less than 10 mL/min, 10% of the usual dose.

Is this a safe order for Mr. Peron? If not, what order would be safe?

CASE STUDY

Mrs. Bell came in for her 3-month checkup for chronic congestive heart failure. The medical assistant noted that her blood pressure was higher than usual and that her feet and ankles are swollen. He asked Mrs. Bell if she had been taking the Lasix 20 mg that the physician had prescribed. She admitted that she has not been taking it on weekdays, but that she took a double dose on Saturday and Sunday.

Further investigation revealed that she was told she must take Lasix in the morning. She said she did not take it weekdays because she spends the day at the Senior Center; she cannot always get to the bathroom frequently. Because Lasix makes her urinate more often, she simply skipped it on Senior Center days, then took twice as much on weekends, when she would be at home and close to the bathroom.

What can the medical assistant do to promote Mrs. Bell's compliance with the prescribed diuretic therapy?

To check your answers, see page 368.

INTERNET ACTIVITY

Note: The Internet is a research tool from which to get basic information. Validate the accuracy of all Internet information.

You work in a long term care facility and are preparing for a state survey. The surveyors are paying close attention to psychotropic drugs. You are asked to review psychotropic drug use for compliance with HCFA guidelines. Check the Internet to learn about the criteria for evaluating the use of these drugs. Suggested key words include HCFA, Health Care Financing Administration, and psychotropic drugs. You may also check the following web site: http://www.ascp.com/public/pubs/tcp/1996/feb/qualityindic2.html

COMPREHENSIVE EVALUATION

The following test will help you check your dosage calculation skills. Throughout the book you have learned a variety of methods for calculating dosages. In these questions, you should use the methods with which you are most comfortable and competent.

In Exercises 1–8, refer to MAR 1.

1. What dose of Neurontin should be administered?

2. By what route should Desyrel be administered?

3. When should Reglan be administered?

4. Why are no times listed for Ativan?

5. Are any of the orders incomplete? If so, what information is missing?

6. What is the likely reason that Reglan is administered half an hour before Neurontin?

7. If the order for Neurontin read q8h instead of TID, when would the second and third doses be administered?

8. If Ativan is administered at 1330, when can the patient receive another dose?

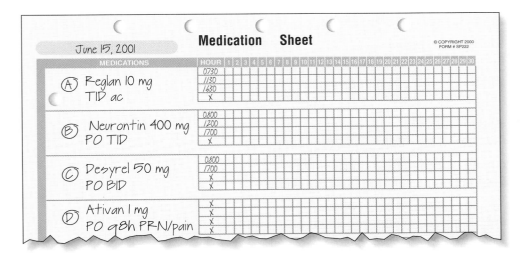

In Exercises 9–12, refer to Label A.

A

9. What is the generic name of the drug?

10. At what temperature should the drug be stored?

11. What is the dosage strength?

12. If an adult took twice the usual adult dose, how long would the container last?

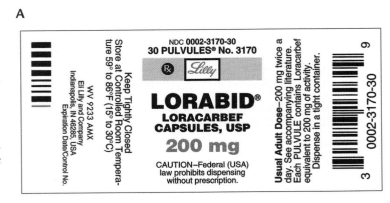

B

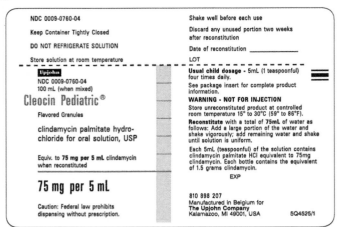

Shake well before each use

Discard any unused portion two weeks after reconstitution

Date of reconstitution _____

LOT

Usual child dosage - 5mL (1 teaspoonful) four times daily.

See package insert for complete product information.

WARNING - NOT FOR INJECTION

Store unreconstituted product at controlled room temperature 15° to 30°C (59° to 86°F).

Reconstitute with a total of **75mL** of water as follows: Add a large portion of the water and shake vigorously; add remaining water and shake until solution is uniform.

Each 5mL (teaspoonful) of the solution contains clindamycin palmitate HCl equivalent to 75mg clindamycin. Each bottle contains the equivalent of 1.5 grams clindamycin.

EXP

810 898 207
Manufactured in Belgium for
The Upjohn Company
Kalamazoo, MI 49001, USA   5Q4525/1

C

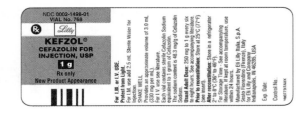

In Exercises 13–14, refer to Label B.

13. How much fluid is used to reconstitute the entire container of granules?

14. If the usual dosage is prescribed for a child, how many days will the container last?

In Exercises 15–16, refer to Label C.

15. How much fluid is used to reconstitute the entire vial for IM use?

16. If *Kefzol 300 mg IM tid* is prescribed for a patient, how many doses are available from one vial?

In Exercises 17–32, calculate the amount to administer.

17. Ordered: *Zoloft 75 mg po qd*
On hand: Zoloft 50 mg scored tablets

18. Ordered: *Zovirax 0.2 g po q4h 5x/day*
On hand: Zovirax suspension 200 mg/5 mL

19. Ordered: *nitroglycerin gr* $\frac{1}{200}$ *SL stat*
On hand: nitroglycerin 0.3 mg tablets

20. Ordered: *morphine sulfate gr* $\frac{1}{4}$ *sc q4h prn/pain*
On hand: morphine sulfate 10 mg/mL vial

21. Ordered: *Claforan 0.6 g IM 30 min pre-op*
On hand: Claforan 300 mg/mL when reconstituted

22. Ordered: *Sandostatin 0.3 mg sc tid*
On hand: Sandostatin 200 mcg/mL multi-dose vial

23. The patient is 14 years old and weighs 97 pounds.
Ordered: *Agenerase sol 17 mg/kg po tid*
On hand: Agenerase Oral Solution, 15 mg/mL

24. The patient is 10 years old and weighs 62 pounds.
Ordered: *Nebcin 1.7 mg/kg IM q6h*
On hand: Nebcin 40 mg/mL multiple-dose vial

25. Ordered: *Follistim 200 IU sc qd*
On hand: Follistim reconstituted to 225 IU/mL

26. The patient is 7 years old and weighs 49 pounds.
Ordered: *Zinacef 20 mg/kg IM q6h*
On hand: Zinacef 220 mg/mL when reconstituted

27. Ordered: *Prilosec 40 mg po qd*
On hand: Refer to Label D.

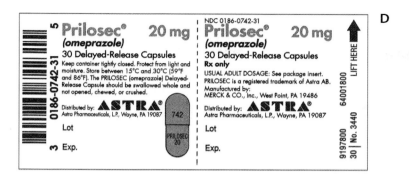

28. Ordered: *Univasc 7.5 mg po qd*
1 hour ac
On hand: Refer to Label E.

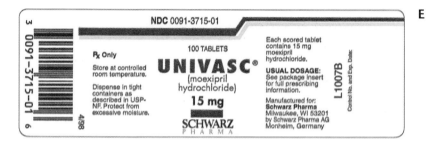

29. Ordered: *Megace 800 mg po qd*
On hand: Refer to Label F.

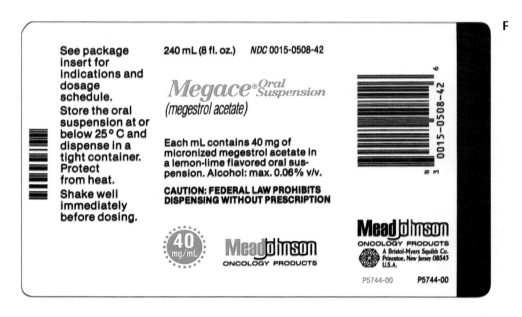

30. The patient is 7 years old and weighs 55 pounds.
Ordered: *Lanoxin Pediatric elix 7 mcg/kg po bid*
On hand: Refer to Label G.

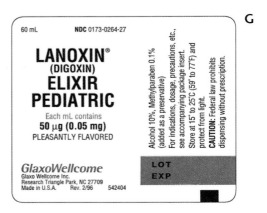

G

31. Ordered: *Haldol 3 mg IM q8h*
On hand: Refer to Label H.

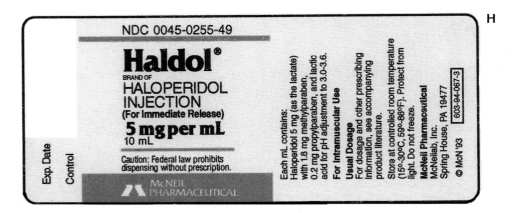

H

32. Ordered: *Vistaril 60 mg IM stat and q6h PRN/emotion*
On hand: Refer to Label I.

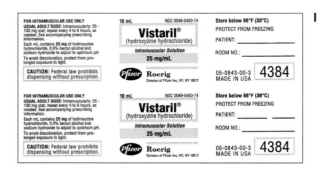

I

33. Which of the following insulins is rapid-acting?
Refer to Labels J and K.

J

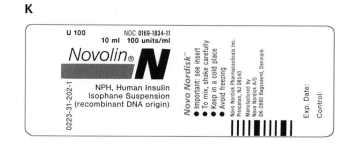

K

34. In what order will you draw the insulin into the syringe for the following order?
Ordered: *Humulin N 46 units and Humulin R 8 units sc ac breakfast*

In Exercises 35–42, find the flow rate.

35. Ordered: *1000 mL RL over 8 hours, using an infusion pump*

36. Ordered: *600 mL 5%D NS over 4 h, 15 gtt/mL tubing*

37. Find the flow rate for an adult who weighs 147 lb.
Ordered: *Garamycin 1.2 mg/kg IV q8h over 45 min*
On hand: Garamycin injectable, 2 mL vial with 40 mg/mL, and 15 gtt/mL tubing; the injection is diluted with 68 mL of D5W.

38. Find the flow rate for a child who weighs 68 lb.
Ordered: *Zofran 0.1 mg/kg IV over 4 min*
On hand: Zofran, premixed with 32 mg in 5% Dextrose, 50 mL, and 10 gtt/mg tubing

39. Find the flow rate for an adult who weighs 134 lb.
Ordered: *Cytoxan 15 mg/kg IV over 30 min tid*
On hand: Refer to Label L. Tubing is 20 gtt/mL.

40. Ordered: *Vasotec 1.25 mg IV over 5 min q6h*
On hand: Refer to Label M. Tubing is microdrip.

L

M

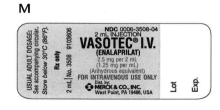

41. Ordered: *Heparin 1300 U/h IV*
On hand: 50,000 U in 1000 mL D5W, 20 gtt/mL tubing

42. Ordered: *Heparin 850 U/h IV*
On hand: 40,000 U in 500 mL D5W via infusion pump

43. Find the amount of medication that has already been administered to the patient.
Ordered: *nitroprusside 40 mg in 500 mL D5W*
The patient has received 175 mL.

44. Calculate the original flow rate for the following order. Then determine if an adjustment is necessary and calculate the adjusted flow rate.
    Ordered: *650 mL NS over 8 h* (15 gtt/mL tubing)
    With five hours remaining, 490 mL of NS remains in the IV bag.

45. The patient's height is 59 inches and weight is 93 pounds. What is the patient's BSA?

46. The patient's height is 150 cm and weight is 61 kg. What is the patient's BSA?

47. The adult patient's height is 66 inches and weight is 125 pounds.
    Ordered: *BiCNU 200 mg/m^2 IV over 2 hr*
    How many mg of BiCNU should be administered?

48. The adult patient's height is 60 inches and weight is 103 pounds. What is the flow rate?
    Ordered: *Leucovorin Calcium 200 mg/m^2 IV over 6 min*
    On hand: Refer to Label N. Tubing is 10 gtt/mL

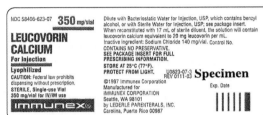

N

49. Find the daily maintenance fluid needs for a child who weighs 18 kg. Then find the microdrip tubing flow rate for DMFN.

50. The patient: 78-year-old male, 5′ 7″ tall, 148 lb, CL_{CR} of 48 mL/min. Determine if the order is safe. If it is, then find the amount to administer.
    Ordered: *Timentin 1.7 g IV q4h*
    On hand: Timentin reconstituted to 20 mg/mL
    According to the package insert, for patients with renal impairment, the following maintenance dosages are recommended: for creatinine clearance over 60 mL/min, 3.1 g q4h; for 30 to 60 mL/min, 2 g q4h; for 10 to 30 mL/min, 2 g q8h; for less than 10 mL/min, 2 g q12h. For patients with more advanced impairments, lower dosages are recommended.

Score 2 points for each exercise you have answered correctly. Your score should be no less than 90. To check your answers, see page 369.

PRETEST ANSWERS

1. 27
2. XIV
3. $4\frac{2}{3}$
4. $\frac{31}{8}$
5. 6
6. 18
7. $\frac{2}{5}$
8. $\frac{3}{8}$
9. $1\frac{7}{40}$
10. $2\frac{1}{21}$
11. $\frac{9}{20}$

12. $5\frac{11}{12}$
13. $\frac{1}{15}$
14. 14
15. $\frac{5}{6}$
16. 2
17. 1.009
18. 14
19. 6.1
20. 19.20
21. 3.8
22. $\frac{9}{200}$

23. 15.3
24. 5.112
25. 14.7
26. 99.43
27. 0.224
28. 20
29. 0.008
30. 99%
31. $2\frac{3}{5}$
32. 112.5%
33. $7:12 = \frac{7}{12}$

34. 1:5
35. 0.08
36. 2:5
37. 38%
38. 1:200
39. true
40. not true
41. ? = 6
42. ? = 8

43. The nurse gives the patient 6 teaspoons each day.

44. The desired supply is short by $2\frac{1}{2}$ bottles. The technician will order 3 bottles.

45. 58.7 milliliters remain in the bottle.

46. The patient receives 1.875 milligrams over five days.

47. 40 grams of medication remain in the bag.

48. The solution contains 6 mL of active drug.

49. 5 mg:500 mL = 1 mg:100 mL

50. 25 mg:1 tablet

CHAPTER 1 ANSWERS

REVIEW AND PRACTICE:
Roman Numerals

1. 6
2. 12
3. 9
4. 14
5. 24

6. 18
7. XIII
8. VIII
9. XXIII
10. XVII

11. xxix
12. xxiv
13. 21
14. 26
15. 11

16. 10
17. 16
18. 7
19. 18
20. 25

REVIEW AND PRACTICE:
Working With Common Fractions

1. 17

2. 8

3. 100

4. 1

5. a, d

6. a, b, d

7. a. $\frac{4}{12}$ b. $\frac{8}{12}$

8. a. $\frac{6}{20}$ b. $\frac{14}{20}$

9. $\frac{16}{3}$

10. $\frac{4}{15}$

11. a. =   b. <   c. >

12. a. >   b. <   c. =

13. $7\frac{1}{6}$

14. $5\frac{2}{3}$

15. 5

16. 1

17. $1\frac{3}{5}$

18. $6\frac{17}{25}$

19. $\frac{50}{17}$

20. $\frac{80}{9}$

21. $\frac{11}{10}$

22. $\frac{33}{8}$

23. $\frac{311}{3}$

24. $\frac{55}{8}$

REVIEW AND PRACTICE:
Equivalent Fractions

For exercises 1–8, answers may vary.

1. $\frac{8}{10}, \frac{16}{20}, \frac{20}{25}$

2. $\frac{2}{20}, \frac{3}{30}, \frac{10}{100}$

3. $\frac{2}{1}, \frac{8}{4}, \frac{16}{8}$

4. $\frac{5}{3}, \frac{30}{18}, \frac{45}{27}$

5. $\frac{18}{2}, \frac{27}{3}, \frac{81}{9}$

6. $\frac{48}{2}, \frac{72}{3}, \frac{96}{4}$

7. $\frac{14}{6}, \frac{21}{9}, \frac{28}{12}$

8. $\frac{11}{3}, \frac{66}{18}, \frac{99}{27}$

9. 6

10. 9

11. 4

12. 6

13. 12

14. 60

15. 210

16. 17

REVIEW AND PRACTICE:
Simplifying Fractions to Lowest Terms

1. $\frac{5}{6}$

2. $\frac{1}{2}$

3. $\frac{1}{3}$

4. $\frac{1}{2}$

5. $\frac{1}{10}$

6. $\frac{11}{20}$

7. $\frac{4}{5}$

8. $\frac{6}{17}$

9. $\frac{7}{9}$

10. $\frac{7}{10}$

11. $\frac{8}{15}$

12. $\frac{7}{12}$

REVIEW AND PRACTICE:
Finding Common Denominators

1. LCD: 21

   $\frac{7}{21}$ and $\frac{3}{21}$

2. LCD: 40

   $\frac{8}{40}$ and $\frac{5}{40}$

3. LCD: 200

   $\frac{8}{200}$ and $\frac{5}{200}$

4. LCD: 72

   $\frac{3}{72}$ and $\frac{2}{72}$

5. LCD: 12

   $\frac{6}{12}$ and $\frac{1}{12}$

6. LCD: 18

   $\frac{3}{18}$ and $\frac{1}{18}$

7. LCD: 42

   $\frac{35}{42}$ and $\frac{24}{42}$

8. LCD: 8

   $\frac{6}{8}$ and $\frac{5}{8}$

9. LCD: 240

$\frac{88}{240}$ and $\frac{63}{240}$

10. LCD: 144

$\frac{15}{144}$ and $\frac{14}{144}$

11. LCD: 12

$\frac{6}{12}, \frac{4}{12},$ and $\frac{3}{12}$

12. LCD: 72

$\frac{12}{72}, \frac{32}{72},$ and $\frac{39}{72}$

13. LCD: 45

$\frac{30}{45}, \frac{20}{45},$ and $\frac{21}{45}$

14. LCD: 48

$\frac{12}{48}, \frac{40}{48},$ and $\frac{21}{48}$

REVIEW AND PRACTICE:
Comparing Fractions

1. <

2. >

3. =

4. >

5. =

6. >

7. >

8. >

9. <

10. >

11. <

12. <

13. >

14. =

15. $\frac{5}{6}, \frac{3}{4}, \frac{4}{7}, \frac{2}{5}$

16. $\frac{4}{7}, \frac{5}{9}, \frac{1}{2}, \frac{1}{3}$

17. $\frac{5}{2}, 2\frac{1}{10}, 1\frac{3}{16}, \frac{9}{8}$

18. $2\frac{1}{2}, 1\frac{5}{6}, \frac{5}{3}, \frac{12}{9}$

19. too little

20. yes, $\frac{25}{125} = \frac{1}{5}$

21. north wing

22. Martha

REVIEW AND PRACTICE:
Adding Fractions

1. $\frac{1}{2}$

2. $\frac{4}{7}$

3. $\frac{2}{7}$

4. $\frac{2}{3}$

5. $\frac{13}{24}$

6. $\frac{12}{25}$

7. $1\frac{5}{24}$

8. $1\frac{11}{18}$

9. $2\frac{4}{5}$

10. $3\frac{8}{11}$

11. $1\frac{5}{6}$

12. $2\frac{23}{40}$

13. $5\frac{29}{35}$

14. $3\frac{5}{8}$

15. $\frac{33}{40}$

16. $\frac{47}{60}$

17. $1\frac{17}{24}$

18. $1\frac{23}{30}$

19. $160\frac{1}{4}$ pounds

20. $2\frac{2}{3}$ cups

21. 2 tablespoons

22. 12 hours

REVIEW AND PRACTICE:
Subtracting Fractions

1. $3\frac{1}{5}$

2. $\frac{1}{5}$

3. $3\frac{1}{3}$

4. $\frac{3}{7}$

5. $\frac{7}{18}$

6. $\frac{7}{12}$

7. $1\frac{5}{8}$

8. $2\frac{1}{8}$

9. $5\frac{1}{2}$

10. $3\frac{3}{4}$

11. $11\frac{17}{30}$

12. $4\frac{9}{35}$

13. $20\frac{15}{16}$

14. $4\frac{19}{20}$

15. $5\frac{1}{3}$

16. $6\frac{4}{7}$

17. $\frac{3}{8}$ cup

18. $\frac{5}{8}$ cup

19. $3\frac{3}{4}$ bottles

20. $143\frac{3}{4}$ pounds

REVIEW AND PRACTICE:
Multiplying Fractions

1. $\frac{1}{48}$
2. $\frac{6}{35}$
3. $\frac{3}{8}$
4. $\frac{1}{9}$
5. $\frac{1}{6}$
6. $\frac{1}{6}$
7. 1

8. $1\frac{1}{2}$
9. $4\frac{1}{2}$
10. $2\frac{1}{2}$
11. $1\frac{1}{2}$
12. 2
13. $19\frac{7}{12}$
14. $14\frac{3}{10}$

15. $\frac{7}{24}$
16. $\frac{9}{56}$
17. $\frac{3}{4}$
18. $\frac{1}{2}$
19. $\frac{2}{5}$
20. 1
21. 234 doses

22. $1\frac{1}{8}$ grains
23. a. $1\frac{1}{3}$ tablespoons
    b. $\frac{3}{4}$ tablespoon
    c. $\frac{7}{12}$ tablespoon
24. 30 ounces

REVIEW AND PRACTICE:
Dividing Fractions

1. $\frac{28}{45}$
2. $\frac{15}{44}$
3. $\frac{3}{4}$
4. $\frac{2}{9}$
5. $2\frac{2}{5}$

6. $1\frac{7}{15}$
7. $1\frac{1}{2}$
8. 1
9. $2\frac{5}{8}$
10. $\frac{1}{2}$

11. $1\frac{7}{9}$
12. $2\frac{4}{5}$
13. $\frac{5}{24}$
14. $9\frac{3}{5}$
15. $1\frac{1}{8}$

16. $1\frac{7}{9}$
17. 160 doses
18. 60 doses
19. 16 times
20. 48 vials

REVIEW AND PRACTICE:
Working With Decimals

1. 0.2
2. 0.17
3. 6.5

4. 7.19
5. 0.003
6. 0.023

7. >
8. >
9. <

10. >
11. <
12. >

REVIEW AND PRACTICE:
Rounding Decimals

1. 14.3
2. 3.5
3. 0.9
4. 0.2
5. 1.0

6. 0.2
7. 9.29
8. 55.17
9. 4.01
10. 2.21

11. 5.52
12. 12.00
13. 11
14. 20
15. 2

16. 51
17. 3.8 milliliters
18. 0.38 milliliters

REVIEW AND PRACTICE:
Converting Fractions Into Decimals

1. 0.4	5. 0.333	9. 1.5	13. 1.8
2. 0.35	6. 0.444	10. 2.2	14. 2.1
3. 0.75	7. 0.556	11. 2.333	15. 6.75
4. 0.5	8. 0.583	12. 1.125	16. 3.5

REVIEW AND PRACTICE:
Converting Decimals Into Fractions

1. $1\frac{1}{5}$	3. $\frac{3}{10}$	5. $5\frac{3}{100}$	7. $100\frac{1}{25}$
2. $98\frac{3}{5}$	4. $\frac{221}{500}$	6. $\frac{301}{1000}$	8. $206\frac{7}{100}$

REVIEW AND PRACTICE:
Adding and Subtracting Decimals

1. 10.82	6. 2.305	11. 5.57	16. 11.98
2. 165.12	7. 0.805	12. 13.8	17. 1.9 degrees
3. 13.66	8. 4.025	13. 0.82	18. $7.45
4. 26.512	9. 14.25	14. 11.228	19. 2.25 grains
5. 2.51	10. 14.625	15. 7.924	20. 37.4 mL

REVIEW AND PRACTICE:
Multiplying Decimals

1. 60.68	5. 0.275	9. 14.42	13. 37.5 milliliters
2. 9.031	6. 0.0108	10. 1.08	14. 4.48 milliliters
3. 1.26	7. 0.00006	11. 0.062	15. 1.125 milligrams
4. 0.1216	8. 0.1875	12. 0.16004	16. 0.2 milligrams

REVIEW AND PRACTICE:
Dividing Decimals

1. 2	6. 0.4	11. 0.2905	16. 80 doses
2. 27	7. 0.0125	12. 0.00348	17. 0.25 grains per dose
3. 122.5	8. 3.15	13. 1322.2	18. 3.75 pounds per month
4. 2	9. 50	14. 6060	
5. 2.5	10. 0.1	15. 80 doses	

CHAPTER 1 REVIEW

1. 24

2. 9

3. 18

4. 29

5. $\frac{19}{8}$

6. $\frac{9}{7}$

7. $\frac{99}{10}$

8. $\frac{155}{12}$

9. $\frac{1}{3}$

10. $\frac{13}{16}$

11. 5

12. $7\frac{1}{8}$

13. LCD: 10

  $\frac{3}{10}$ and $\frac{8}{10}$

14. LCD: 18

  $\frac{15}{18}$ and $\frac{8}{18}$

15. LCD: 24

  $\frac{9}{24}, \frac{18}{24},$ and $\frac{4}{24}$

16. LCD: 60

  $\frac{42}{60}, \frac{15}{60},$ and $\frac{40}{60}$

17. >

18. <

19. =

20. <

21. $2\frac{11}{12}$

22. 2

23. $\frac{29}{100}$

24. $7\frac{3}{8}$

25. $\frac{8}{9}$

26. $\frac{1}{20}$

27. $1\frac{3}{8}$

28. $2\frac{5}{7}$

29. $\frac{5}{9}$

30. $\frac{1}{6}$

31. 8

32. $4\frac{1}{8}$

33. $\frac{4}{21}$

34. 16

35. $15\frac{3}{4}$

36. $\frac{4}{15}$

37. >

38. >

39. =

40. <

41. 0.23

42. 7.09

43. 46.00

44. 9.89

45. 4.3

46. 3.7

47. 7.0

48. 0.1

49. 9

50. 21

51. 1

52. 12

53. 0.5

54. 0.625

55. 2.6

56. 8

57. $\frac{41}{50}$

58. $\frac{13}{20}$

59. $3\frac{1}{2}$

60. $1\frac{1}{1000}$

61. 19.61

62. 4.79

63. 1.021

64. 13.704

65. 7.11

66. 0.89

67. 0.242

68. 13.222

69. 11.27

70. 0.00066

71. 4.995

72. 12.07005

73. 18.5

74. 1.5

75. 20

76. 20

77. Type O — $\frac{4}{9}$

  Type A — $\frac{5}{18}$

  Type AB — $\frac{1}{9}$

  Type B — $\frac{1}{6}$

78. receives $\frac{2}{3}$ cup; amount is $\frac{5}{6}$ cup less than the patient should receive

79. $8\frac{3}{4}$

80. a. 64 doses

  b. 40 doses

Critical Thinking

$\frac{1}{16}, \frac{1}{8}, \frac{3}{16}, \frac{1}{4}, \frac{5}{16}, \frac{7}{16}, \frac{1}{2}$

$\frac{3}{8}$–diameter instrument is missing.

Case Study

Day 2, 8:00 A.M. $+1\frac{1}{2}$ pounds

Day 3, 8:00 A.M. $+1\frac{3}{4}$ pounds

Day 3, 2:00 P.M.	$-1\frac{1}{2}$ pounds
Day 4, 8:00 A.M.	$-1\frac{1}{2}$ pounds
Day 4, 4:00 P.M.	$-2\frac{1}{4}$ pounds

Internet Activity

Pages on the Internet change frequently. Any URLs listed may have been removed from the Internet by the time you use this text.

http://www.meds.com

CHAPTER 2 ANSWERS

REVIEW AND PRACTICE:
Working With Percents

1. 0.14	10. 0.038	19. 1500%	28. $\frac{7}{500}$
2. 0.3	11. 0.045	20. 3200%	29. 75%
3. 0.02	12. 2.5075	21. $\frac{11}{50}$	30. 80%
4. 0.09	13. 404%	22. $\frac{1}{25}$	31. 17%
5. 1.03	14. 230%	23. $1\frac{29}{50}$	32. 56%
6. 3	15. 70%	24. 3	33. 110%
7. 0.00021	16. 33%	25. $\frac{1}{1000}$	34. 225%
8. 0.004	17. 6%	26. $\frac{1}{125}$	35. 175%
9. 0.425	18. 1.3%	27. $\frac{9}{1000}$	36. 40%

REVIEW AND PRACTICE:
Solution Strengths

1. 5 grams	3. 10 grams	5. 100 grams
2. 6 grams	4. 10 grams	6. 25 grams

REVIEW AND PRACTICE:
Working With Ratios

1. $\frac{3}{4}$	4. $\frac{10}{1}$	7. 2:3	10. 7:3
2. $\frac{4}{9}$	5. $\frac{1}{20}$	8. 6:7	11. 15:8
3. $1\frac{2}{3}$	6. $\frac{1}{250}$	9. 5:4	12. 10:3

13. 3:5

14. 2:3

15. 1:50

16. 1:75

17. 0.25

18. 0.13

19. 0.75

20. 0.4

21. 50

22. 12.5

23. 2.67

24. 0.83

25. 9:10

26. 3:10

27. 1:100

28. 9:20

29. 6:1

30. 12:5

31. 25%

32. 4%

33. 22%

34. 41%

35. 2000%

36. 750%

37. 7:50

38. 13:20

39. 4:1

40. 7:4

41. 3:500

42. 9:5000

REVIEW AND PRACTICE:
Ratio Strengths

1. 1 g:20 mL

2. 1 g:20 mL

3. 5 mg:1 capsule

4. 40 mg:1 tablet

5. 1 mg:5 mL

6. 1 mg:10 mL

7. 30 mg:1 tablet

8. 10 mg:1 tablet

9. 1 mL:5 mL

10. 1 mL:2 mL

11. 5 grains:1 tablet

12. 1 g:4 tablets

REVIEW AND PRACTICE:
Writing Proportions

1. $\frac{4}{5} = \frac{8}{10}$

2. $\frac{5}{12} = \frac{10}{24}$

3. $\frac{1}{10} = \frac{100}{1000}$

4. $\frac{2}{3} = \frac{20}{30}$

5. $\frac{50}{25} = \frac{10}{5}$

6. $\frac{6}{4} = \frac{18}{12}$

7. 3:4::75:100

8. 1:5::3:15

9. 8:4::2:1

10. 8:7::24:21

11. 18:16::9:8

12. 10:1::40:4

REVIEW AND PRACTICE:
Means and Extremes

1. True

2. Not true

3. Not true

4. True

5. 16

6. 8

7. 100

8. 20

9. 35

10. 4

11. 9

12. 65

13. 150 milligrams

14. 40 grams

15. 15 milligrams

16. 300 milliliters

REVIEW AND PRACTICE:
Cross-Multiplying

1. Not true	5. 1	9. 200	13. 42 tablets
2. True	6. 25	10. 1	14. 300 milligrams
3. True	7. 24	11. 1	15. 24 hours
4. Not true	8. 150	12. 9	16. 250 milligrams

CHAPTER 2 REVIEW

Exercise	Fraction	Decimal	Ratio	Percent
1.	$\frac{2}{3}$	0.67	2:3	66%
2.	$\frac{5}{4}$	1.25	5:4	125%
3.	$\frac{7}{25}$	0.28	7:25	28%
4.	$\frac{3}{100}$	0.03	3:100	3%
5.	$\frac{40}{8}$	5	40:8	500%
6.	$\frac{4}{12}$	0.33	4:12	33%
7.	$\frac{9}{27}$	0.33	9:27	33%
8.	$\frac{7}{5}$	1.4	7:5	140%
9.	$\frac{1}{200}$	0.005	1:200	0.5%
10.	$\frac{3}{50}$	0.06	3:50	6%
11.	$\frac{1}{4}$	0.25	1:4	25%
12.	$\frac{6}{1}$	6	6:1	600%
13.	$\frac{1}{9}$	0.11	1:9	11%
14.	$\frac{3}{2}$	1.5	3:2	150%
15.	$\frac{6}{97}$	0.06	6:97	6%
16.	$\frac{64}{5}$	12.8	64:5	1280%

17. 40	21. 48	25. 75 milligrams	29. 2 milliliters
18. 1	22. 1	26. 300 milliliters	30. 30 g:100 mL
19. 4	23. 2	27. 25 grams	
20. 25	24. 5	28. 150 milliliters	

Critical Thinking

5 grams

Case Study

a. 250 milligrams

b. 10 milliliters

Internet Activity

Pages on the Internet change frequently. Any URLs listed may have been removed from the Internet by the time you use this text.

http://www.scholarnet.com

http://www.mathleague.com/help/help.htm

CHAPTER 3 ANSWERS

REVIEW AND PRACTICE:
Understanding Metric Notation

1. D	4. D	7. 4.5 mL	10. 0.7 m
2. D	5. B	8. 0.62 g	11. 12 L
3. C	6. C	9. 0.75 mL	12. 0.75 kg

REVIEW AND PRACTICE:
Converting Within the Metric System

1. 7000 mg	6. 0.1 L	11. 250 mcg	16. 500,000 mcg
2. 1.2 g	7. 3600 mm	12. 462,000 mcg	17. 0.008 g
3. 0.023 kg	8. 5.233 m	13. 0.25 mg	18. 0.02 g
4. 8000 g	9. 0.5 km	14. 0.075 mg	
5. 8010 mL	10. 3250 m	15. 60,000 mcg	

REVIEW AND PRACTICE:
Other Systems of Measurement

1. m or ♏

2. dr or ʒ

3. gr

4. oz or ℥

5. gtt

6. tsp or t

7. tbs or T

8. pt

9. mEq

10. U

11. gr vii or gr $\overline{vii}$

12. ʒ v or ʒ $\overline{v}$

13. 3 oz or ℥ iii or ℥ $\overline{iii}$

14. 8 oz or ℥ viii or ℥ $\overline{viii}$

15. gr 14

16. gr 17

17. $\frac{1}{2}$ tsp

18. $\frac{1}{2}$ tbs

19. gr ss

20. $\frac{1}{2}$ oz or ℥ ss

21. $2\frac{1}{2}$ oz or ℥ iiss

22. $5\frac{1}{2}$ oz or ℥ vss

23. 2000 U

24. 40 mEq

REVIEW AND PRACTICE:
Converting Among Metric, Apothecary, and Household Systems

1. 3 tsp

2. 125 cc

3. 24 tsp

4. 8 oz

5. gr $\frac{1}{4}$

6. 900 mg

7. gr $\frac{1}{6}$

8. gr 37ss

9. 92.4 lb

10. 19.1 kg

11. $1\frac{1}{2}$ pt

12. 10 mL of syrup

13. 143 lb

14. 85 kg

15. 2 tbs

16. 960 mL

17. 0.2 g

18. gr ss

REVIEW AND PRACTICE:
Temperature

1. 93.2°F

2. 105.8°F

3. 35°C

4. 38.9°C

5. 7.4°C

6. 100°C

7. 77°F

8. 212°F

REVIEW AND PRACTICE:
Time

1. 0235

2. 0757

3. 0008

4. 0055

5. 1349

6. 1514

7. 2354

8. 2219

9. 12:11 A.M.   11. 3:25 A.M.   13. 1:13 P.M.   15. 9:45 P.M.

10. 12:36 A.M.   12. 8:49 A.M.   14. 3:27 P.M.   16. 11:59 P.M.

CHAPTER 3 REVIEW
Check Up

1. 25.5 kg	14. 8 mL	27. gr ix	40. 28.2°C
2. 0.45 cm	15. 320 g	28. 45 mg	41. 75.2°F
3. 40 mcg	16. 50 mcg	29. 81 kg	42. 110.8°F
4. 0.75 L	17. 0.988 km	30. 103.4 lb	43. 60.1°F
5. 0.9 mg	18. 0.01725 km	31. 325 mg	44. 47.8°F
6. gr iss	19. 0.368 g	32. 20 kg	45. 0321
7. 0.375 g	20. 0.247 kg	33. 15 mL	46. 1642
8. 12 mL	21. gr 120	34. 45 mL	47. 2247
9. 60 mg	22. 150 mg	35. $2\frac{1}{2}$ qt	48. 1120
10. 0.125 mg	23. 6 tbs	36. 90 kg	49. 12:29 A.M.
11. 4 m	24. 25 mL	37. 36.4°C	50. 2:17 P.M.
12. 7.5 mm	25. 30 mL	38. 22.2°C	51. 8:53 P.M.
13. 0.965 L	26. 40 oz	39. 14.1°C	52. 9:12 A.M.

Critical Thinking

1. preferably a calibrated or baking tablespoon, or a calibrated or baking teaspoon

2. 1 tbs of medication every 8 hours

3. two half-pint bottles

Case Study

between 2.22°C and 5°C

Internet Activity

Pages on the Internet change frequently. Any URLs listed may have been removed from the Internet by the time you use this text. The many sites available include:

http://lamar.colostate.edu/~hillger/
http://www.metricusa.com
http://www.neonatology.org/ref/conv.html
http://www.dot.state.al.us/Boards_Committees/metrication/ primer/primer.htm
http://www.agiweb.org/labman/pages/measures.html

CHAPTER 4 ANSWERS

REVIEW AND PRACTICE:
Oral Administration

1. False	5. False	9. False	13. D
2. False	6. False	10. False	14. B
3. False	7. True	11. D	
4. True	8. True	12. C	

REVIEW AND PRACTICE:
Hypodermic Syringes

1. Tenths of a cc (0.1 cc)
2. Units (1 Unit or 0.01 cc)
3. Hundredths of a cc (0.01 cc)
4. Two-tenths of a cc (0.2 cc)
5. True
6. True
7. False
8. True
9. False
10. False
11. False

12. False
13. Type: Standard   Volume: 1 cc
14. Type: Insulin   Volume: 49 Units
15. Type: Tuberculin   Volume: 0.05 cc
16. Type: Large-capacity   Volume: 4.2 cc
17. Type: Standard   Volume: 2.2 cc
18. Type: Insulin   Volume: 22 Units
19. Type: Tuberculin   Volume: 0.8 cc
20. Type: Standard   Volume: 3.0 cc
21. Type: Large-capacity   Volume: 9.5 cc
22. Type: Insulin   Volume: 1 Unit

CHAPTER 4 REVIEW
Check Up

1. A and C	6. A	11. True	16. False
2. C	7. C	12. False	17. True
3. D	8. B	13. False	18. False
4. C and D	9. A	14. True	19. False
5. D	10. D	15. True	20. False

21.

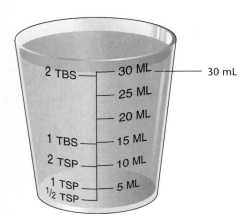

30 mL

22.

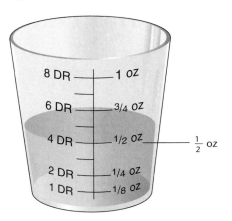

$\frac{1}{2}$ oz

23.

1 mL

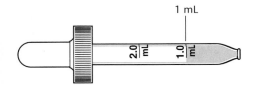

24.

0.6 mL

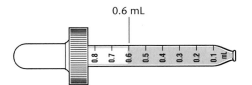

25.

2 mL

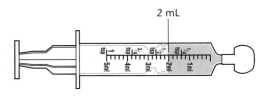

26.

$1\frac{1}{2}$ tsp

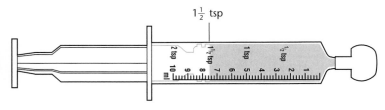

27.

1.5 cc

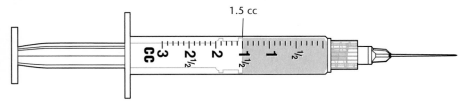

28.

2.3 cc

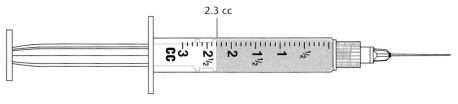

29.

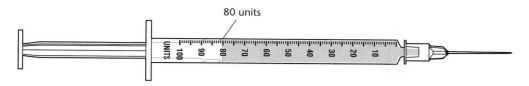

80 units

30.

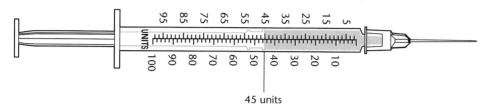

45 units

31.

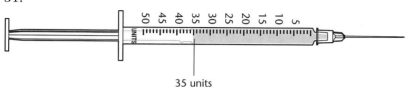

35 units

32.

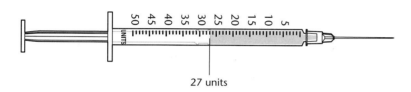

27 units

33.

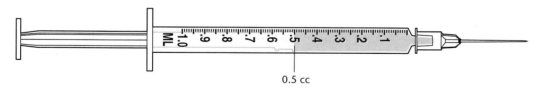

0.5 cc

34.

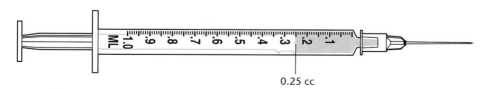

0.25 cc

35.

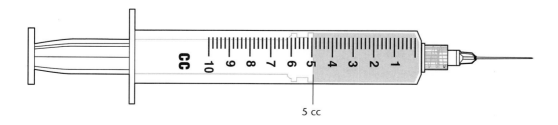

5 cc

36.

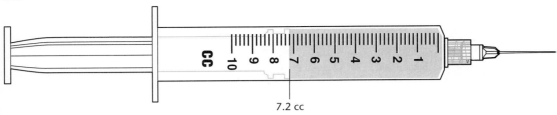

7.2 cc

Critical Thinking

A. standard, safety, or needleless syringe

B. insulin syringe

C. tuberculin syringe

D. oral syringe

E. medicine cup, calibrated spoon, or oral syringe

F. standard, safety, or needleless syringe

G. medicine cup, calibrated spoon, or oral syringe

H. large-capacity syringe

I. transdermal patch

J. dropper or oral syringe

Case Study

The dose to be administered is 0.75 tsp. It could be measured in a calibrated spoon. Another acceptable form of administration would be 3.75 cubic centimeters in an oral syringe.

Internet Activity

Pages on the Internet change frequently. Any URLs listed may have been removed from the Internet by the time you use this text. Answers include:
http://www.cyberlution.com
http://www.new-medical-technology.com
http://www.safetysyringes.com

CHAPTER 5 ANSWERS

REVIEW AND PRACTICE:
Physicians' Orders and Prescriptions

1. The card is complete.

2. 90

3. three times a day

4. 50 mg

5. 180 days or approximately 6 months

6. The strength of the oral suspension is not listed.

7. 100 mL; however, the pharmacy technician still needs to know the solution strength.

8. One teaspoon (i tsp)

9. It cannot be refilled.

10. Every 8 hours (q8h)

11. Three times a day (TID) before meals (AC)

12. Instilled into the left eye (OS)

13. Once a day (qd)

14. 0.4 mg

15. Orally (po)

16. Twice a day (BID)

17. 0.25 mg

18. At bedtime (HS)

19. Sublingually (SL)

20. Seven

REVIEW AND PRACTICE:
Medication Administration Systems

1. Check if the patient's systolic blood pressure is below 110.

2. 5 mg

3. 0630 (6:30 A.M.)

4. sc, or subcutaneous injection

5. The Maalox is administered two hours after meals and at bedtime.

6. 30 cc

7. immediately (card J)

8. instilled into both eyes (card I)

9. The time is based on the patient's needs (card C).

10. IVPB, or intravenous piggyback (card H)

11. A, D, E, F, G, H, and I

12. Card B (no route listed) and Card C (no dose listed nor reason for prn order)

13. three times a day

14. by mouth

15. Dilantin

16. 24 units

17. MDI, metered dose inhaler

18. 500 mg

19. twice a day

20. three doses

CHAPTER 5 REVIEW
Check Up

1. Administer one 2-mg tablet of Dilaudid orally when necessary, as often as every four hours.

2. Administer one 30-mg tablet of Codeine orally four times a day.

3. Instill 2 drops in the right eye 4 times a day.

4. twice

5. instilled into the right eye

6. "for ophthalmic use"

7. every 8 hours

8. by inhalation, using a metered dose inhaler

9. 1000

10. 8 tablets

11. 200 mg

12. twice a day

13. intravenous

14. 10 mg

15. Trental and Rocephin

16. three times a day

17. 8:00 A.M.

18. Order B (the Right Time rule), Order C (does not list a specified route), Order D (does not list the frequency)

19. instilled into the right eye

20. 1.25 mg

21. 0800, 1400, and 2000

22. A and D

23. 0600

24. every 8 hours

25. the doses would be spaced evenly throughout the entire 24-hour period, e.g., 0200, 0800, 1400, 2000

26. Card B (does not list the dose), Card C (does not list the route)

27. Determine if the patients ate at lunchtime. Determine if any medications have to be taken on an empty stomach. Double-check your calculations to ensure that they are correct and that your answers make sense. Make sure you use the appropriate measuring device to administer medications. Finally, ensure that there are no time considerations for administering these medications after a meal.

28. Ask patients their names; verify their names with their patient identification bracelets. Do not administer drugs prescribed for the elderly to children or vice versa.

Critical Thinking

Contact the physician to find the strength that should be given. Administer the tablet immediately. Be sure that the revised order is signed.

Case Study

1. Tell Mr. Burke to take one Tagamet tablet half an hour before each meal and at bedtime.

2. Give 120 tablets at one time. You may refill the prescription once.

Internet Activity

According to the article on cephalexin, the usual adult dose of cephalexin is 1 to 4 g daily, in divided doses. If the patient receives 500 mg q6h, the patient will receive 500 mg every 6 hours or 4 times a day. Four doses of 500 mg is a total of 2000 mg, or 2 g per day. This amount is within the acceptable range. You may want to check for more information by using "cephalexin" as your search word.

CHAPTER 6 ANSWERS

REVIEW AND PRACTICE:
Locating Information on Drug Labels and Package Inserts

1. Amoxil

2. amoxicillin

3. multiple doses, 60 chewable tablets

4. SmithKline Beecham Pharmaceuticals

5. 125 mg/tablet

6. room temperature

7. Clorazepate dipotassium

8. Tranxene

9. 7.5 mg/tablet

10. peach-colored, distinctive T-shape, marked with a code for product identification

11. 03-2192-3/R9

12. protected from moisture, stored below 77°F (25°C), bottle kept tightly closed

13. IntronA

14. 6 doses

15. 3 million IU/0.2 mL

16. injection

17. refrigerate between 2° and 8°C (36° and 46°F)

18. to learn about the usual dose of the medication or how to inject the drug

19. albuterol sulfate

20. orally

21. label does not state; refer to the package insert

22. 2 mg/5 mL

23. 3 teaspoons

24. almost 11 days. The total amount in the bottle is 16 fl. oz. If 1 oz = 30 mL, then 16 oz = 480 mL. Three doses of 15 mL = 45 mL. If you administered 45 mL daily, the bottle would have enough for 10 full days and two doses on the 11th day.

25. kanamycin sulfate

26. Kantrex

27. intramuscular (IM) or intravenous (IV) injection

28. The Kantrex injection should not be physically mixed with other antibacterial agents. The maximum daily dose is 1.5 g.

29. 500 mg/2 mL

30. if the standard dose is 500 mg of Kantrex, then three times daily

31. Augmentin combines amoxicillin and clavulanate potassium.

32. Tap the bottle until all the powder flows freely. Add $\frac{2}{3}$ of the total water (67 mL) and shake vigorously. Add remaining water and shake vigorously.

33. approximately 45 mL

34. 125 mg/5 mL

35. if the drug was not stored in the refrigerator, if more than 10 days had passed since it was reconstituted, if inner seal is not intact, if the container is not tightly closed, and if the powder is not stored at room temperature

36. 15 doses

37. A, B

38. A, B, D, F   39. F   40. C, F   41. C, E

42. Amoxicillin, it is the only drug present in Drug A, as a chewable tablet. It is one of two drugs present in Drug F and must be reconstituted.

REVIEW AND PRACTICE:
Oral Drugs

1. yes

2. 250 mcg/tablet or 0.25 mg/tablet

3. yes

4. You would give the patient $1\frac{1}{2}$ tablets.

5. Lamictal

6. orally to be chewed

7. 5 mg/tablet

8. The label does not provide the usual dosage but refers you to the package outsert.

9. Theophylline Anhydrous

10. 100

11. Each capsule provides 24 hours of medication.

12. No

13. 23 mL

14. 50 mg/mL

15. 30 mL

16. 14 days

17. A and D. A is scored; D is a liquid.

18. D

19. A, B, C, D

20. C

REVIEW AND PRACTICE:
Parenteral Drugs

1. 20 mcg/mL

2. intramuscular injection only

3. Do not dilute; shake well before using.

4. Engerix-B

5. 100 mcg/1mL or 0.1 mg/1 mL

6. Store at 15° to 25° C (59° to 77° F). Protect from light.

7. digoxin

8. No, the label does not indicate the specific route by which the injection is administered.

9. may be habit forming

10. 500 mg/50 mL

11. injection

12. 1

13. rDNA (human origin)

14. 100 units/mL

15. insulin lispro injection

16. 100 doses

REVIEW AND PRACTICE:
Drugs Administered by Other Routes

1. albuterol sulfate

2. 2.5 mg/3 mL

3. 0.083%

4. No further dilution is necessary.

5. topically

6. Store refrigerated 2°–8°C (36°–46°F).

7. 0.01% of the gel

8. becaplermin

9. nasal spray

10. 50 mcg/spray

11. 120

12. no

13. transdermally via a patch on the skin

14. 0.4 mg/hr

15. Each 24-hour period should include a patch-on period of 12 to 14 hours, followed by a patch-free interval.

16. 30

CHAPTER 6 REVIEW
Check Up

1. The generic name is the one official name recognized by the USP and the NF. Brand or trade names can be registered with the U.S. Patent and Trademark Office. A drug may have several different trade names, but only one generic name.

2. when the drug is a combination drug

3. IM means intramuscular, or into the muscle. IV means intravenously, or into the vein.

4. unscored tablets, gelcaps, caplets, enteric-coated tablets, and controlled-, sustained-, or extended-release capsules; breaking them would change the action or absorption of the drug

5. when the label does not have enough information to administer the drug correctly

6. A lot number provides a code that enables a company to know when and where the drug was manufactured. A company can use the lot number to recall a product in the case of contamination.

7. Iberet-Liquid

8. 8 fl oz (236 mL)

9. Abbott Laboratories

10. orally

11. flunisolide

12. by oral inhalation

13. 3.5 g/metered inhalation

14. 50 inhalations

15. no

16. 300 mg/geldose capsule

17. Protect from light. Store between 2° and 25°C (36° and 77°F), in a dry place.

18. 30

19. rDNA origin

20. regular, which means fast-acting

21. by injection

22. 100 units/mL

Critical Thinking

The capsules would probably be preferable for an adult homeless patient. The oral suspension needs refrigeration, a condition that would not be available to someone living on the streets or in a shelter. In addition, a homeless person might not have adequate facilities to wash the medicine cup. Finally, the capsules can be stored in a much smaller container than the liquid and are, therefore, more portable.

Case Study

a. Read the package insert, check any warnings on the package insert, and note any warnings on the label.

b. by intramuscular injection (see the label or package insert)

c. This is a single-dose vial. Dispose of the container, following the guidelines at your facility. Destroy leftover medication, with a co-worker as a witness, following facility guidelines.

Internet Activity

Pages on the Internet change frequently. Any URLs listed may have been removed from the Internet by the time you use this text. By doing a search using words such as coumadin and interactions, you will find a variety of sites. Sample sites include:

http://www.druginfonet.com/faq/faqcouma.htm
http://www.thriveonline.com/medical
http://www.healthtouch.com

CHAPTER 7 ANSWERS

REVIEW AND PRACTICE:
Calculating the Desired Dose

1. Desired dose: 250 mg
2. Desired dose: 500 mg
3. Desired dose: 30 mg
4. Desired dose: 150 mcg
5. Desired dose: 1 tsp

6. Desired dose: 10 cc
7. Desired dose: 300 mg
8. Desired dose: 15 mg
9. Desired dose: 50 mcg
10. Desired dose: 90 mcg

REVIEW AND PRACTICE:
The Proportion Method

1. Amount to administer: 2 tablets
2. Amount to administer: 10 mL
3. Amount to administer: 10 mL
4. Amount to administer: 2 tablets
5. Amount to administer: 5 mL

6. Amount to administer: 1 capsule
7. Amount to administer: 2 capsules
8. Amount to adminster: 2 tablets
9. Amount to administer: 2 tablets
10. Amount to administer: 2 tablets

REVIEW AND PRACTICE:
The Formula Method

1. Amount to administer: 10 mL
2. Amount to administer: $1\frac{1}{2}$ mL or 1.5 mL
3. Amount to administer: $\frac{1}{2}$ tablet
4. Amount to administer: $\frac{1}{2}$ mL or 0.5 mL
5. Amount to administer: $7\frac{1}{2}$ mL or 7.5 mL

6. Amount to administer: 2 tablets
7. Amount to administer: $\frac{4}{5}$ mL = 0.8 mL
8. Amount to administer: $\frac{28}{100}$ mL = 0.28 mL or 28 Units
9. Amount to administer: 3 tablets
10. Amount to administer: $\frac{1}{2}$ tablet

CHAPTER 7 REVIEW
Check Up

1. Desired dose: 5 mg

   Amount to administer: $2\frac{1}{2}$ tablets

2. Desired dose: 16 mg

   Amount to administer: 2 tablets

3. Desired dose: 400 mg

   Amount to administer: 2 tablets

4. Desired dose: 800 mg

   Amount to administer: 2 tablets

5. Desired dose (D): 2 mg

    Amount to administer: 2 tablets

6. Desired dose (D): 7.5 mg

    Amount to administer: 2 tablets

7. Desired dose (D): 0.1 mg

    Amount to administer: 2 tablets

8. Desired dose (D): 250 mg

    Amount to administer: $2\frac{1}{2}$ tablets

9. Desired dose (D): 500 mg

    Amount to administer: 2 tablets

10. Desired dose (D): 20 mg

    Amount to administer: 2 capsules

11. Desired dose (D): 200 mg

    Amount to administer: 8 mL

12. Desired dose (D): 400 mg

    Amount to administer: 10 mL

13. Desired dose: 4 mg

    Amount to administer: 10 mL

14. Desired dose: 60 mg

    Amount to administer: 12 mL

Critical Thinking

1. Amount to administer: 10 mL
2. Amount to administer: 20 mL
3. Amount to administer: 25 mL

Case Study

1. Amount to administer: $1\frac{1}{2}$ of the 5 mg tablets

2. The patient should take $1\frac{1}{2}$ tablets three times a day orally for 7 days.
   The tablets are scored. You may need to show the patient how to break a tablet in half to fill the order properly. Most pharmacies will break the tablets for the patient.

3. The order now calls for 7 mg, rather than 7.5 mg. A combination of a 2-mg tablet and a 5-mg tablet will provide 7 mg of medication.

Internet Activity

Pages on the Internet change frequently. Any URLs listed may have been removed from the Internet by the time you use this text. You can find numerous web sites with information about chemotherapy, both drugs and treatment. Government agencies such as the National Institutes of Health (NIH) and organizations such as the American Cancer Society sponsor many sites. Other sites are sponsored by universities, hospitals, and medical centers. Many individuals, including those who have had cancer, sponsor their own sites. As always, evaluate the quality of the information from each site. Some places to begin include:
http://www.nci.nih.gov (National Cancer Institute)
http://www.cancer.org (American Cancer Society)

CHAPTER 8 ANSWERS

REVIEW AND PRACTICE:
Introducing Dimensional Analysis

1. *dosage ordered:* mg
   amount to administer: chewable tablet

2. *dosage ordered:* mg
   amount to administer: capsule

3. *dosage ordered:* mg
   amount to administer: mL

4. *dosage ordered:* mg
   amount to administer: mL

5. *dosage ordered:* Units
   amount to administer: mL

6. *dosage ordered:* Units
   amount to administer: mL

7. *dosage ordered:* mg
   amount to administer: mL

8. *dosage ordered:* mcg
   amount to administer: mL

9. *dosage ordered:* mg
   amount to administer: tablet

10. *dosage ordered:* mg
    amount to administer: tablet

11. *dosage ordered:* mg
    amount to administer: mL

12. *dosage ordered:* mg
    amount to administer: mL

13. $\dfrac{30 \text{ mL}}{1 \text{ oz}}$

14. $\dfrac{1 \text{ kg}}{2.2 \text{ lb}}$

15. $\dfrac{1000 \text{ mL}}{1 \text{ L}}$

16. $\dfrac{1 \text{ g}}{\text{gr xv}}$

17. 0.7 g

18. 300 mg

19. 0.15 mg

20. 600 mcg

21. 4 tsp

22. 60 mL

23. 3 mg

24. gr iss

25. 88 lb

26. 55 kg

REVIEW AND PRACTICE:
Dimensional Analysis with One Conversion Factor

1. 2 tablets

2. 2 capsules

3. 5 mL

4. 0.5 mL

5. 0.5 mL

6. 0.8 mL

7. 2 mL (injection)

8. $\dfrac{1}{2}$ mL = 0.5 mL (injection)

9. 2 tablets

10. 2 tablets

11. 1.25 mL

12. 1 mL

REVIEW AND PRACTICE:
Calculating the Desired Dose with the One-Step Method

1. 400 mcg

2. 0.25 g

3. 0.2 mg

4. 150 mg

5. 500 mg

6. 0.75 mg

7. 50 mg

8. 0.25 g

9. 600 mg

10. 30 mg

REVIEW AND PRACTICE:
Calculating the Amount to Administer

1. 2 tablets
2. $1\frac{1}{2}$ tablets
3. 10 mL
4. 1.5 mL
5. 3 mL
6. 2.5 mL

7. 2 inhalations
8. 2 inhalations
9. 0.8 mL
10. 12.5 mL
11. 2 tablets
12. $\frac{1}{2}$ tablet

13. 10 mL
14. 10 mL
15. 1.5 mL
16. 0.5 mL
17. 2 puffs
18. 2 mL

19. 2 tablets
20. 2 tablets
21. 7.5 mL
22. 10 mL
23. 3 mL
24. 0.5 mL

CHAPTER 8 REVIEW
Check Up

1. 2 capsules
2. $2\frac{1}{2}$ tablets
3. 20 mL
4. 7.2 mL
5. 4 mL
6. 10 mL

7. 6 mL
8. 10 mL
9. 2 tablets
10. 1 tablet
11. 15 mL
12. 16 mL

13. 0.5 mL
14. 0.5 mL
15. 2 tablets
16. 2 tablets
17. 10 mL
18. 30 mL

19. 10 mL
20. 10 mL
21. 1 vial
22. 0.5 mL

Critical Thinking

$\frac{1}{4}$ tsp

Case Study

1. First patient: $2\frac{1}{2}$ 250-mcg tablets
   Second patient: $1\frac{1}{2}$ 1-mg tablets
   Third patient: $2\frac{1}{2}$ 500-mcg tablets
2. Third patient: 1 250-mcg tablet and 1 1-mg tablet
3. Second patient: 3 500-mcg tablets

Internet Activity

Pages on the Internet change frequently. Any URLs listed may have been removed from the Internet by the time you use this text. The following are among the web sites you might find:
http://www.the-thyroid-society.org   The Thyroid Society
http://www.tsh.org   The Thyroid Foundation of America

CHAPTER 9 ANSWERS

REVIEW AND PRACTICE:
Tablets and Capsules

1. 2 tablets
2. $1\frac{1}{2}$ tablets
3. 3 tablets
4. $1\frac{1}{2}$ tablets

5. $1\frac{1}{2}$ tablets
6. $1\frac{1}{2}$ tablets
7. 2 tablets
8. $2\frac{1}{2}$ tablets

9. $1\frac{1}{2}$ tablets
10. $1\frac{1}{2}$ tablets
11. 2 tablets
12. $\frac{1}{4}$ tablet

13. 2 tablets
14. 2 tablets
15. 2 tablets
16. $1\frac{1}{2}$ tablets

REVIEW AND PRACTICE:
Liquid Medications

1. 4 mL
2. 7.5 mL
3. 5 mL

4. 0.78125 mL = 0.8 mL
5. 10 mL
6. 30 mL

7. 20 mL
8. 15 mL
9. 12.5 mL

10. 20 mL

CHAPTER 9 REVIEW
Check Up

1. $\frac{1}{2}$ tablet
2. 2 tablets
3. $\frac{3}{4}$ tablet
4. 6 mL
5. 7.5 mL

6. 2 tablets
7. 2.5 mL
8. $1\frac{1}{2}$ tablets
9. 10 mL
10. $1\frac{1}{2}$ tablets

11. 2 tablets
12. $\frac{1}{2}$ tablet
13. $\frac{1}{2}$ tablet
14. 3.3 mL
15. 1 tablet

16. 2 tablets
17. 2 capsules
18. 5 mL

19. 2 2-mg tablets and 1 1-mg tablet

20. 2000 mg = 2 g

21. Use: J
    Administer: 7.5 mL

22. Use: E
    Administer: $\frac{1}{2}$ tablet

23. Use: G
    Administer: 2 capsules

24. Use: F
    Administer: 4 mL

25. Use: H
    Administer: 2 tablets

26. Use: Q
    Administer: 3 tablets

27. Use: L
    Administer: 2 tablets

28. Use: O
    Administer: 3 tablets

29. Use: N
    Administer: 12.5 mL

30. Use: M
    Administer: $\frac{1}{2}$ tablet

Critical Thinking

1. a. Isoptin SR: 1 tablet

   b. Valium: 2 tablets

   c. Dilaudid: $\frac{3}{4}$ tablet

   d. Keflex: 2 capsules

2. Isoptin SR and Dilaudid

3. Valium would be crushed and dissolved in water. The Keflex capsules would be opened and the powder dissolved in water. Both would then be administered through the tube.

4. Consult either the pharmacist or a drug reference. Isoptin is now available only in SR form. Dilaudid is available in a liquid form, allowing the precise dose to be measured. With this information, consult the physician about how to handle the Isoptin SR. You would also ask if the Dilaudid liquid could replace the tablets. In some cases, you may need to have the physician's authorization to crush any medication.

Case Study

1. First add half of 55 mL of water to the powdered drug, and shake. Then add the other half of the water, and shake again.

2. 7.5 mL

3. An oral syringe marked in tenths of a milliliter

Internet Activity

Pages on the Internet change frequently. Any URLs listed may have been removed from the Internet by the time you use this text.

http://www.pharmasave.com

http://ohioline.ag.ohio-state.edu/ss-fact/0132.html

http://www.ntl.sympatico.ca/healthyway/HEALTHYWAY/com_4.html

CHAPTER 10 ANSWERS

REVIEW AND PRACTICE:
Calculating Parenteral Dosages

1. Administer: 3.8 mL   Syringe: 2 standard syringes

2. Administer: 2 mL   Syringe: standard syringe

3. Administer: 0.3 mL   Syringe 0.5-mL tuberculin syringe

4. Administer: 0.5 mL   Syringe: 0.5-mL tuberculin syringe

5. Administer: 1 mL   Syringe: 1-mL tuberculin syringe

6. Administer: 1 mL   Syringe: 1-mL tuberculin syringe

7. Administer: 1.6 mL   Syringe: standard syringe

8. Administer: 0.5 mL   Syringe: 0.5-mL tuberculin syringe

9. Administer: 2.5 mL   Syringe: standard syringe

10. Administer: 2 mL   Syringe: standard syringe

11. Administer: 2 mL   Syringe: standard syringe

12. Administer: 0.2 mL   Syringe: 0.5-mL tuberculin syringe

13. Administer: 0.6 mL   Syringe: 1-mL tuberculin syringe

14. Administer: 0.8 mL   Syringe: 1-mL tuberculin syringe

15. Administer: 0.35 mL   Syringe: 0.5-mL tuberculin syringe

16. Administer: 0.3 mL   Syringe: 0.5-mL tuberculin syringe

17. Administer: 0.2 mL   Syringe: 0.5-mL tuberculin syringe

18. Administer: 0.4 mL   Syringe: 0.5-mL tuberculin syringe

19. Administer: 1.5 mL   Syringe: standard syringe

20. Administer: 0.38 mL   Syringe: 0.5-mL tuberculin syringe

21. Administer: 0.75 mL   Syringe: 1-mL tuberculin syringe

22. Administer: 1.2 mL   Syringe: standard syringe

REVIEW AND PRACTICE:
Reconstituting Powdered Medication

1. 17 mL of sterile diluent

2. 20 mg/mL

3. 7 days

4. Store at 25°C (77°F). Keep within a range of 15–30°C (59–86°F). Protect from light.

5. sterile water for injection

6. 2.5 mL

7. Exp. 1/13/2002 1000, 330 mg/mL, with your initials, on the label

8. 0.76 mL

9. sterile water for injection

10. 2 vials

11. 1 mL

12. 1 mL

13. No expiration date. Use reconstituted Follistim immediately and discard the remainder.

14. one injection

15. sterile water for injection

16. 3.0 mL

17. 220 mg/mL

18. *Exp. 6/6/2002 2400*

19. *Exp. 6/7/2002 2400*

20. 3.6 mL

21. 8.2 mL

22. 750,000 Units/mL

23. *Exp. 11/27/02 1200*

24. 2 mL

REVIEW AND PRACTICE:
Insulin

1. vial D

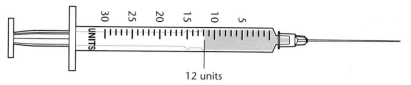

12 units

2. vial A

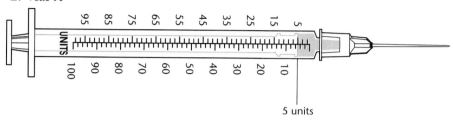

5 units

3. vial C

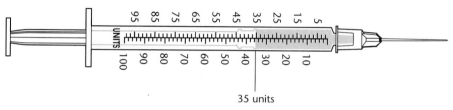

35 units

4. vial B

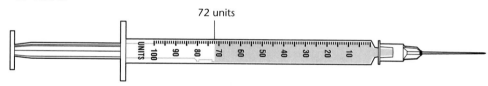

72 units

5. vial G

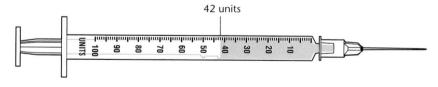

42 units

6. vial E

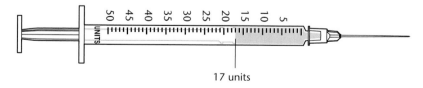

17 units

7. vial F

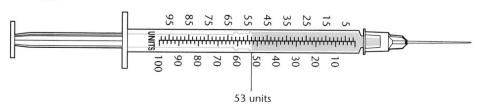

53 units

8. vial F

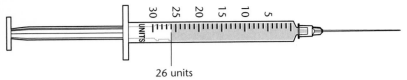

26 units

9. vial B

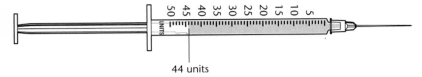

44 units

10. vial A

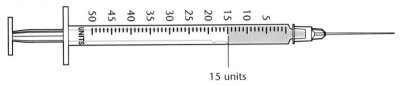

15 units

11. vial C

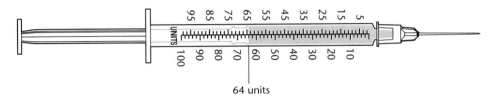

64 units

12. vial G

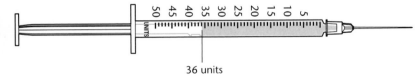

36 units

13. vial E

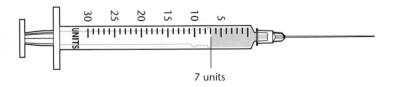

7 units

14. vial D

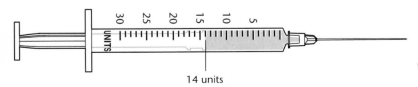

14 units

15.

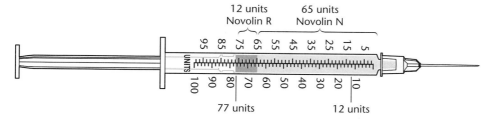

16.

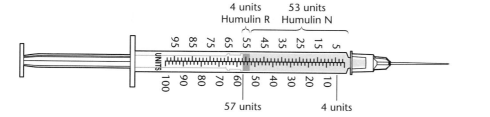

REVIEW AND PRACTICE:
Other Medication Routes

1. 5 mL

2. 0.5 mL

3. 2 supp

4. one 10-mg and one 5-mg suppository

5. 2 patches

6. one TTS-3 patch and one TTS-2 patch

7. one 0.1 mg/day patch with one 0.05 mg/day patch, or two 0.75 mg/day patches

8. one 0.2 mg/hr patch with one 0.1 mg/hr patch

CHAPTER 10 REVIEW

1. Administer: 2 mL   Syringe: standard syringe

2. Administer: 1.2 mL   Syringe: standard syringe

3. Administer: 0.6 mL   Syringe: 1-mL tuberculin syringe

4. Administer: 0.7 mL   Syringe: 1-mL tuberculin syringe

5. Administer: 1.5 mL   Syringe: standard syringe

6. Administer: 2.5 mL   Syringe: standard syringe

7. Administer: 0.8 mL   Syringe: 1-mL tuberculin syringe

8. Administer: 0.75 mL   Syringe: 1-mL tuberculin syringe

9. Administer: 0.75 mL   Syringe: 1-mL tuberculin syringe

10. Administer: 0.1 mL   Syringe: 0.5-mL tuberculin syringe

11. Administer: 0.4 mL   Syringe: 0.5-mL tuberculin syringe

12. Administer: 0.24 mL   Syringe: 0.5-mL tuberculin syringe

13. Administer: 0.375 mL   Syringe: 0.5-mL tuberculin syringe

14. Administer: 0.3 mL   Syringe: 0.5-mL tuberculin syringe

15. Administer: 0.4 mL   Syringe: 0.5-mL tuberculin syringe

16. Administer: 0.25 mL   Syringe: 0.5-tuberculin syringe

17. Administer: 0.42 mL   Syringe: 0.5-mL tuberculin syringe

18. Administer: 0.9 mL   Syringe: 1-mL syringe

19. Administer: 0.625 mL   Syringe: 1-mL syringe

20. Administer: 0.5 mL   Syringe: 1-mL tuberculin syringe

21. 0.1 mL should be discarded.

22. The medication represented by label H should be used. It requires a smaller volume to fill the physician's order.

23. sterile water for injection, bacteriostatic water for injection, or 0.5% or 1% lidocaine hydrochloride injection

24. 1.5 mL   26. 24 hours at room   28. 250 mg/mL   30. 4 mL
                          temperature

25. 280 mg/mL   27. 3.0 mL   29. *Exp. 2000 8/30/2002*

31. Q

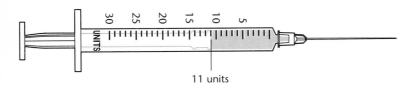

11 units

32. O

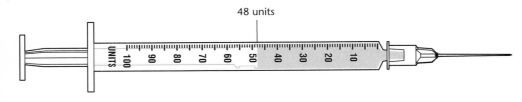

48 units

33. P

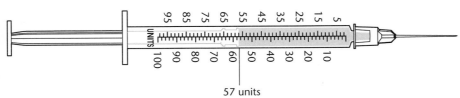

57 units

34. M

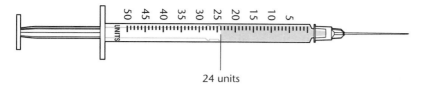

24 units

35. L

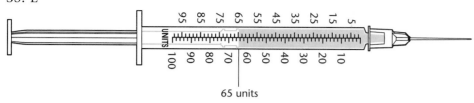

65 units

36. N

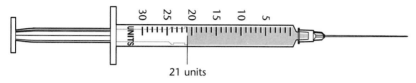

21 units

37.

8 units | 27 units
Humulin R | Humulin N

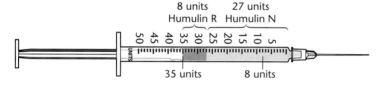

35 units | 8 units

38.

13 units | 57 units
Novolin R | Novolin N

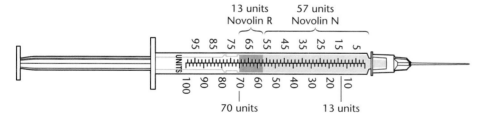

70 units | 13 units

39. 8 mL

40. 0.25 mL

41. two 25-mg suppositories

42. 2 supp

43. 2 patches

44. one 0.2 mg/hr patch with one 0.1 mg/hr patch

Critical Thinking

1. The contents of one vial of the drug should be dissolved in 1 to 2 mL of sterile saline and administered immediately through IM injection.

2. 1 to 2 mL

3. The prepared solution should be discarded. A new solution must be prepared when the patient returns.

Case Study

She would first check whether the patient had any hypersensitivity to any component of the drug or its diluent. If not, she would then check the package insert or PDR and according to what she read, prepare the medication by mixing the entire contents of the vial with 3 mL of lidocaine hydrochloride and shaking it to form a suspension. She would then withdraw the entire suspension and inject it intramuscularly within an hour of its preparation, using a 3 mL standard syringe.

Internet Activity

Pages on the Internet change frequently. Any URLs listed may have been removed from the Internet by the time you use this text. You may come up with web sites similar to those that follow when using the keywords insulin + injection sites:

http://www.merck.com
http://www.diabetes.org/diabetescare/supplement/s31.htm
http://www.diabetesdigest.com
You may come up with web sites similar to the one below when using the keywords insulin + site selection:
http://www.diabetes.ca

CHAPTER 11 ANSWERS

REVIEW AND PRACTICE:
IV Equipment

1. injection port

2. roller or screw clamp

3. slide clamp

4. infusion pump

5. microdrip tubing

6. PCA pump

7. syringe pump

8. ADD-Vantage® system

9. if a patient needed a large amount of fluids, a rapid infusion of medication, an infusion of highly concentrated solutions, or long-term IV therapy

10. flow rate, whether an ordered medication has been infused properly, times at which an IV bag needs to be changed, and signs of infiltration or phlebitis

11. swelling, coolness, or discomfort at the IV site

12. irritation of the vein by IV additives, movement of the needle or catheter, and long-term IV therapy

REVIEW AND PRACTICE:
Calculating Flow Rates

1. 167 mL/h

2. 150 mL/h

3. 125 mL/h

4. 133 mL/h

5. 125 mL/h

6. 83 mL/h

7. 94 mL/h

8. 100 mL/h

9. 75 mL/h

10. 83 mL/h

11. 14 gtt/min

12. 8 gtt/min

13. 31 gtt/min

14. 14 gtt/min

15. 50 gtt/min

16. 16 gtt/min

17. 21 gtt/min

18. 50 gtt/min

19. 50 gtt/min

20. 50 gtt/min

21. 28 gtt/min

22. 23 gtt/min

23. original flow: 21 gtt/min

    adjusted flow rate: 17 gtt/min

24. original flow rate: 33 gtt/min

    adjusted flow rate: 37 gtt/min

REVIEW AND PRACTICE:
Infusion Time and Volume

1. 12 h 3 min

2. 4 h

3. 8 h 4 min

4. 7 h 34 min

5. The infusion will be finished at 2225.

6. The infusion will be finished the next day at 1154.

7. The infusion will be finished at 1402.

8. The infusion will be finished at 0355.

9. 187.5 mL

10. 360 mL

11. 1500 mL

12. 30 mL

REVIEW AND PRACTICE:
Heparin Calculations

1. 75 mL/h

2. $\dfrac{25 \text{ gtt}}{\text{min}}$

3. $\dfrac{8 \text{ gtt}}{\text{min}}$

4. $\dfrac{4 \text{ gtt}}{\text{min}}$

5. The hourly dose is 1000 U/h. This dosage is within the safe daily rate of heparin.

6. The hourly dose is 450 U/h. This dosage lies below (and therefore, within) the safe daily rate.

7. The hourly dose is 3333 U/h. This dosage is well above the safe daily rate of heparin. It would not be safe to administer.

8. The hourly dose is 2400 U/h. This dosage lies above the safe daily rate of heparin. It would not be safe to administer.

REVIEW AND PRACTICE:
Critical Care IV

1. a. $\dfrac{100 \text{ mL}}{\text{h}}$
   b. $\dfrac{33 \text{ gtt}}{\text{min}}$

2. a. $\dfrac{18 \text{ mL}}{1 \text{ h}}$
   b. $\dfrac{18 \text{ gtt}}{1 \text{ min}}$

3. a. $\dfrac{30 \text{ mL}}{\text{h}}$
   b. $\dfrac{5 \text{ gtt}}{1 \text{ min}}$

4. a. $\dfrac{45 \text{ mL}}{\text{h}}$
   b. $\dfrac{11 \text{ gtt}}{\text{min}}$

5. 15 gtt/min

6. 18 gtt/min

7. 21 gtt/min

8. 31 gtt/min

9. The patient has received 0.8 g of Lidocaine.

10. The patient has received 180 mg of Remicade.

11. The patient has received 120 mg of Dobutrex.

12. The patient has received 56 mg of Gentamicin.

CHAPTER 11 REVIEW
Check Up

1. Flow rate = 125 mL/h

2. Flow rate = 62.5 mL/h

3. Flow rate = 100 mL/h

4. Flow rate = 62.5 mL/h

5. Flow rate = 66.7 mL/h

6. Flow rate = 100 mL/h

7. 23 gtt/min

8. 6 gtt/min

9. 42 gtt/min

10. 50 gtt/min

11. 31 gtt/min

12. 50 gtt/min

13. original flow rate: 31 gtt/min
    adjusted flow rate: 36 gtt/min

14. original flow rate: 17 gtt/min
    adjusted flow rate: 18 gtt/min

15. 8 h

16. 4 h

17. 14 h 17 min

18. 17 h 9 min

19. The infusion will be finished at 1714.

20. The infusion will be finished the next day at 0220.

21. The infusion will be finished the next day at 0551.

22. The infusion will be finished the next day at 1326.

23. 688 mL

24. 816 mL

25. 540 mL

26. 398 mL

27. 8 gtt/min

28. 5 gtt/min

29. 15 mL/h

30. 40 gtt/min

31. $\dfrac{1800 \text{ U}}{\text{h}}$
    This dosage lies above the safe daily rate of heparin. It would not be safe to administer.

32. $\dfrac{1260 \text{ U}}{\text{h}}$
    This dosage is within the safe daily rate of heparin.

33. $\dfrac{1600 \text{ U}}{\text{h}}$
    This dosage is within the safe daily rate of heparin.

34. $\dfrac{1000 \text{ U}}{\text{h}}$
    This dosage is within the safe daily rate of heparin.

35. a. $\dfrac{210 \text{ mL}}{\text{h}}$

    b. $\dfrac{53 \text{ gtt}}{1 \text{ min}}$

36. a. $\dfrac{34 \text{ mL}}{\text{h}}$

    b. $\dfrac{34 \text{ gtt}}{\text{min}}$

37. a. $\dfrac{45 \text{ mL}}{\text{h}}$

    b. $\dfrac{8 \text{ gtt}}{\text{min}}$

38. a. $\dfrac{45 \text{ mL}}{\text{h}}$

    b. $\dfrac{15 \text{ gtt}}{\text{min}}$

39. 12 gtt/min

40. 12 gtt/min

41. The patient has received 8 g of magnesium sulfate.

42. The patient has received 3 mg of nitroprusside.

Critical Thinking

1. Set the initial rate at 48 mL/h.
2. The maximum safe rate is 480 mL/h.
3. The infusion rate has not yet reached the maximum safe dose. Therefore, it may be increased in an attempt to lower the patient's systolic pressure.
4. The injection is now running at the maximum safe rate and cannot be raised further. Because the patient's systolic pressure is still above the one desired, you should contact the patient's physician for further instructions.

Case Study

The patient received 4.5 mg of morphine sulfate during the shift.

Internet Activity

1. 5–10 mg/kg in 5 min
2. a. 5–10 mcg

   b. every 5–10 minutes
3. Mechanical ventilatory support should be in place.

CHAPTER 12 ANSWERS

REVIEW AND PRACTICE:
Dosages Based on Body Weight

1. 30 kg
2. 35 kg
3. 24.55 kg
4. 16.82 kg
5. 7.39 kg
6. 5.28 kg
7. 4.49 kg
8. 6.51 kg

9. Two doses of 5 mg, or 10 mg/day is within a safe range.
   Amount to administer: 0.5 mL

10. The order is above the appropriate starting dosage. Consult the physician.

11. The order of 225 mg per dose is above the maximum safe dose for a child with a severe infection. The order should not be administered.

12. The ordered dose of 175 mg is within a safe range. The original solution is mixed with diluent so that its dosage strength is 500 mg/100 mL.
    Amount to administer: 35 mL over 60 minutes.

13. The ordered dose is safe to administer to this child.
    Amount to administer: 2.5 mL

14. The safe range is 300-600 mg/day or 75-150 mg/dose qid. This order is within the safe range.
    Amount to administer: $\frac{1}{2}$ tablet

15. The order is consistent with the recommended dose in the package insert. Therefore, you can calculate the amount to administer directly.
    Amount to administer: 38.16 mL over 30 minutes

16. This order exceeds the safe upper range of 159 mg/dose for this product. It should not be administered. Consult the physician.

17. The maximum safe dose is 102.25 mg/dose. The ordered dose of 150 mg exceeds this amount and may not be safely administered. Consult the physician.

18. The maximum safe dose is 54.5 mg/dose. The ordered dose of 50 mg may be administered safely. Amount to administer: 2 mL

REVIEW AND PRACTICE:
Dosages Based on Body Surface Area (BSA)

1. 0.57 m^2
2. 0.82 m^2
3. 0.25 m^2
4. 0.37 m^2
5. 1.03 m^2
6. 0.69 m^2
7. 0.36 m^2
8. 0.42 m^2
9. 143.5 mcg
10. 0.26 mg
11. 14.65 mcg
12. 0.18 mg

REVIEW AND PRACTICE:
IM and IV Medications

1. 0.64 mL/dose

2. 5.4 mL/dose

3. 14.65 mL/dose

4. 1.68 mL/dose

5. This order is safe.

    Amount to administer: 0.7 mL

6. Upper range: 1109 mg per dose

    Lower range: 832 mg per dose

    The ordered dose of 1 g falls within this range and is safe.

    Amount to administer: 25 mL

7. The ordered amount, 700 mg per dose, is safe to administer.

    Amount to administer: 7 mL

8. The ordered dose of 3.3 mg is consistent with the recommended dose and is safe.

    Amount to administer: 1.65 mL over 4 minutes

9. The dosage ordered is the same as the recommended pediatric dosage.

    Amount to administer: 1.09 mL

10. The order is consistent with the recommended dosage.

    Amount to administer: 2.59 mL

11. Upper range: 1.14 mg

    Lower range: 0.86 mg

    The ordered dose of 1 mg is within this range and is safe.

    Amount to administer: 1 mL

12. Upper range: $1.184 \text{ m}^2 \times \dfrac{75\text{mg}}{\text{m}^2} = 88.8 \text{ mg}$

    Lower range: $1.184 \text{ m}^2 \times \dfrac{60\text{mg}}{\text{m}^2} = 71.04 \text{ mg}$

    The ordered dose of 80 mg is within this range and is safe.

    Amount to administer: 40 mL

13. The flow rate is 12 gtt/min.

14. The flow rate is 11 gtt/min.

15. 800 mL

16. 1760 mL

17. 1341 mL

18. 1628 mL

19. Flow rate: $\dfrac{63 \text{ gtt}}{1 \text{ min}}$

20. Flow rate: $\dfrac{52 \text{ gtt}}{1 \text{ min}}$

21. Flow rate: $\dfrac{32 \text{ gtt}}{1 \text{ min}}$

22. Flow rate: $\dfrac{60 \text{ gtt}}{1 \text{ min}}$

CHAPTER 12 REVIEW
Check Up

1. 22.27 kg

2. 27.73 kg

3. 2.98 kg

4. 5.82 kg

5. 0.74 m²

6. 0.5 m²

7. 0.66 m²

8. 0.47 m²

9. $\dfrac{66 \text{ gtt}}{1 \text{ min}}$

10. $\dfrac{58 \text{ gtt}}{1 \text{ min}}$

11. The ordered dose of 100 mg may be administered safely.
    Amount to administer: 2 mL

12. The usual dose corresponds to the dosage ordered. The order of 1.6 mg may be administered safely.
    Amount to administer: 4 mL

13. The maximum safe dose is 7.04 mg/dose. The ordered dose of 7.5 mg exceeds this amount and may not be safely administered. Consult the physician.

14. The ordered dose is 1300, slightly less than the recommended dosage and, therefore, is safe to administer.
    Amount to administer: 1.73 mL

15. The maximum safe dose is 232.5 mg/dose. The ordered dose of 225 mg may be administered safely.
    Amount to administer: 4.5 mL

16. The ordered dose matches the recommended dosage and, therefore, is safe to administer.
    Amount to administer: 15 mL

17. Upper range: 4219 mg/day
    Lower range: 2110 mg/day

    The ordered dose is for 1 g administered four times a day, or 4 g (4000 mg) per day. This quantity is within the recommended dosage and is safe to administer.

    Amount to administer: 5.56 mL

18. Amount to administer: 0.42 mL

Critical Thinking

1. First patient: Her order is for 90 mg, slightly under the recommended dose of 91 mg, and is, therefore, safe to administer.

   Second patient: His order is for 180 mg, which is about 1% above the recommended dose. In most cases, especially given the relative maturity of the youngster, this dose will be considered safe to administer, though you should check your facility's policy.

2. 2 40-mg and 1 10-mg capsules

3. 1 100-mg capsule and 2 40-mg capsules

Case Study

1. Upper range: 1364 mg/day

   Lower range: 909 mg/day

2. The hourly flow rate is 60 mL/h.

3. The order for 1200 mg is within the accepted range of 909-1364 mg. It may be administered safely. If the infection has not been resolved, you may consult the physician. The physician may order that the dose be increased to the upper range.

Internet Activity

Pages on the Internet change frequently. Any URLs listed may have been removed from the Internet by the time you use this text. Your search on the Internet using keywords such as *leukemia* and *pediatric leukemia* may yield the following Web sites:

http://www.meds.com/leukemia/leukemia.html
http://www.oncolink.upenn.edu/disease/leukemia
http://www.leukemia.org

CHAPTER 13 ANSWERS

REVIEW AND PRACTICE:
Age-Related Changes

1. safe 　　　　2. safe 　　　　3. safe 　　　　4. safe

5. safe; the amount to administer is $\frac{1}{2}$ tablet.

6. safe; the amount to administer is 10 mL every 4 hours.

CHAPTER 13 REVIEW
Check Up

1. safe; amount to administer: 1 tablet

2. safe; amount to administer: 1.67 mL

3. safe; amount to administer: 9 mL

4. safe; amount to administer: 100 mL

5. not safe; consult the physician

6. safe; amount to administer: 100 mL

Critical Thinking

The order of 100 mg is not safe. The safe dose is 80 mg.

Case Study

Mrs. Bell must be taught about the dangers of the way she is using her medication. She must be told that doubling her doses of medication can cause adverse effects, such as a drastic drop in blood pressure, which might make her fall. Telling her exactly what might happen may help her understand the importance of compliance. Point out her symptoms (high blood pressure and swollen feet and ankles) and mention others she might notice, such as fatigue and shortness of breath. Make the connection between these symptoms and not taking the medication.

Ask her more about her schedule to determine whether there is a better way to schedule her Lasix. Patients are often automatically told to take diuretics in the morning, to avoid multiple wakenings at night to urinate. However, most of the urinary urgency and frequency from diuretics occurs in the first two or three hours after taking the medication. Mrs. Bell may spend the evening at home, where she can easily reach the bathroom. If she takes her Lasix with dinner, she will have easy access to the bathroom in the evening, and probably will not experience sleep disturbance because the effects will diminish before she goes to bed.

Internet Activity

The suggested web site includes an article by pharmacist, Michael Posey, with a table that shows how quality indicators related to psychotropic drugs are calculated. The author notes that one problem in state surveys would be lack of documentation of a psychiatric diagnosis to support use of psychotropic drugs. The article also includes a table with the maximum recommended doses of antipsychotic drugs for the elderly. The author explains the inappropriateness of long acting benzodiazepines in treating anxiety in the elderly.

COMPREHENSIVE EVALUATION ANSWERS

1. 400 mg

2. Orally (*po*)

3. 0730, 1130, and 1630

4. The order indicates that Ativan should be administered when necessary for pain, rather than according to a set schedule.

5. The order for Reglan is incomplete. It does not list the route.

6. Reglan is administered before meals (*ac*).

7. 1600 and 2400. If the order was for *q8h*, Neurontin would be administered every 8 hours.

8. 2130. The order indicates that Ativan may be administered every 8 hours. If Ativan is administered at 1330, then the patient may not receive another dose for another 8 hours, at 2130.

9. Loracarbef

10. The drug should be stored at controlled room temperature, 59° to 86°F.

11. 200 mg/capsule (pulvule)

12. The usual adult dose is 200 mg (one capsule or pulvule) twice a day. Therefore, the usual adult dose is two capsules (pulvules) a day. Twice the usual dose, then, is four capsules a day. The container has 30 capsules. At the rate of four capsules a day, the container would last $30 \div 4$ or $7\frac{1}{2}$ days.

13. According to the drug label, 75 mL of water are used to reconstitute the container of granules.

14. The usual child dosage is 5 mL of solution four times a day, for a total of 20 mL per day. The fully reconstituted container will have 100 mL of solution. At the rate of 20 mL per day, 100 mL will last 5 days ($100 \div 20$).

15. According to the drug label, 2.5 mL of Sterile Water for Injection are used. (The total volume of solution, once reconstituted, is approximately 3.0 mL.)

16. The vial contains 1 g or 1000 mg of medication. Three doses is 3 x 300 mg, or 900 mg. (Four doses would require more than one vial.)

17. Desired dose (D): 75 mg

    Dose on hand (H): 50 mg

    Dosage unit (Q): 1 tablet

    $75 \text{ mg} \times \dfrac{1 \text{ tablet}}{50 \text{ mg}} = {}^{3}\cancel{75 \text{ mg}} \times \dfrac{1 \text{ tablet}}{{}_{2}\cancel{50 \text{ mg}}}$

    $= 3 \times \dfrac{1}{2} \text{ tablet}$

    $= \dfrac{3}{2} \text{ tablets}$

    Amount to administer: $1\dfrac{1}{2}$ tablets

18. $0.2 \text{ g} \times \dfrac{1000 \text{ mg}}{1 \text{ g}} \times \dfrac{5 \text{ mL}}{200 \text{ mg}}$

    $= 0.2 \cancel{\text{g}} \times \dfrac{{}^{5}\cancel{1000 \text{ mg}}}{1 \cancel{\text{g}}} \times \dfrac{5 \text{ mL}}{{}_{1}\cancel{200 \text{ mg}}}$

    $= 0.2 \times 5 \times 5 \text{ mL} = 5 \text{ mL}$

    Amount to administer: 5 mL

19. First convert gr $\dfrac{1}{200}$ to mg.

    gr $\dfrac{1}{200}$:? mg::1 gr:60 mg

    $? \times 1 = \dfrac{1}{200} \times 60$

    $? = \dfrac{60}{200} = 0.3$

    Desired dose (D): 0.3 mg

    Dose on hand (H): 0.3 mg

    Dosage unit (Q): 1 tablet

    $0.3 \text{ mg} \times \dfrac{1 \text{ tablet}}{0.3 \text{ mg}} = {}^{1}\cancel{0.3 \text{ mg}} \times \dfrac{1 \text{ tablet}}{{}_{1}\cancel{0.3 \text{ mg}}}$

    $= 1 \times 1 \text{ tablet}$

    $= 1 \text{ tablet}$

    Amount to administer: 1 tablet

20. gr $\dfrac{1}{4} \times \dfrac{60 \text{ mg}}{1 \text{ gr}} \times \dfrac{1 \text{ mL}}{10 \text{ mg}}$

    $= \text{gr } \dfrac{1}{4} \times \dfrac{{}^{6}\cancel{60 \text{ mg}}}{1 \cancel{\text{gr}}} \times \dfrac{1 \text{ mL}}{{}_{1}\cancel{10 \text{ mg}}}$

    $= \dfrac{1}{4} \times 6 \times 1 \text{ mL} = \dfrac{6}{4} \text{ mL}$

    Amount to administer: 1.5 mL

21. $0.6 \text{ g} \times \dfrac{1000 \text{ mg}}{1 \text{ g}} \times \dfrac{1 \text{ mL}}{300 \text{ mg}}$

    $= 0.6 \cancel{\text{g}} \times \dfrac{{}^{10}\cancel{1000 \text{ mg}}}{1 \cancel{\text{g}}} \times \dfrac{1 \text{ mL}}{{}_{3}\cancel{300 \text{ mg}}}$

    $= 0.6 \times 10 \times \dfrac{1 \text{ mL}}{3} = 2 \text{ mL}$

    Amount to administer: 2 mL

22. $0.3 \text{ mg} \times \dfrac{1000 \text{ mcg}}{1 \text{ mg}} \times \dfrac{1 \text{ mL}}{200 \text{ mcg}}$

    $= 0.3 \cancel{\text{mg}} \times \dfrac{{}^{5}\cancel{1000 \text{ mcg}}}{1 \cancel{\text{mg}}} \times \dfrac{1 \text{ mL}}{{}_{1}\cancel{200 \text{ mcg}}}$

    $= 0.3 \times 5 \times 1 \text{ mL} = 1.5 \text{ mL}$

    Amount to administer: 1.5 mL

23. $97 \cancel{\text{lb}} \times \dfrac{1 \text{ kg}}{2.2 \cancel{\text{lb}}} = 44 \text{ kg}$

    $44 \cancel{\text{kg}} \times \dfrac{17 \text{ mg}}{1 \cancel{\text{kg}}} = 748 \text{ mg}$

    $748 \cancel{\text{mg}} \times \dfrac{1 \text{ mL}}{15 \cancel{\text{mg}}} = \dfrac{748}{15} \text{ mL} = 49.9 \text{ mL}$

    The amount to administer is 50 mL.

24. $62 \cancel{\text{lb}} \times \dfrac{1 \text{ kg}}{2.2 \cancel{\text{lb}}} = 28.2 \text{ kg}$

    $28.2 \cancel{\text{kg}} \times \dfrac{1.7 \text{ mg}}{1 \cancel{\text{kg}}} = 48 \text{ mg}$

    $^{6}\cancel{48 \text{ mg}} \times \dfrac{1 \text{ mL}}{{}_{5}\cancel{40 \text{ mg}}} = 6 \times \dfrac{1}{5} \text{ mL} = \dfrac{6}{5} \text{ mL}$

    The amount to administer is 1.2 mL.

25. Desired dose (D): 200 IU

    Dose on hand (H): 225 IU

    Dosage unit (Q): 1 mL

    $200 \text{ IU} \times \dfrac{1 \text{ mL}}{225 \text{ IU}} = {}^{8}\cancel{200 \text{ IU}} \times \dfrac{1 \text{ mL}}{{}_{9}\cancel{225 \text{ IU}}}$

    $= 8 \times \dfrac{1}{9} \text{ mL} = \dfrac{8}{9} \text{ mL}$

    Amount to administer: 0.89 mL

26. $49 \cancel{\text{lb}} \times \dfrac{1 \text{ kg}}{2.2 \cancel{\text{lb}}} = 22.3 \text{ kg}$

    $22.3 \cancel{\text{kg}} \times \dfrac{20 \text{ mg}}{1 \cancel{\text{kg}}} = 446 \text{ mg}$

    $446 \cancel{\text{mg}} \times \dfrac{1 \text{ mL}}{220 \cancel{\text{mg}}} = 446 \times \dfrac{1}{220} \text{ mL}$

    $= \dfrac{446}{220} \text{ mL}$

    The amount to administer is 2 mL.

27. Desired dose (D): 40 mg

    Dose on hand (H): 20 mg

Dosage unit (Q): 1 capsule

$$40 \text{ mg} \times \frac{1 \text{ capsule}}{20 \text{ mg}} = {}^{2}\cancel{40} \cancel{\text{mg}} \times \frac{1 \text{ capsule}}{_{1}\cancel{20} \cancel{\text{mg}}}$$

$$= 2 \times 1 \text{ capsule}$$

$$= 2 \text{ capsules}$$

Amount to administer: 2 capsules

28. Desired dose (D): 7.5 mg

Dose on hand (H): 15 mg

Dosage unit (Q): 1 tablet

$$7.5 \text{ mg} \times \frac{1 \text{ tablet}}{15 \text{ mg}} = {}^{1}\cancel{7.5} \cancel{\text{mg}} \times \frac{1 \text{ tablet}}{_{2}\cancel{15} \cancel{\text{mg}}}$$

$$= 1 \times \frac{1}{2} \text{ tablet}$$

$$= \frac{1}{2} \text{ tablet}$$

Amount to administer: $\frac{1}{2}$ tablet

29. Desired dose (D): 800 mg

Dose on hand (H): 40 mg

Dosage unit (Q): 5 mL

$$800 \text{ mg} \times \frac{1 \text{ mL}}{40 \text{ mg}} = {}^{20}\cancel{800} \cancel{\text{mg}} \times \frac{1 \text{ mL}}{_{1}\cancel{40} \cancel{\text{mg}}}$$

$$= 20 \times 1 \text{ mL}$$

$$= 20 \text{ mL}$$

Amount to administer: 20 mL

30. $55 \cancel{\text{lb}} \times \dfrac{1 \text{ kg}}{2.2 \cancel{\text{lb}}} = 25 \text{ kg}$

$25 \cancel{\text{kg}} \times \dfrac{7 \text{ mcg}}{1 \cancel{\text{kg}}} = 175 \text{ mcg}$

$${}^{7}\cancel{175} \cancel{\text{mcg}} \times \frac{1 \text{ mL}}{_{2}\cancel{50} \cancel{\text{mcg}}} = \frac{7}{2} \text{ mL}$$

The amount to administer is 3.5 mL.

31. Desired dose (D): 3 mg

Dose on hand (H): 5 mg

Dosage unit (Q): 1 mL

$$3 \text{ mg} \times \frac{1 \text{ mL}}{5 \text{ mg}} = 3 \cancel{\text{mg}} \times \frac{1 \text{ mL}}{5 \cancel{\text{mg}}}$$

$$= 3 \times \frac{1}{5} \text{ mL} = \frac{3}{5} \text{ mL}$$

Amount to administer: 0.6 mL

32. Desired dose (D): 60 mg

Dose on hand (H): 25 mg

Dosage unit (Q): 1 mL

$$60 \text{ mg} \times \frac{1 \text{ mL}}{25 \text{ mg}} = {}^{12}\cancel{60} \cancel{\text{mg}} \times \frac{1 \text{ mL}}{_{5}\cancel{25} \cancel{\text{mg}}}$$

$$= 12 \times \frac{1}{5} \text{ mL} = \frac{12}{5} \text{ mL}$$

Amount to administer: 2.4 mL

33. Novolin R is a rapid-acting insulin. Novolin N is an intermediate-acting insulin.

34. Draw the rapid-acting insulin into the syringe first, then the intermediate-acting insulin. In this case, draw Humulin R first, then Humulin N.

35. $\dfrac{1000 \text{ mL}}{8 \text{ h}} = \dfrac{125 \text{ mL}}{1 \text{ h}}$

Administer: 125 mL/h

36. $\dfrac{15 \text{ gtt}}{1 \text{ mL}} \times \dfrac{600 \text{ mL}}{4 \text{ h}} \times \dfrac{1 \text{ h}}{60 \text{ min}}$

$$\frac{{}^{1}\cancel{15} \text{ gtt}}{1 \cancel{\text{mL}}} \times \frac{{}^{150}\cancel{600} \cancel{\text{mL}}}{_{1}\cancel{4} \cancel{\text{h}}} \times \frac{1 \cancel{\text{h}}}{_{4}\cancel{60} \text{ min}}$$

$$= 1 \text{ gtt} \times 150 \times \frac{1}{4} \text{ min}$$

$$= \frac{150 \text{ gtt}}{4 \text{ min}} = 37.5 \text{ gtt/min}$$

Flow rate: 38 gtt/min

37. $147 \cancel{\text{lb}} \times \dfrac{1 \text{ kg}}{2.2 \cancel{\text{lb}}} = 66.8 \text{ kg}$

$66.8 \cancel{\text{kg}} \times \dfrac{1.2 \text{ mg}}{1 \cancel{\text{kg}}} = 80 \text{ mg}$

You want to administer 80 mg of Zofran over 45 minutes. The vial had 2 mL of 40 mg/mL injection, or 80 mg/2 mL. It is mixed with 68 mL of D5W, leading to a solution with 80 mg/70 mL.

$$\frac{80 \text{ mg}}{? \text{ mL}} = \frac{80 \text{ mg}}{70 \text{ mL}}$$

No further calculation is needed to see that you will need to administer 70 mL over 45 minutes. The tubing is calibrated for 15 gtt/mL. Therefore,

$$\frac{15 \text{ gtt}}{1 \text{ mL}} \times \frac{70 \text{ mL}}{45 \text{ min}}$$

$$= \frac{{}^{1}\cancel{15} \text{ gtt}}{1 \cancel{\text{mL}}} \times \frac{70 \cancel{\text{mL}}}{_{3}\cancel{45} \text{ min}} = 1 \text{ gtt} \times \frac{70}{3 \text{ min}} = \frac{23 \text{ gtt}}{1 \text{ min}}$$

Flow rate: 23 gtt/min

38. $68 \cancel{\text{lb}} \times \dfrac{1 \text{ kg}}{2.2 \cancel{\text{lb}}} = 31 \text{ kg}$

$31 \cancel{\text{kg}} \times \dfrac{0.1 \text{ mg}}{1 \cancel{\text{kg}}} = 3.1 \text{ mg}$

You want to administer 3.1 mg of Zofran.

$$\frac{3.1 \text{ mg}}{? \text{ mL}} = \frac{32 \text{ mg}}{50 \text{ mL}}$$

$$3.1 \text{ mg} \times 50 \text{ mL} = ? \text{ mL} \times 32 \text{ mg}$$

$$4.8 = ?$$

You want to administer 4.8 mL of Zofran over 4 minutes. The tubing is calibrated for 10 gtt/mL. Therefore,

$$\frac{10 \text{ gtt}}{1 \text{ mL}} \times \frac{4.8 \text{ mL}}{4 \text{ min}}$$

$$= \frac{^5\cancel{10} \text{ gtt}}{1 \text{ mL}} \times \frac{4.8 \text{ mL}}{_2\cancel{4} \text{ min}} = 5 \text{ gtt} \times \frac{4.8}{2 \text{ min}} = \frac{12 \text{ gtt}}{1 \text{ min}}$$

Flow rate: 12 gtt/min

39. $134 \text{ lb} \times \dfrac{1 \text{ kg}}{2.2 \text{ lb}} = 61 \text{ kg}$

$61 \text{ kg} \times \dfrac{15 \text{ mg}}{1 \text{ kg}} = 915 \text{ mg}$

You want to administer 915 mg of Cytoxan. According to the drug label, the reconstituted vial will have 1 g (or 1000 mg) per 50 mL of solution.

$$\frac{915 \text{ mg}}{? \text{ mL}} = \frac{1000 \text{ mg}}{50 \text{ mL}}$$

$$915 \text{ mg} \times 50 \text{ mL} = ? \text{ mL} \times 1000 \text{ mg}$$

$$45.75 = ?$$

You want to administer 45.75 mL of Cytoxan over 30 minutes. The tubing is calibrated for 20 gtt/mL. Therefore,

$$\frac{20 \text{ gtt}}{1 \text{ mL}} \times \frac{45.75 \text{ mL}}{30 \text{ min}}$$

$$= \frac{^2\cancel{20} \text{ gtt}}{1 \text{ mL}} \times \frac{45.75 \text{ mL}}{_3\cancel{30} \text{ min}} = 2 \text{ gtt} \times \frac{45.75}{3 \text{ min}}$$

$$= \frac{30.5 \text{ gtt}}{1 \text{ min}}$$

Flow rate: 31 gtt/min

40. You want to administer 1.25 mg of Vasotec I.V. According to the drug label, the vial contains 1.25 mg per mL of solution. Therefore, you want to administer 1.25 mL of Vasotec over 5 minutes. The tubing is microdrip, 60 gtt/mL.

$$\frac{60 \text{ gtt}}{1 \text{ mL}} \times \frac{1 \text{ mL}}{5 \text{ min}}$$

$$= \frac{^{12}\cancel{60} \text{ gtt}}{1 \text{ mL}} \times \frac{1 \text{ mL}}{_1\cancel{5} \text{ min}} = 12 \text{ gtt} \times \frac{1}{1 \text{ min}}$$

$$= \frac{12 \text{ gtt}}{1 \text{ min}}$$

Flow rate: 12 gtt/min

41. $\dfrac{20 \text{ gtt}}{1 \text{ mL}} \times \dfrac{1300 \text{ U}}{1 \text{ h}} \times \dfrac{1000 \text{ mL}}{50,000 \text{ U}} \times \dfrac{1 \text{ h}}{60 \text{ min}}$

$$= \frac{9 \text{ gtt}}{1 \text{ min}}$$

42. $\dfrac{850 \text{ U}}{1 \text{ h}} \times \dfrac{500 \text{ mL}}{40,000 \text{ U}} = \dfrac{11 \text{ mL}}{\text{h}}$

43. $\dfrac{40 \text{ mg}}{500 \text{ mL}} = \dfrac{? \text{ mg}}{175 \text{ mL}}$

$$40 \text{ mg} \times 175 \text{ mL} = 500 \text{ mL} \times ? \text{ mg}$$

$$14 = ?$$

The patient has received 14 mg of nitroprusside.

44. $\dfrac{15 \text{ gtt}}{1 \text{ mL}} \times \dfrac{650 \text{ mL}}{8 \text{ h}} \times \dfrac{1 \text{ h}}{60 \text{ min}} = F$

$$\frac{^1\cancel{15} \text{ gtt}}{1 \text{ mL}} \times \frac{^{325}\cancel{650} \text{ mL}}{_4\cancel{8} \text{ h}} \times \frac{1 \text{ h}}{_4\cancel{60} \text{ min}} = \frac{20.31 \text{ gtt}}{\text{min}}$$

The original flow rate is 20 gtt/min. The amount that should have infused in the first three hours is

$$3 \text{ h} \times \frac{60 \text{ min}}{1 \text{ h}} \times \frac{20 \text{ gtt}}{1 \text{ min}} \times \frac{1 \text{ mL}}{15 \text{ gtt}} = 240 \text{ mL}$$

The amount that has infused is 650 mL − 490 mL = 160 mL. The solution has been infusing too slowly and needs to be adjusted.

The amount of solution remaining is 490 mL. Recalculate the flow rate for 490 mL over 5 h.

$$\frac{15 \text{ gtt}}{\text{mL}} \times \frac{490 \text{ mL}}{5 \text{ h}} \times \frac{1 \text{ h}}{60 \text{ min}} = F$$

$$\frac{^1\cancel{15} \text{ gtt}}{1 \text{ mL}} \times \frac{^{98}\cancel{490} \text{ mL}}{_{1}5 \text{ h}} \times \frac{1 \text{ h}}{_4\cancel{60} \text{ min}} = \frac{24.5 \text{ gtt}}{\text{min}}$$

The adjusted flow rate should be 25 gtt/min. Checking if it is within 25% of the original flow rate,

$$25\% \times 20 = 5$$

Because 25 gtt/min is 5 gtt/min more than the original flow rate, 25 gtt/min is within the acceptable range.

45. $\text{BSA} = \sqrt{\dfrac{59 \times 93}{3131}} \text{ m}^2 = \sqrt{\dfrac{5487}{3131}} \text{ m}^2 = 1.324 \text{ m}^2$

46. $\text{BSA} = \sqrt{\dfrac{150 \times 61}{3600}} \text{ m}^2 = \sqrt{\dfrac{9150}{3600}} \text{ m}^2 = 1.594 \text{ m}^2$

47. $\text{BSA} = \sqrt{\dfrac{66 \times 125}{3131}} \text{ m}^2 = \sqrt{\dfrac{8250}{3131}} \text{ m}^2 = 1.623 \text{ m}^2$

$$1.623 \text{ m}^2 \times \frac{200 \text{ mg}}{\text{m}^2} = 324.7 \text{ mg}$$

Administer: 324.7 mg

48. $BSA = \sqrt{\dfrac{60 \times 103}{3131}}\ m^2 = \sqrt{\dfrac{6180}{3131}}\ m^2 = 1.4\ m^2$

$1.4\ m^2 \times \dfrac{200\ mg}{m^2} = 280\ mg$

You want to administer 280 mg of Leucovorin Calcium. According to the label, the reconstituted Leucovorin will have a dosage strength of 20 mg/mL.

$\dfrac{280\ mg}{?\ mL} = \dfrac{20\ mg}{1\ mL}$

$280\ mg \times 1\ mL = ?\ mL \times 20\ mg$

$14 = ?$

You want to administer 14 mL of Leucovorin Calcium over 6 minutes. The tubing is calibrated for 10 gtt/mL. Therefore,

$\dfrac{10\ gtt}{1\ mL} \times \dfrac{14\ mL}{6\ min}$

$= \dfrac{{}^5\cancel{10}\ gtt}{1\ \cancel{mL}} \times \dfrac{14\ \cancel{mL}}{{}_3\cancel{6}\ min} = 5\ gtt \times \dfrac{14}{3\ min} = \dfrac{23\ gtt}{1\ min}$

Flow rate: 23 gtt/min

49. $1000\ mL + [\dfrac{50\ mL}{1\ kg} \times (18 - 10)]$

$= 1000\ mL + [\dfrac{50\ mL}{1\ kg} \times 8] = 1000\ mL + 400\ mL = 1400\ mL$

DMFN = 1400 mL; for microdrip tubing,

$\dfrac{1400\ mL}{1\ \cancel{day}} \times \dfrac{1\ \cancel{day}}{24\ h} = \dfrac{1400\ mL}{24\ h} = \dfrac{58\ gtt}{1\ min}$

50. The patient's CL_{CR} is 48 mL/min. The recommended maintenance dosage is 2 g q4h. This amount is more than the order, which is safe to administer.

$1.7\ \cancel{g} \times \dfrac{1000\ \cancel{mg}}{1\ \cancel{g}} \times \dfrac{1\ mL}{20\ \cancel{g}} = 85\ mL$

INDEX

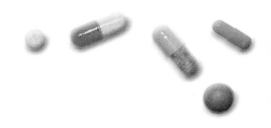

Photo Credits

Abbott Laboratories, 269; ALARIS Medical Sytems, 268 (top left, right); Roche Laboratories, Inc., 99; Medex, 268 (bottom left); Medical Images Inc., 107, 268 (bottom right); © Claire Paxton & Jacqui Farrow/Science Photo Library/Photo Researchers Inc., 266 (bottom left); Retractable Technologies, Inc., 101 (bottom left, right); SGM Photography, iii, xiv, 5, 46, 71, 93, 95 (top, bottom), 100 (all), 101 (top), 102 (both), 103, 114, 137, 161, 185, 205, 206 (both), 211 (both), 228, 262, 266 (bottom right), 267 (both), 281, 292, 312, 317, 375; The Terry Wild Studio, 6, 34, 42, 51, 58, 67, 68, 77, 86, 95 (middle), 97, 104, 108, 116, 120, 122, 129, 145, 150, 154, 179, 196, 209, 212, 216, 217, 232, 234, 239, 243, 245, 266 (top), 275, 280, 293, 299, 313